AF612575

A COMPUTER-AIDED DESIGN AND SYNTHESIS ENVIRONMENT FOR ANALOG INTEGRATED CIRCUITS

THE KLUWER INTERNATIONAL SERIES IN ENGINEERING AND COMPUTER SCIENCE

ANALOG CIRCUITS AND SIGNAL PROCESSING

Consulting Editor*: Mohammed Ismail. *Ohio State University

Related Titles:

A DESIGN AND SYNTHESIS ENVIRONMENT FOR ANALOG INTEGRATED CIRCUITS
G. Van der Plas, G. Gielen and W. Sansen
ISBN: 0-7923-7697-8

COMPLEXITYOF LATTICE PROBLEMS: A Cryptographic Perspective
D. Micciancio and S. Goldwasser
ISBN: 0-7923-7688-9

ON-CHIP ESD PROTECTION FOR INTEGRATED CIRCUITS
A. Wang
ISBN: 0-7923-7647-1

POWER TRADE-OFFS AND LOW POWER IN ANALOG CMOS ICS
M.Samduleanu and Ed A.J.M.van Tuijl
ISBN: 0-7923-7642-0

DOPPLER APPLICATIONS IN LEO SATELLITE COMMMUNICATION SYSTEMS
I.Ali, P. Bonanni, N. Al-Dhahir and J. Hersey
ISBN: 0-7923-7616-1

HIGH PERFORMANCE COMPUTING SYSTEMS AND APPLICATIONS
N. Dimopoulos and K. Li
ISBN: 0-7923-7617-X

COMPUTAIONAL METHODS FOR LARGE SPARSE POWER SYSTEMS ANALYSIS
S.Soman, S.Khaparde and S.Pandit
ISBN: 0-7923-7591-2

POWER TRADE-OFFS AND LOW POWER IN ANALOG CMOS ICS
M. Sanduleanu, van Tuijl
ISBN: 0-7923-7643-9

RF CMOS POWER AMPLIFIERS: THEORY, DESIGN AND IMPLEMENTATION
M.Hella, M.Ismail
ISBN: 0-7923-7628-5

WIRELESS BUILDING BLOCKS
J.Janssens, M. Steyaert
ISBN: 0-7923-7637-4

CODING APPROACHES TO FAULT TOLERANCE IN COMBINATION AND DYNAMIC SYSTEMs
C. Hadjicostis
ISBN: 0-7923-7624-2

DATA CONVERTERS FOR WIRELESS STANDARDS
C. Shi, M. Ismail
ISBN: 0-7923-7623-4

STREAM PROCESSOR ARCHITECTURE
S. Rixner
ISBN: 0-7923-7545-9

LOGIC SYNTHESIS AND VERIFICATION
S. Hassoun, T. Sasao
ISBN: 0-7923-7606-4

VERILOG-2001-A GUIDE TO THE NEW FEATURES OF THE VERILOG HARDWARE DESCRIPTION LANGUAGE
S. Sutherland
ISBN: 0-7923-7568-8

IMAGE COMPRESSION FUNDAMENTALS, STANDARDS AND PRACTICE
D. Taubman, M. Marcellin
ISBN: 0-7923-7519-X

ERROR CODING FOR ENGINEERS
A.Houghton
ISBN: 0-7923-7522-X

MODELING AND SIMULATION ENVIRONMENT FOR SATELLITE AND TERRESTRIAL COMMUNICATION NETWORKS
A.Ince
ISBN: 0-7923-7547-5

MULT-FRAME MOTION-COMPENSATED PREDICTION FOR VIDEO TRANSMISSION
T. Wiegand, B. Girod
ISBN: 0-7923-7497-5

A COMPUTER-AIDED DESIGN AND SYNTHESIS ENVIRONMENT FOR ANALOG INTEGRATED CIRCUITS

by

Geert Van der Plas
KU Leuven

Georges Gielen
KU Leuven

and

Willy Sansen
KU Leuven

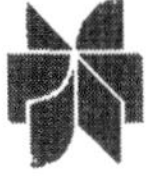

SPRINGER SCIENCE+BUSINESS MEDIA, LLC

A C.I.P. Catalogue record for this book is available from the Library of Congress.

DOI 10.1007/978-0-306-47913-7

Printed on acid-free paper

Abstract

Due to the ever decreasing feature size of silicon technology the complexity that can be integrated on a single chip has reached the system level. Soon, as much as 100 million transistors will be integrated on one ICs. We have truly entered the System-on-a-Chip (SoC) era. The existing design methodologies are insufficient for handling these designs, hence a growing design productivity gap develops: design productivity can not keep up with the design needs created by SoCs. Although these SoCs are primarily digital, they interface to the real world, which is analog. Analog building blocks thus become increasingly more important in a world dominated by digital techniques. In this work, research into design automation for analog circuits has been carried out. Two complementary approaches have been investigated.

Firstly, an automatic analog synthesis system, **AMGIE**, has been built. The **AMGIE** system is targeted towards the automatic synthesis from specifications down to layout of moderate-complexity analog circuits (device count lower than 100) that have a high reuse factor. It uses a performance-driven, hierarchical top-down refinement, bottom-up assembly design methodology. Two libraries are required for its operation: (1) a cell (topology) library containing a set of alternative implementation templates and (2) a technology library containing technology parameters. Five design tools automate the different design tasks. Topology selection selects among the topologies in the library the most likely candidate using a sequence of three filters. The sizing and optimization tool determines the sizes and biasing of the selected schematic by using a (modified) equation-based optimization methodology. The derivation of the sizing plan has been automated using a setup environment supported by design tools. The layout tool LAYLA [Lam 99] uses a direct performance-driven macro-cell place & route methodology to generate the layout of the sized schematic. Verification steps after sizing and layout extraction verify the design. Potential design problems are dispatched to the redesign wizard. The redesign wizard provides corrective design procedures to help the designer resolve the detected problem.

A comparison experiment between different sizing approaches indicates that the implemented *modified equation-based optimization* approach is the most appropriate when a high reuse factor is to be expected. A second experiment, the design of an OTA circuit by EE Master students, indicates that the **AMGIE** system creates a new breed of analog designers: system-level designers or less experienced analog designers that are capable of successfully designing moderate-complexity analog circuits in a few hours. The **AMGIE** system can however also handle more complex circuits, as has been demonstrated by the design, fabrication and measurement of an analog signal processing building block: a charge-sensitive amplifier – pulse-shaping amplifier combination.

The design automation approach used in the **AMGIE** approach, however, relies on accumulated design expertise under the form of a cell library which is reused by less experienced designers. Sometimes, the performance specifications of an analog block can not be obtained using existing analog design knowledge and techniques: these are high-challenge designs that require design creativity. In this case full automation is not possible, but the designer can still be supported. The systematic design methodology that is presented in this work is targeted towards the design of these high-performance analog blocks. It leaves room for analog design creativity: coming up with new ideas to solve hard design problems. The methodology steers this creativity to be productive, by linking every design choice that has to be made to the requested specifications. The design productivity is further increased by support through analog CAD tools.

The **Mondriaan** tool presented in this work is such a tool. It automates the layout generation of the highly-regular analog blocks often found in high-speed converter architectures. It automates the back-end process of routing and technology mapping while giving the designer a more abstract view of the layout problem: a floorplan which determines the final position and connectivity of the cell array.

The presented systematic design methodology has then been applied to the design of high-speed current-steering D/A-converters. The first phase in the design flow is the specification phase. Using behavioral modeling and simulation the specification of the D/A-converter functionblock have been derived. The second phase in the design flow is the synthesis of the converter. A top-down refinement, bottom-up, mixed-signal design strategy has been adopted. In the bottom-up path, **Mondriaan** was used to generate the layout of the analog modules, while a standard cell place & route tool was used to create the digital layout. In the last phase of the design a behavioral model is extracted that mimics the actual silicon part. This research has resulted in the first 14-bit accurate current-steering D/A-converter in CMOS technology that does not require trimming or tuning. This performance was obtained by creating the novel Q^2 random walk switching scheme.

Both presented approaches increase analog design productivity. This is demonstrated in the text with design time reports for all the experiments that have been carried out.

List of Abbreviations

1P2M	single poly, double metal
1P3M	single poly, triple metal
2P2M	double poly, double metal
AC	alternating current
A/D-converter	analog to digital converter
ADSL	asymmetric digital subscriber line
AHDL	analog hardware description language
AMS	analog and mixed-signal
A/MS	analog / mixed-signal
ASIC	application-specific integrated circuit
ASSP	application-specific standard parts
AWE	asymptotic waveform evaluation
BC	boundary checking
BiCMOS	bipolar complementary metal-oxide semiconductor
CAD	computer-aided design
CD	compact disc
CMOS	complementary metal-oxide semiconductor
CNN	cellular neural network
CPU	central processing unit
CSA	charge-sensitive amplifier
CSA-PSA	charge-sensitive amplifier – pulse-shaping amplifier
CUD	cell under design
D/A-converter	digital to analog converter
dB	deciBel
DC	direct current *or* design controller
DIFF	differentiator
DLL	delay-locked loop
DNL	differential non-linearity
DRC	design rule check
DRI	data representation interface
DSP	digital signal process(ing/or)
DVD	digital versatile disc
EDA	electronic design automation
EE	electrical engineering
ERC	electrical rule check

ET	extraction tool
GaAs	Gallium-Arsenide
GCM	geometrical calculation model
GP	geometric program(ming)
GUI	graphical user interface
HDL	hardware description language
IC	integrated circuit
INL	integral non-linearity
INT	integrator
IP	intellectual property
ITRS	international technology roadmap for semiconductors
LC-VCO	inductor-capacitor tank VCO
LNA	low-noise amplifier
low-IF	low intermediate-frequency
LSB	least significant bit
LSI	large-scale integration
LT	layout generation tool
LVS	layout versus schematic
MMPRE	mismatch preprocessor
MOS	metal-oxide semiconductor
MSB	most significant bit
NMOS	n-type MOS transistor
OPAMP	operational amplifier
OTA	operational transconductance amplifier
OTA-C	operational transconductance amplifier - capacitor
PC	personal computer
PCA	principal components analysis
PDFE	particle detector front-end
PLL	phase-locked loop
PMOS	p-type MOS transistor
PSA	pulse-shaping amplifier
PSRR	power-supply rejection ratio
PWL	piecewise-linear
Q^2	quad quadrant
RC	resistor-capacitor
RF	radio-frequency
RGB	red green blue
ROM	read-only memory
S/H	sample-and-hold
S&O	sizing and optimization tool
SFDR	spurious-free dynamic range
SIA	semiconductor industry association
SiGe	silicon-germanium
SNDR	signal-to-noise-and-distortion ratio
SNR	signal-to-noise ratio

SoC	system-on-a-chip
SQP	sequential quadratic programming
SVD	singular value decomposition
SWITCAP	switched-capacitor
TS	topology selection
VCO	voltage-controlled oscillator
VFSR	very fast simulated re-annealing
VGA	variable-gain amplifier
VLSI	very large-scale integration
VSI	virtual socket interface
VT	verification tool
xDSL	any type of digital subscriber line
zero-IF	zero intermediate-frequency

List of Symbols

Notation:

∞	infinity
$\emptyset$	the empty set
$\propto$	proportional to
$=$	equal to
$\neq$	not equal to
$\approx$	approximately equal to
$a_0, a_1, \ldots, a_n$	coefficients of polynomial
$i, j, \ldots$	integer counters
$f, g, \ldots$	scalar functions
$x, y, \ldots$	scalar variables
$\mathbf{f}, \mathbf{g}, \ldots$	vector functions
$\mathbf{x}, \mathbf{y}, \ldots$	vector variables
$f_i, g_i, \ldots$	scalar subfunctions of vector function
$x_i, y_i, \ldots$	scalar subvariables of vector variable
α_{ij}	exponent
$E\{x\}$	expected value of x
$\overline{x}$	average value of x

List:

A	context dependent parameter
$\mathbf{A}$	set of design parameters, input specs and technology parameters
A_{glitch}	the amplitude of the glitch

A_{v0}	low-frequency gain
A_{V_T}, A_β	MOS mismatch model parameters [Laksh 86, Pel 89]
β	scaling parameter for scalar cost function
$\beta()$	beta function
BW	bandwidth
C_d	detector capacitance
C_f	(CSA) feedback capacitance
cgs, cgd, ...	gate source, gate drain, etc. capacitance of transistor
C_{load}	load capacitance
C_{out}	output capacitance
C_p, C_{pk}	statistical indices for design centering
C_{par}	parasitic capacitance
ΔP	performance specification margin or range
DNL	differential non-linearity
$\epsilon^{(i)}$	ith order error profile
E_{glitch}	glitch energy
ENC	equivalent noise charge
ENC_{tot}	total equivalent noise charge
$\Phi(\mathbf{x})$	scalar cost function
f_{in}	input signal frequency
$f_{p\|z}$	frequency of pole or zero
$f_{routing}$	routing overhead factor
f_s	sampling frequency
γ	scaling parameter for scalar cost function
GBW	gainbandwidth
gm, go, ...	transconductance and output conductance of MOS transistor
$i_n(f)$	noise spectral density
INL	integral non-linearity
IR	input range
I_{gm}	MOS DC current generating transconductance
I_{LSB}	LSB current
I_{tot}	total DC current
I_{out}	full-scale output current
k	Boltzmann's constant (1.38e-23 J/K)
KP	transistor transconductance factor, μC_{ox}
l	loop counter or number of binary bits in a D/A-converter
λ_i	ith eigenvalue
Λ	eigenvalue matrix
L_{m1}	length of transistor $m1$
$level_i$	output value of code level in a D/A-converter
$LMIN$, $LGRID$, $LMAX$	length related technology parameters
$logL$, $logW$	process independent values of length and width of transistors
m	number of unary bits in a D/A-converter
n	PSA order, number of bits
OR	output range

P	performance specification
PM	phase margin
$\psi_{lb,ub}$	topology performance region lower- or upperbound
q	elementary electron charge (1.602e-19 C)
rf	reuse factor
R_f	(CSA) feedback resistance
R_{gnd}	ground line resistance
R_{load}	load resistance
ro	output resistance of MOS transistor
R_{output}	output resistance of a D/A-converter
R_{par}	parasitic resistance
rv	topology ranking value
$\mathbf{S}$	subblock specification set (estimators)
$\sigma(x)$	standard deviation of a quantity x
Σ	singular value decomposition matrix
S_b^a	sensitivity of a to variable b
SNR	signal to noise rate
SR	slew rate
S_{V_T}, S_β	MOS mismatch model parameters [Laksh 86, Pel 89]
T	Temperature
τ	time constant
Θ	technology parameter set
τ_p	peaking time constant
τ_{pz}	pole zero time constant
τ_r	rise time constant
t_{glitch}	glitch duration time
$u()$	step function
V_{dd}, V_{ss}	power supply voltages
$V_{gs}, V_{ds}, V_{bs}, \ldots$	device terminal voltage differences
V_{gst}	transistor overdrive voltage, $V_{gs} - V_T$
V_{off}	offset voltage due to random and systematic effects
V_{out}	full-scale output voltage
V_T	threshold voltage
$\sharp\, wires$	number of wires
w_j	weight of constraint in cost function
W_{m1}	width of transistor $m1$
$WMIN, WGRID, WMAX$	width related technology parameters

Contents

List of Figures

List of Tables

Chapter 1

Introduction

The micro-electronics market and in particular the markets for application-specific integrated circuits (ASICs), application-specific standard parts (ASSPs) and high-volume commodity ICs are characterized by an ever increasing level of integration complexity, now featuring multi-million transistor ICs. In recent years, complete systems that previously occupied one or more boards are being integrated on a few chips or even one single chip. Examples of such *Systems on a Chip* (SoC) are the single-chip television or the single-chip camera [EDTN 99] or new generations of integrated telecommunication systems that include analog, digital and eventually radio-frequency (RF) sections on one chip [OtEy 01] or completely integrated LSIs for DVD systems [Mats 01]. The technology of choice for these systems is CMOS, because of the good digital scaling, but also BiCMOS is used when needed for the analog or radio-frequency circuits. Although most functions in such integrated systems are implemented with digital or digital signal processing (DSP) circuitry, the analog circuits needed at the interface between the electronic system and the *real* world are also being integrated on the same die for reasons of cost and performance. A typical future SoC might look like figure 1.1, containing several embedded processors, several chunks of embedded memory, some reconfigurable logic and a few analog interface circuits to communicate with the continuous-valued external world.

Despite the trend previously to replace analog circuit functions with digital computations (for instance digital signal processing in place of analog filtering), there are some typical functions that will always remain analog:

- The first typically analog function is on the input side of a system: signals from a sensor, microphone, antenna, wireline and the like, must be sensed or received and then amplified and filtered up to a level that allows digitization with sufficient signal-to-noise-and-distortion ratio (SNDR). Typical analog circuits used here are low-noise amplifiers (LNA), variable-gain amplifiers (VGA), filters, oscillators and mixers (in case of down-conversion). Applications are, for instance, instrumentation (e.g., data and biomedical), sensor interfaces (e.g., airbag accelerometers), process control loops, telecommunication receivers (e.g., telephone or cable modems, wireless phones, set-top boxes, etc.), recording (e.g., speech recognition, cameras), and smart cards.

- The second typically analog function is on the output side of a system: the signal is reconverted from digital to analog form and it has to be strengthened so that it can drive the outside load (e.g., actuator, antenna, loudspeaker, wireline) without too much

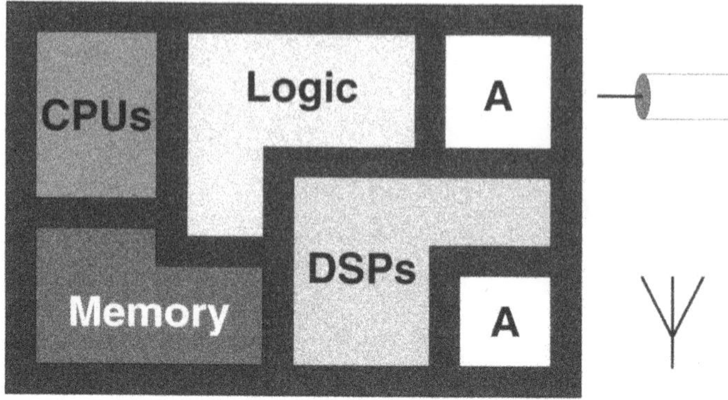

Figure 1.1: Typical floorplan of a System-on-a-Chip (SoC).

distortion. Typical analog circuits used here are drivers and buffers, filters, oscillators and mixers (in case of upconversion). Applications are, for instance, process control loops (e.g., voltage regulators for engines), telecommunication transmitters, audio and video (e.g., CD, DVD, loudspeakers, TV, PC monitors, etc.), and biomedical actuation (e.g., hearing aids).

- The third type of blocks are the true mixed-signal circuits that interface the above analog circuits with the DSP part of the system. Typical circuits used here are the sample-and-hold (S/H) circuits for signal sampling, analog-to-digital converters (A/D-converters) for amplitude discretization, digital-to-analog converters (D/A-converters) for signal reconstruction, phase-locked loops (PLL), delay-locked loops (DLL) and frequency synthesizers to generate a timing reference or perform timing synchronization.
- In addition, the above circuits need stable absolute references for their operation, which are generated by voltage and current reference circuits, crystal oscillators, etc.

Clearly, analog circuits are indispensable in all electronic applications that interface with the outside world, and will even be more prevalent in our lives if we move towards the intelligent homes, the mobile road/air offices and the wireless workplaces of the future.

When both analog (possibly RF) and digital circuits are needed in a system, it becomes obvious to integrate them together to reduce cost and improve performance, provided the technology allows one to do so. The growing market share of integrated mixed-signal ICs observed today in modern electronic systems for telecommunications, consumer, computing, and automotive applications, among many others, is a direct result of the need for higher levels of integration. Since the early 1990s, the average growth rate of the mixed-signal IC market has been between 15 and 20% per year [Liang 98], and has reached $29 billion in the year 2000 according to the Semiconductor Industry Association (SIA) [Curr 01]. Recent developments in CMOS technology have offered the possibility to combine good and scalable digital performance with adequate analog performance on the same die. The shrinking of CMOS device sizes down to the deep submicron regime (essentially in line with or even ahead of the predicted technology roadmaps [SIA 97, ITRS 99, ITRS 00]) makes higher levels of system integration possible and also offers analog MOS transistor performance that approaches the performance of a bipolar transistor.

This explains why CMOS is the technology of choice today, and why other technologies like BiCMOS are only used when more aggressive bipolar device characteristics (e.g., power, noise or distortion) are really needed. The technology shift from bipolar to CMOS (or BiCMOS) has been apparent in most applications. Even fields like RF, where traditionally GaAs and bipolar were the dominant technologies, now show a trend towards BiCMOS (preferably with a SiGe bipolar option) and even plain CMOS for reasons of higher integration and cost reduction. These higher levels of mixed-signal integration however also introduce a whole new set of problems and design effects that need to be accounted for in the design process.

Indeed, together with the increase in circuit complexity, the design complexity of today's ICs has increased drastically: (1) due to integration, more and more transistors are combined per IC, performing both analog and digital functions, to be co-designed together with the embedded software; (2) new signal processing algorithms and corresponding system architectures are developed to accommodate new required functionalities and performance requirements (including power) of emerging applications; and (3) due to the rapid evolution of process technologies, the expectation for changing process technology parameters needs to be accounted for in the design cycle. At the same time, many ASIC and ASSP application markets are characterized by shortening product life cycles and tightening time-to-market constraints. The time-to-market factor is really critical for ASICs and ASSPs that eventually end up in consumer, telecom or computer products: if one misses the initial market window relative to the competition, prices and therefore profit can be seriously eroded.

Key to manage this increased design complexity while meeting the shortening time-to-market factor is the use of computer-aided design (CAD) and verification tools. Today's high-speed workstations provide ample power to make large and detailed computations possible. What is needed to expedite the analog and mixed-signal design process is a structured methodology and supporting CAD tools to manage the entire design process and design complexity. CAD tools are also needed to assist or automate many of the routine and repetitive design tasks, taking away the tedium of manually designing these sections and providing the designer with more time to focus on the creative aspects of design. ICs typically are composed of many identical circuit blocks used across different designs. The design of these repetitive blocks can be automated to reduce the design time. In addition, CAD tools can increase the productivity of designers, even for non-repetitive analog blocks. Therefore, analog CAD and circuit design automation are likely to play a key role in the design process of the next generation of mixed-signal ICs and ASICs. And although the design of mixed-signal ASICs served as the initial impetus for stepping up the efforts in research and development of analog design automation tools, the technology trend towards integrating complete systems on a chip in recent years has provided yet another driving force to bolster analog CAD efforts. In addition, for such systems new design paradigms are being developed that greatly affect how we will design analog blocks. One example is the macro-cell design reuse methodology of assembling a system by reusing soft or hard macro-cells ("virtual components") that are available on the intellectual property (IP) market and that can easily be mixed and matched in the "silicon board" system if they comply with the Virtual Socket Interface (VSI) standard [VSI 97]. This methodology again poses many new constraints, also on the analog blocks. Platform-based design is another emerging system-level design methodology [Chang 99, Claas 00].

In the digital domain, CAD tools are fairly well developed and commercially available today, certainly for the lower levels of the design flow. First of all, the digital IC market is much larger than the analog IC market. In addition, unlike analog circuits, a digital system can naturally be represented in terms of Boolean representation and programming language constructs, and its functionality can easily be represented in algorithmic form, thus paving the way for a logical transition into automation of many aspects of digital system design. At the present time many lower-level aspects of the digital design process are fully automated. The hardware is described in a hardware description language (HDL) such as VHDL or Verilog, either at the behavioral level or most often at the structural level. High-level synthesis tools attempt to synthesize the behavioral HDL description into a structural representation. Logic synthesis tools then translate the structural HDL specification into a gate-level netlist and semi-custom layout tools (place & route) map this netlist into a correct-by-construction mask-level layout based on a cell library specific for the selected technology process. Research interest is now moving in the direction of system synthesis where a system-level specification (in languages such as C/C++, SystemC or SpecC, ...) is translated into a hardware-software co-architecture with high-level specifications for both the hardware, the software and the interfaces. Reuse methodologies and platform-based design methodologies are being developed to further reduce the design effort for complex systems. Of course, the level of automation is far from the push-button stage, but the developments are keeping up reasonably well with the chip complexity offered by the technology.

Unfortunately, the story is quite different on the analog side. There are not yet any robust commercial CAD tools to support or automate analog circuit design apart from circuit simulators (in most cases some flavor of the ubiquitous SPICE simulator [Nagel 75, Vlad 94]) and layout editing environments and their accompanying tools (e.g., some limited optimization capabilities around the simulator, or layout verification tools). Some of the main reasons for this lack of automation are that analog design in general is perceived as less systematic and more heuristic and knowledge-intensive in nature than digital design, and that it has not yet been possible for analog designers to establish a higher level of abstraction that shields all the device-level and process-level details from the higher-level design. Analog IC design is a complex endeavor, requiring specialized knowledge and circuit design skills acquired through many years of experience. The variety of circuit schematics and the number of conflicting requirements and corresponding diversity of device sizes is also much larger. In addition, analog circuits are more sensitive to nonidealities and all kinds of higher-order effects and parasitic disturbances (resistive and capacitive layout parasitics, crosstalk, substrate noise, supply noise, device matching, ...). These differences from digital design also explain why analog CAD tools cannot simply adapt the existing digital algorithms, but why specific analog solutions need to be developed that are targeted to the analog design paradigm and complexity.

As a result, due to the lack of adequate and mature commercial analog CAD tools, analog designs today are still largely being handcrafted with only a SPICE-like simulation shell and an interactive layout environment as supporting facilities. The design cycle for analog and mixed-signal ICs remains long and error-prone. Therefore, although analog circuits typically occupy only a small fraction of the total area of mixed-signal ICs, their design is often the bottleneck in mixed-signal systems, both in design time and effort as well as test cost, and they are often responsible for design errors and expensive reruns.

This situation, however, can no longer be accepted today. The economic pressure for high-quality yet cheap electronic products and the decreasing time-to-market constraints have clearly revealed the need in the present micro-electronics industry for analog CAD tools to assist designers with fast and first-time-correct design of analog circuits, or even to automate certain tasks of this design process where possible. The push for more and more integrated systems (SoCs) containing both analog and digital circuitry heavily constrains analog designers. To keep pace with the digital world and to fully exploit the potential offered by the present deep submicron VLSI technologies, boosting analog design productivity is a major concern in the industry today. The goals of analog CAD tools are therefore the following.

Firstly the design time and cost for analog circuits from specification to successful silicon has to be reduced drastically. The risk for design errors impeding first-pass functional (and possibly also parametrically correct) chips has to be eliminated. Secondly, analog CAD tools can also help to increase the quality of the resulting designs. Before starting detailed circuit implementation, more higher-level explorations and optimizations should be performed at the system architectural level, preferably across the analog-digital boundary, since decisions at those levels have a much larger impact on key overall system parameters such as power consumption and chip area.

Likewise, designs at lower levels should be *automated* where possible. Designers find difficulty in considering multiple conflicting trade-offs at the same time — computers don't. Computers are adept at trying out and exploring large numbers of competing alternatives. Typical examples are fine-tuning through optimization of an initial handcrafted design and improving design robustness with respect to operating parameter variations (temperature, supply voltage) and/or with respect to manufacturing tolerances (inter-die technology variations) and mismatches (intra-die technology variations).

Thirdly, the continuous pressure of technology updates and process migrations is a large burden on analog designers. CAD tools could take over large part of the technology retargeting effort, and could make analog design easier to port or migrate to new technologies. Finally, the systems-on-a-chip design reuse methodology also requires executable models and other information for the analog macro-cells to be used in system-level design and verification. Tools and modeling techniques have to be developed to make this possible.

This need for analog CAD tools beyond simulation has also clearly been identified in the MEDEA EDA roadmap, as indicated in figure 1.2, where analog synthesis is predicted to take off somewhere beyond the year 2002 [Medea 00].

Despite the lack of commercial analog CAD tools, analog CAD and design automation over the past fifteen years has been a field of profound academic and industrial research activity; although with not quite as many researchers as in the digital world, resulting in a slow but steady progress [Carl 96]. Some of the aspects of the analog CAD field are fairly mature, some are ready for commercialization, while others are still in the process of exploration and development. The simulation area has been particularly well developed since the advent of the SPICE simulator, which has led to the development of many simulators including timing simulators in the digital field and the newer generation of mixed-signal and multi-level commercial simulators. Analog circuit and layout synthesis has recently shown promising results at the research level, but commercial solutions are only starting to appear on the marketplace. The development of analog and mixed-signal hardware description languages like VHDL-AMS [VHDL-AMS 99] and Verilog-A/MS [Verilog-AMS 98] is intended to provide a unify-

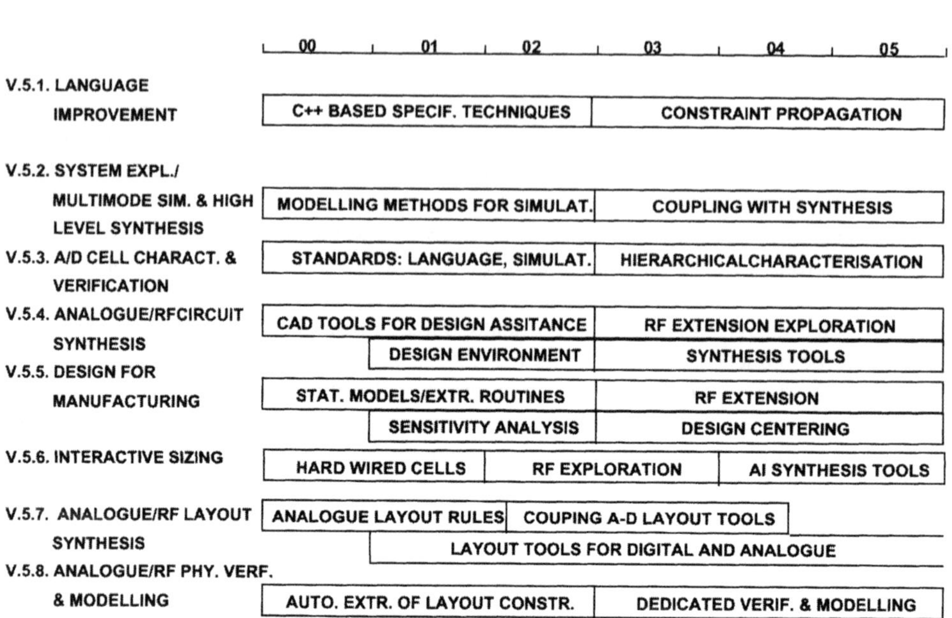

Figure 1.2: European Medea EDA roadmap [Medea 00] for mixed analog/digital and RF design.

ing trend that will link the various analog design automation tasks in a coherent framework that supports a more structured analog design methodology from the design conceptualization stage to the manufacturing stage. They also provide a link between the analog and the digital domains, as needed in designing mixed analog-digital ICs and the Systems-on-a-Chip (SoC) of the future.

If we zoom in on the analog part of these mixed-signal ICs and early SoCs, we can distinguish a number of abstraction levels. At the highest level of the SoC functionblock hierarchy, as shown in figure 1.3, is the system. At the highest level the system is partitioned in digital, DSP and analog implementation parts. This partitioning is up till now largely a manual operation, automating it is currently the subject of intensive research work. Hardware description languages link the different views of the system: the behavior and the structure at the level of top-level digital, DSP and analog blocks. The refinement of digital and DSP parts is not the subject of this work and will thus not further be discussed. The analog parts of a mixed-signal IC or SoC are further composed, at what we call the architectural level. As an example, an RF receiver could be considered an integral analog part. An architectural implementation could for instance be a low-IF or a zero-IF receiver. The mapping of analog function to architecture has been studied extensively in [Don 98]. At a certain level in the abstraction hierarchy one reaches the module and/or circuit level: the synthesis of these blocks is the subject of this thesis. A tentative, but surely incomplete list of analog functionblocks frequently encountered in these chips is given next:

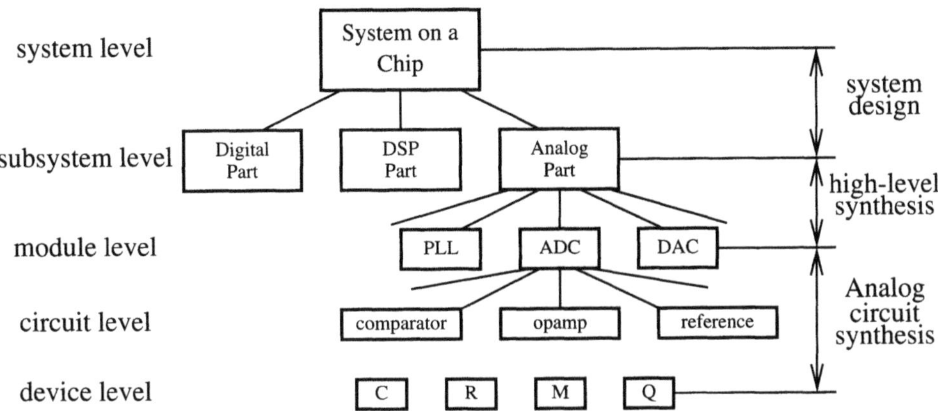

Figure 1.3: System-on-a-Chip functionblock hierarchy: the analog part has been refined down to the device level.

- amplifiers (linear circuits)
  - operational amplifiers (OPAMPs)
  - operational transconductance amplifiers (OTAs)
  - buffers
- converters (A/D- and D/A-converters):
  - flash A/D-converter
  - folding/interpolating A/D-converter
  - pipelined A/D-converter
  - Δ / Σ A/D-converter
  - Δ / Σ D/A-converter
  - current-steering D/A-converter
  - resistor string D/A-converter
- RF circuits:
  - low-noise amplifiers (LNAs)
  - voltage-controlled oscillators (VCOs)
  - mixers
  - RF filters
  - phase-locked loops (PLLs)
  - delay-locked loops (DLLs)
  - power amplifiers
  - receivers
  - transmitters
- filters:
  - OTA-C (or gm-C) filters
  - OPAMP RC filters
  - Switched-capacitor (SWITCAP) filters
  - Switched-current filters
- reference generators
  - crystal oscillators
  - bandgap references
  - biasing structures
  - clock generators and drivers

The first entries in this list are typical (linear) amplifier circuits. OPAMPs, OTAs and buffers are among the most frequently used building blocks of analog circuits. A lot of effort has gone into the modeling of these fundamental building blocks.

Next on the list are probably the most important (from a SoC standpoint) analog building blocks: A/D- and D/A-converters. The importance of these analog circuits is that they are indispensable in this digital era. The performance limits of the system are often deter-

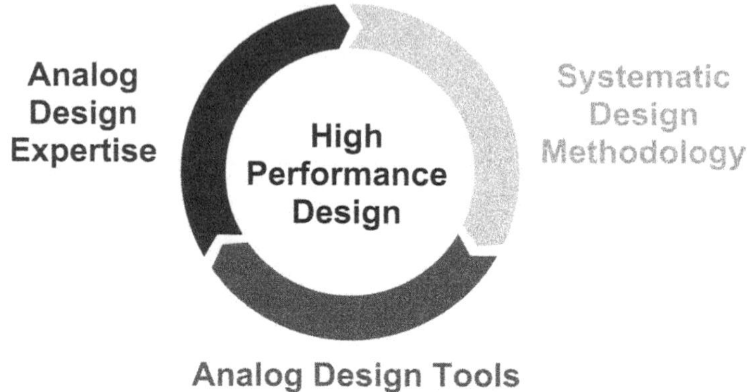

Figure 1.4: High-performance analog design.

mined by the quality of the conversion from analog to digital and digital to analog. In the converter circuits a number of architectures, are distinguished: flash type A/D-converters, including interpolating and folding subarchitectures, are aiming at the higher conversion speeds at moderate to medium accuracy (6 – 10 bits), pipelined converters are aiming at medium to higher accuracies (8 – 14 bits). The Δ/Σ-converter class of converters cover the higher-accuracy applications (10 – 24 bits) with moderate-speed requirements (due to the oversampling requirement). The successive approximation converters also provide high accuracy, at even more moderate speeds. For D/A-converters also different architectures exist that target different application areas in terms of speed, accuracy and power specifications.

RF circuits have been added since they form a separate category, not overlapping much with the other categories. The requirements for these circuits are different from the more *traditional* analog circuits. The high operating frequencies impede traditional design techniques that ignore parasitic effects such as MOS gate resistance, MOS non-quasi-static effect, wiring inductance, ... At the same time, there is a lot of interest for these circuits, explained by the importance of the wireless telecommunications market.

Filters in the analog domain is another important class of circuits. Continuous-time filters with OTA-C implementations allow the highest operating frequencies, but with limited accuracy (< 60dB). OPAMP-RC implementations have the highest accuracy (up till and more than 90dB), but have a reduced frequency range. Switched-capacitor filters provide an intermediate solution: high accuracy and moderate speed (due to the oversampling requirement).

At the end of the list one finds circuits that provide reference signals for all other types of analog circuits. Crystal oscillators generate accurate timing information and frequency references, bandgap references and biasing structures provide biasing currents and voltages, and clock generators and drivers distribute clocking signals.

Although this list may not be complete, it demonstrates that a wide range of analog circuits exist. Consequently a wide range of design techniques has been devised to design these circuits. Merging all these highly optimized design techniques in one global analog synthesis approach thus does not seem feasible at all. However, as with any design task a number of key elements can be identified. In figure 1.4 high-performance analog design is surrounded by

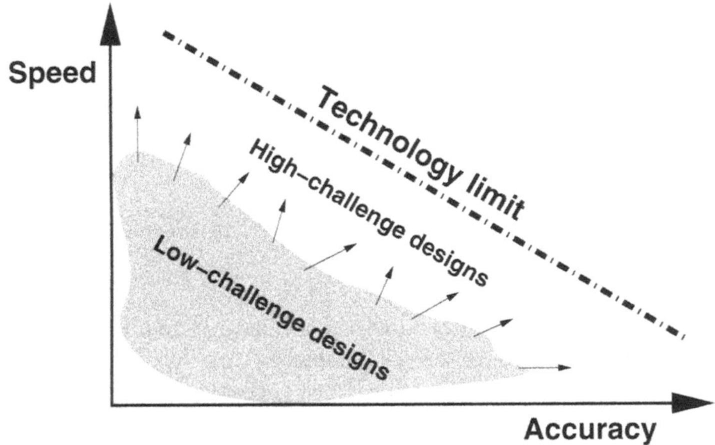

Figure 1.5: View of design space: low-challenge and high-challenge designs and technology limit as a function of speed and accuracy.

these mandatory components. Analog design is not possible without *analog design creativity*. Design is not analysis: somewhere, sometime, someone comes up with an idea, that can be stored and analyzed, but without a steady instream of new ideas no progress can be made. The creativity that delivers new ideas, however, must be harnessed by a *systematic design methodology*. The design methodology guides the designer to create useful designs efficiently. To minimize the design time further the design process has to be supported by *analog design tools*.

1.1 Goals of this Work

If now another look is taken towards the analog synthesis challenge, we can distinguish different types of design problems. Consider the most important design criteria for analog design: speed (operating frequency, bandwidth, ...) and accuracy (noise, distortion, offset, ...). In combination with power consumption (cost) these fundamental specifications form a bounded design space determined by technological constraints as set forward in [Roov 96, King 96a, King 96b]. All known circuit topologies together form this boundary, new circuit schematics and design techniques push the available application area towards this technology-determined limit, as is shown in figure 1.5. However, many of the designs at hand are not situated on this boundary. Otherwise stated, many designs do not challenge the design capabilities of the designer fully. Many designs can be brought back to the same problem over and over again. That's why two major trends in design automation can be recognized, which are complementary to each other: (1) *automated or semi-automated synthesis*: the low-challenge analog design problems, for which known topologies and design procedures suffice and the design problem is reduced to applying them. Automation is feasible and even appreciated by analog designers: analog design experts prefer not to spend time on these repetitive designs anyway. Also the porting of existing designs to a new process often falls in this category. (2) *high-challenge designs*: high-speed or high-accuracy have to be combined or new ideas, architectures and design techniques/methodologies are necessary to push the design closer to the technology limits. This is interesting, creative work, that is by definition not possible with automation, but can be supported by CAD tools. Tools can help push the limits here. In this work both directions will be explored, as summarized in the following two goal statements of this work.

The first goal of this work is to further the research in *automated synthesis of analog integrated circuits*:

- Build a synthesis system (software tool) for the (semi-)automated design of frequently used analog circuits: OTAs, OPAMPs, Comparators, etc. Try to eliminate/avoid the disadvantages of previously tried solutions. The system should be capable of supporting inexperienced designers (novices or system-level digital-oriented designers) to increase analog design productivity and to free up valuable analog design experts for more challenging designs. It should be able to handle sufficiently complex circuits to be useful in practice.

- Investigate and implement new design methodologies, design flows, algorithms and techniques to improve analog synthesis results or speed up analog synthesis. Use the system to explore alternatives, benchmark, demonstrate and get feedback from designers, use as a learning tool etc. We want to go whole the way: make a functional system that can be used in practice, not only a research prototype that can only be run by the creator.

- Verify the effectiveness of the implemented solution by doing experiments. Let inexperienced designers test drive the system and verify the result. Design a circuit with the system and actually fabricate and measure it, closing the loop that is so important for analog: a circuit is only proven to work when it is measured. Verify design quality, etc.

The second goal is to further the research in *systematic design of high-performance analog integrated circuits*:

- Design and implement a layout tool **Mondriaan**, targeted to the automatic layout generation of highly regular array-type analog blocks often found in analog circuits. In this sense it is complementary to the LAYLA tools [Lam 98], which are targeted to device-level layout generation of analog circuits (see figure 1.3 for a definition of module and circuit). Investigate the impact of such tools on design productivity and design quality.

- Apply the *systematic design methodology* to a real-life, high-performance analog circuit of reasonable complexity. In this work the class of high-accuracy, current-steering D/A-converters was chosen to verify the *systematic design* approach. Report the impact on design productivity and design quality. Once again, to close the loop, actual circuits have to be fabricated and measured.

1.2 Outline of this Work

In figure 1.6 an outline of this work is shown.

- In part I the **AMGIE** analog synthesis system will be presented.

    1. In chapter 2 the terminology that is used in this research field will be defined. An overview of the previous research results in the analog synthesis area will be given and a representative set of previously proposed tools will be discussed. The **AMGIE** system will then be introduced, and its main features will be described.
    2. In chapter 3 the **AMGIE** system will be described in detail. First the hierarchy and performance specification concepts will be refined. Next the five subtools automating the design process will be described. Simplified and/or representative examples will illustrate the implemented algorithms and techniques.
    3. Experimental results will be provided in chapter 4, demonstrating the capabilities of the **AMGIE** system. The first reported experiment is a comparison between three different sizing approaches. The aim is to verify if the approach implemented in the **AMGIE** system is indeed the most appropriate solution for the automation of frequently used circuits. The second experiment, a student exercise session, verifies in how far **AMGIE** is capable in supporting unexperienced or novice designers. The last experiment, the design of an analog signal processing chain, stresses the **AMGIE** system with respect to the complexity of circuits it can handle.

- In part II of this work, *systematic design* of analog circuits will be discussed. First a definition will be given for systematic design. The focus of the work is then oriented towards the design of high-performance D/A-converters.

    1. In chapter 5 the **Mondriaan** tool will be presented. **Mondriaan** is a layout tool for the generation of highly regular layout structures as encountered in high-performance D/A-converters. Care has been taken to generalize the implemented approach so that it is useful in a much wider application area (A/D-converters, cellular neural networks, etc.).
    2. The proposed systematic design methodology will then be applied to the design of high-performance current-steering D/A-converter macro-cells in chapter 6. In this chapter the first intrinsically accurate 14-bit current-steering D/A-converter in CMOS technology will be presented.

- In chapter 7 conclusions will be formulated and suggestions for future work will be proposed.

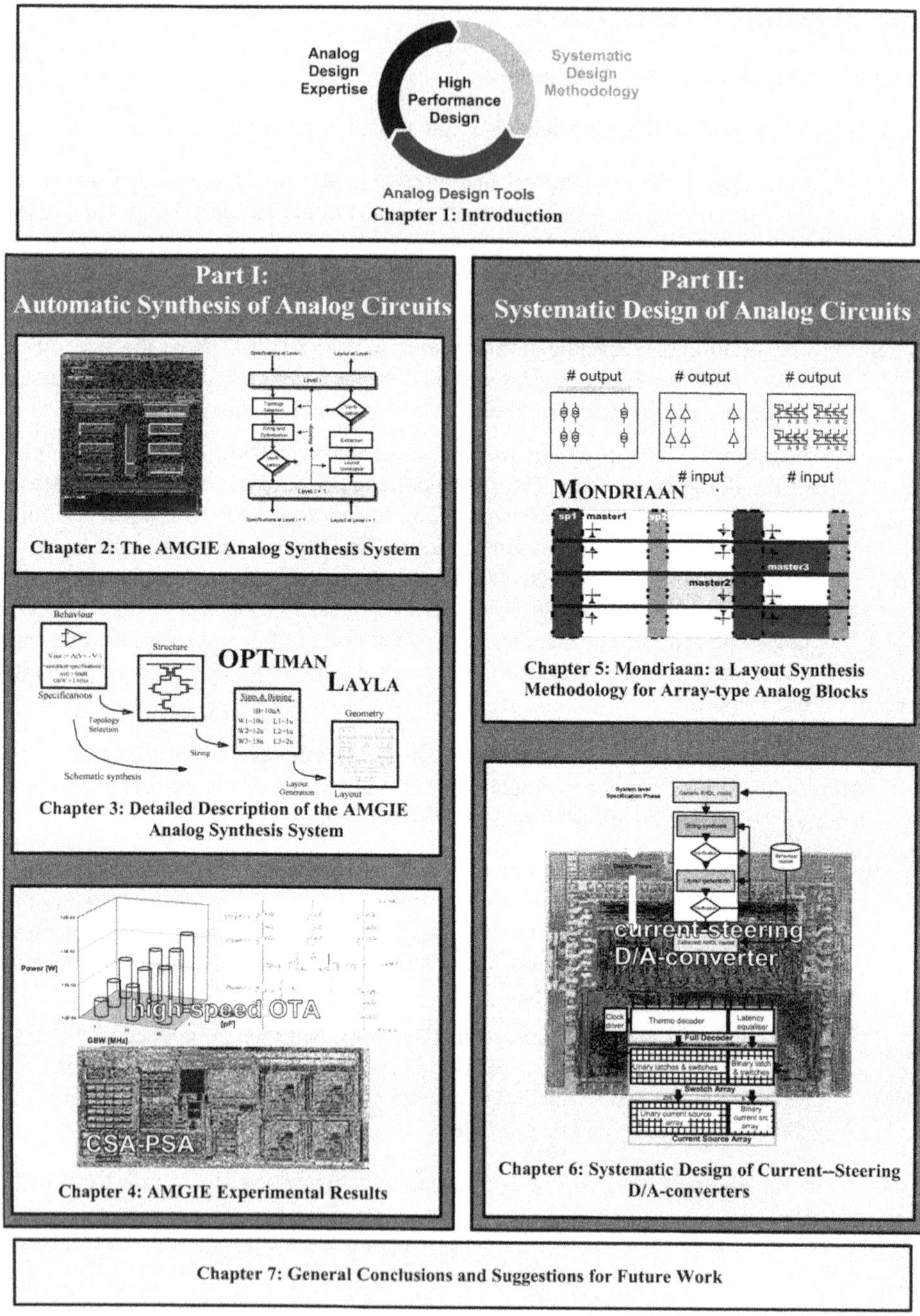

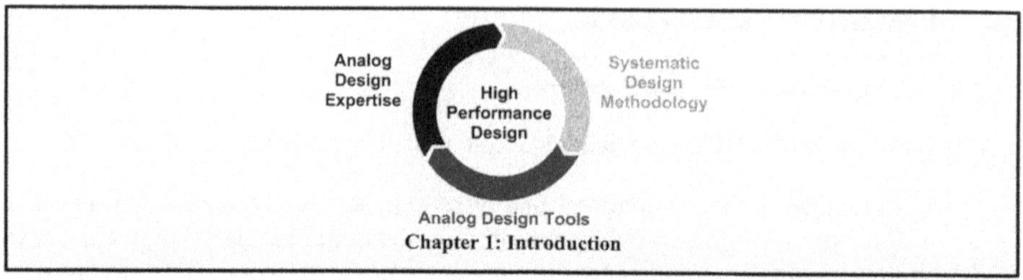

Part I:
Automatic Synthesis of Analog Circuits

Chapter 2: The AMGIE Analog Synthesis System

OPTIMAN
LAYLA

Chapter 3: Detailed Description of the AMGIE Analog Synthesis System

high-speed OTA
CSA-PSA

Chapter 4: AMGIE Experimental Results

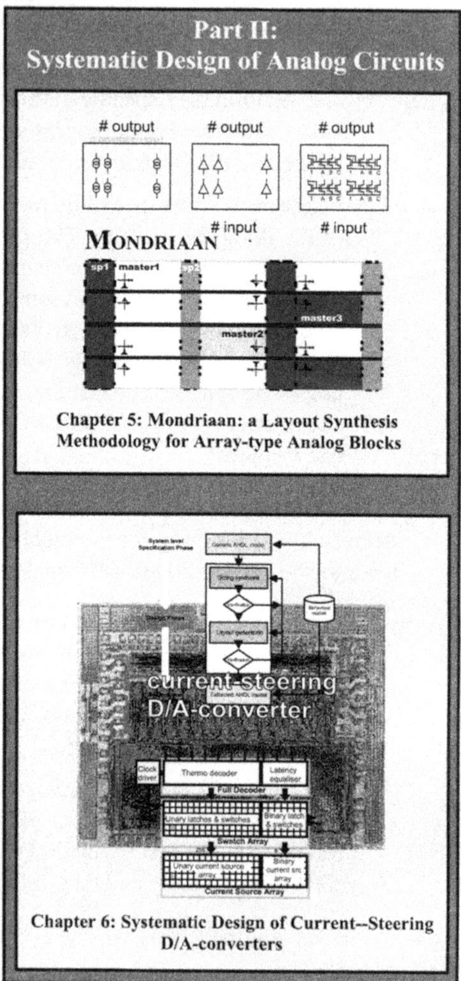

Chapter 7: General Conclusions and Suggestions for Future Work

Figure 1.6: Outline of this work.

Part I

Automatic Synthesis of Analog Circuits

Chapter 2

The AMGIE Analog Synthesis System

2.1 Introduction

In this first part the **AMGIE** analog synthesis system will be presented that can automatically generate fully optimized analog circuits from specifications to layout in a specified technology. In the first chapter the **AMGIE** system will be introduced. In the second chapter the internals of the **AMGIE** system will be discussed in detail, and in the third chapter experimental results obtained with the **AMGIE** system will be presented. Conclusions will be formulated at the end of part I.

This chapter is structured as follows. Firstly, a terminology will be established leading up to the definition of the *analog synthesis* problem. Next a summary of existing analog synthesis approaches will be given: three generations have been identified, their advantages and disadvantages will be summarized. This chapter ends with a description of the features of the **AMGIE** synthesis system that is the subject of this work. The next chapter will then describe the implementation details of the **AMGIE** analog synthesis system.

2.2 Definitions

The aim of this section is to establish a terminology that is clear and unambiguous in defining the different processes and data of an analog synthesis system. Although many of the defined terms are found in literature (which will be discussed in the next section), they do not always have the same meaning or scope. First, a list of unambiguous definitions is provided. These are building blocks to the definition of analog synthesis provided at the end of this section. Examples have been added to clarify some of the concepts.

Analog circuit: any implementation of an analog function. A list of analog circuit types can be found in the introduction, chapter 1.

Functionblock: an analog circuit type. The type is defined by its expected behavior, which is quantified by its behavioral parameters, and an interface. For instance *OPAMP* is a functionblock, which — in the functionblock interpretation — is a single-ended amplifier with relatively low output impedance that has a differential input and a DC gain. The functionblock thus defines an interface (how many inputs, outputs) and a behavior (it amplifies the difference at its inputs to the output). Note that the definition of a specific functionblock is not universal. One could define a *SWITCAP_OPAMP* where in addition to the expected *OPAMP* behavior also some switched-capacitor related behavior is imposed: externally connected capacitor values and clock phase information could for instance be specified.

Behavioral parameters: the values quantifying the behavior of a functionblock. In the *OPAMP* case this is for instance the value of the DC gain or the output impedance. If this value is a value requested by a designer for an implementation, this behavioral parameter is called a *performance specification* [Don 98] or in short a *specification.* If it is a simulated (and thus extracted) behavioral parameter, this is called a *simulated performance.* If it is measured, it is called a *measured performance.* If it is a value input when simulating with a behavioral model, it is called a *behavioral parameter.* For instance a DC gain of at least 60dB is specified, an implementation provides a DC gain of 70dB in simulation and a DC gain of 67dB is measured (after fabrication). Note that a specification is typically a range of values (from 60dB to ∞), while a simulated or measured performance is typically one value, possibly with a variation expressed under the form of a standard deviation σ (if a Gaussian or normal distribution is assumed).

Behavioral model: is a description of a functionblock that can be simulated. It implements the interface and behavior that the functionblock represents and, when given values for the behavioral parameters, it allows a numerical or other simulation to evaluate the behavior. When the behavioral parameters are equal to the simulated or measured performance of an analog circuit, the behavioral model mimics closely the behavior of the designed or fabricated circuit and the behavioral model is called an *extracted* behavioral model.

In figure 2.1 the flow of the analog synthesis process is shown as implemented by a majority of the analog synthesis systems that have been proposed. The abstract behavior, represented by a functionblock together with its performance specifications is the starting point of the process. It expresses what type of function that has to be realized by the implementation and how well it has to be realized. The first step in the process is finding a *topology* (or schematic, netlist), i.e. an interconnection of lower-level instances that is capable of realizing the wanted behavior. This is a mapping of behavior to a suitable structure. This phase of the analog synthesis process is called *topology selection* and/or *generation.* The distinction between topology selection and generation is important: many systems rely on a library of known structures to select a good candidate, while only a few synthesize a custom topology from scratch. The parameters of the structure, which are typically sizes and biasing (when the topology consists of basic devices), are determined during *sizing synthesis* (which is also called *circuit sizing*). In many publications analog synthesis is narrowed down to this subtask of the complete process. When topology generation/selection and sizing synthesis are combined, one speaks of *schematic synthesis.* At the end of this step a complete structure is determined. Remains the mapping to geometry. Actual silicon devices are fabricated through a chemical process. The patterns generated by this processing step are controlled by masks.

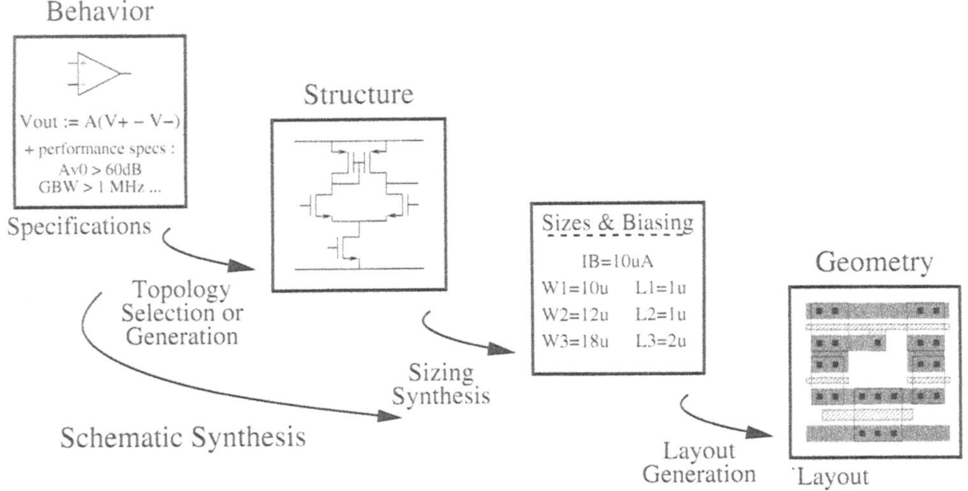

Figure 2.1: Definitions.

The structure (sized schematic) thus needs to be translated to a geometrical pattern defining the devices and interconnections: *(mask-level) layout.* This step is called *layout generation* or *layout synthesis.*

The complete flow (figure 2.1) discussed up till now is referred to in this work by *analog synthesis* at the cell level. The building blocks of the topologies are basic silicon devices. In practice only circuits with limited complexity can be handled by this approach. To enlarge the scope of analog synthesis, the divide and conquer principle is used: split the large problem in more manageable smaller problems. There are different ways of splitting the problem up, as shown in figure 2.2. The most obvious approach is a *functional decomposition.* Complex analog circuits as for instance flash type A/D-converters can be built up out of the (lower-level) functionblocks shown in figure 2.2(a): a resistor ladder (R-LADDER), a pre-amplifier (PREAMP), an input amplifier (AMP), a comparator (COMPARATOR) and encoder (ENCODER) functionblock. The *functional decomposition* naturally fits the analog synthesis flow described in the previous paragraph.

The *functional decomposition* is not the only decomposition used in the design of analog circuits. A decomposition often used in manual design is *structural decomposition.* When drawing schematics, the hierarchy drawn is chosen to reuse structural instances as much as possible, as shown in figure 2.2(b). These primitives or intermediate components do not necessarily have a function (as represented by a functionblock), they can be chosen arbitrarily, to reduce schematic complexity. An example of this approach is for instance the signal processing chain used in a flash-type A/D-converter. The same set of functional blocks is repeated many times. It is thus obvious to draw one signal processing chain: preamplifier, amplifier and comparator and represent it with one symbol. This symbol is instantiated at the higher level a number of times equal to the number of bits. This symbol does not represent a functionblock, it

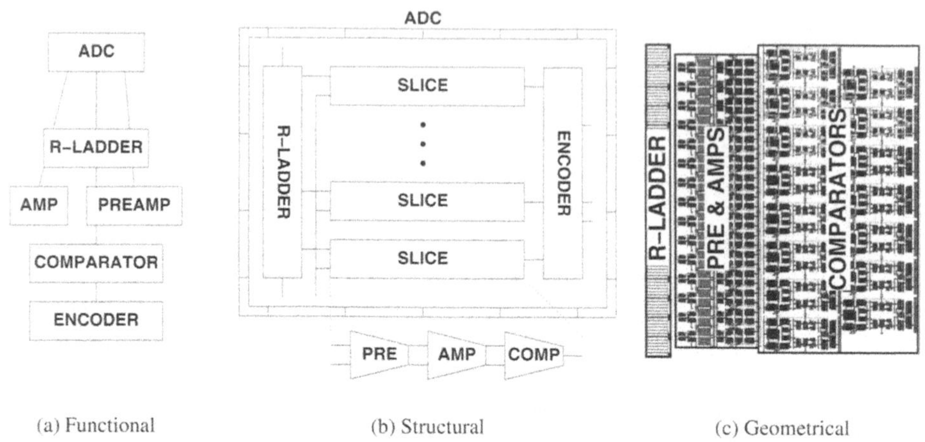

(a) Functional (b) Structural (c) Geometrical

Figure 2.2: Different types of hierarchical decomposition for a flash type A/D-converter.

is an intermediate level between A/D-converter and preamplifier, amplifier, comparator functionblocks to ease schematics drawing. In this case the *structural decomposition* refines the *functional decomposition.*

Geometrical decomposition is also employed in manual analog design. Although the design has been done with a certain structural or functional decomposition, when generating a mask layout a new decomposition is often chosen. When we look at the same A/D-converter as in the *structural decomposition,* a flash type, then we see that instead of grouping into one signal processing chain (as in the schematic), the basic cells are grouped differently, as is shown in figure 2.2(c). The preamplifiers are drawn together with the amplifiers and an array is made of them, while the comparators are placed in a separate array. This is because at the mask layout (geometrical) level other rules govern the choices made: the area is to be minimized, small blocks are merged before they are placed with larger blocks to optimize area. Once again this *geometrical decomposition* refines the *functional decomposition.*

The latter two decompositions are frequently used in analog design. The examples given did not give rise to conflicts with a *functional decomposition.* The *functional decomposition* is the dominant decomposition in analog synthesis tools. This is not always completely understood. When a manually designed analog circuit is inspected, one will often find that the schematics hierarchy (structural decomposition) and layout database (geometrical decomposition) do not coincide and that only at the top-level the functionblock is represented. Intermediate functionblocks cannot be identified, they are not explicitly inserted in the schematic hierarchy and layout database. In the remainder of this work it is assumed that using an identifiable *functional decomposition* is a fundamental component of structured design in general and analog synthesis in particular.

In figure 2.3, a high-level view of the analog design process is shown [Gie 00]. Note that the different design steps reflect a *functional decomposition* of the analog circuit. In addition to the design steps extra checks are built into the design process.

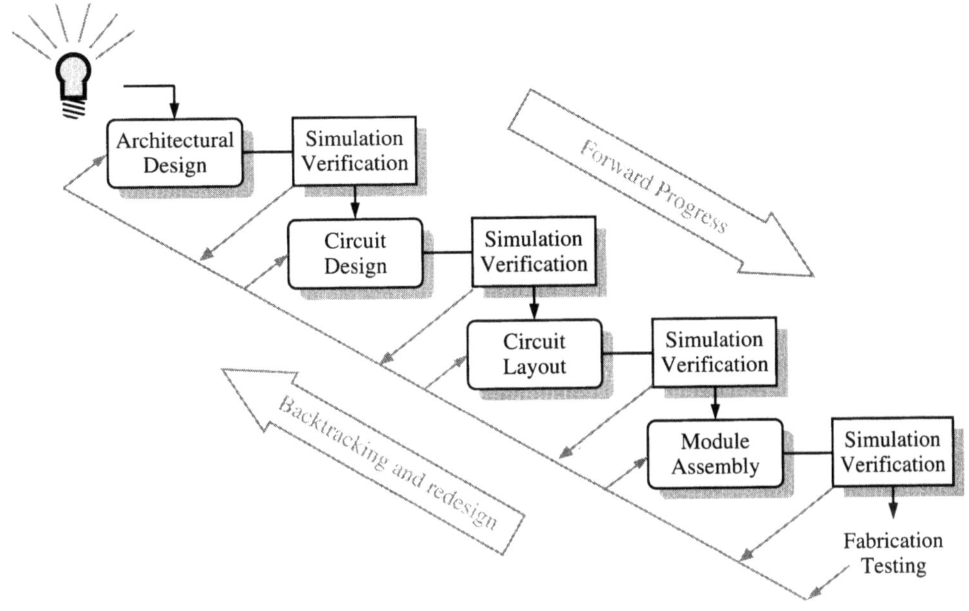

Figure 2.3: Hierarchical view of the design process [Gie 00].

Every design step is followed by a verification step. This step verifies the decisions taken in the design in an independent way. Typically numerical simulations of some kind are used to check the behavior of the design. At the layout level first an extraction of a netlist is required since a numerical circuit simulator does not work directly at the geometrical level. In case a design problem is detected doing this verification step some means of feedback is required to correct the problem by backtracking.

In conclusion we can now give a definition of analog synthesis: **Analog Synthesis** *is the process of designing analog circuits from behavioral specification to mask layout, using functional, structural or geometrical decomposition when required, in an automated or semi-automated way.*

In the next section an overview of the research in the area of analog synthesis will be given.

2.3 Overview of Analog Synthesis Research

Research in analog design automation has been relatively slow, lagging far beyond its digital counterpart. An overview of the recent state of the art is presented in [Carl 96] and [Gie 00]. In this section the emphasis is put on reporting the trends in the analog design automation field, not on giving a complete and detailed overview of all research.

2.3.1 Early Work

2.3.1.1 ADAM: IDAC (Sizing Synthesis) & ILAC (Layout Generation)

IDAC [Degra 87] is a sizing synthesis tool that relies on manually derived design equations. These equations can be compared to the equations a designer uses when deriving an initial design point in a manual design process. The equations, which are typically written from operating point information and small-signal parameters towards specifications (or behavioral parameters), actually need to be inverted for synthesis. Since in many cases the degrees of freedom (the independent design variables) are much higher than the number of specifications, this requires choosing and implementing a set of different design scenarios, depending on the specification values. For every topology this results in a separate hand-crafted design plan that contains all the knowledge of the circuit.

Once this design plan is available and stored in the library, fast execution times are possible and even trade-off analyses and performance space exploration is well within reach in affordable CPU times. At the same time it must be noted that setup times are long and setup cost is high. In [Been 93] it has been reported that the creation of a design plan typically takes 4 times more effort than is needed to actually design the circuit *once*. Considering the large number of circuits in industrial use, only highly reusable topologies are worthwhile to be included in the library. The integration of the tool in a spreadsheet environment, PlanFrame [Hend 93], did not remove this setup handicap. Furthermore, the selection of the topology amongst a set of candidates available in the library, is left to the designer.

IDAC has a companion layout tool set, ILAC [Rijm 89]. Its implementation borrows heavily from digital layout generation: a slicing tree floorplanning with flexible blocks, global maze routing and detailed channel routing followed by compaction. The major problem with this approach is to adapt the digital-oriented algorithms to handle the layout generation of low-level geometric optimizations that characterize expert manual design. ILAC compensates this with an extensive library of primitive device generators, that is however also difficult to maintain and port considering the rapidly evolving silicon technology.

It must also be noted that the two tools (IDAC & ILAC) were not integrated into one fully automated, easy to use environment. Nevertheless a large part of the analog synthesis flow is covered by the two tools.

2.3.1.2 ACACIA: OASYS (Sizing) & ANAGRAM (Layout)

ACACIA [Carl 88, Carl 89] is an analog synthesis environment. It uses the OASYS [Harj 89] and ANAGRAM [Gar 88] tools to automate the schematic synthesis and layout generation of analog circuits.

OASYS [Harj 89] adopts a design plan approach which is similar to IDAC. But instead of using flat schematics, it explicitly introduces hierarchy and also adds a heuristic approach to topology selection. Hierarchy allows the reuse of design plans of lower-level cells while building higher-level cell design plans. One top-level schematic combined with lower-level design plans is thus capable of generating a wide variety of transistor schematics. Collecting and ordering all the design knowledge however still remains a time-consuming task. The hierarchy improves the ratio design plan reuse over design plan creation, since a design plan for a particular lower-level block can be used in multiple higher-level topology templates. At the same time it must be noted that getting design plans right for multiple different applications is not trivial (consider a current source topology that can be used in an OTA, D/A-converter, biasing network, ...), turning the advantage of the hierarchy into an even greater burden when used *too extensively*.

ANAGRAM [Gar 88] uses the macro-cell style of ILAC but removes the necessity to have a large library of device generators by implementing important layout optimizations, such as diffusion-level device mergings, in the placement. The successors of ANAGRAM will be discussed later on.

2.3.1.3 BLADES (Sizing)

BLADES [ElTu 89] approaches the analog sizing problem in a completely different way. It uses artificial intelligence techniques to mimic the analog design expert. An expert system has been built incorporating analog design knowledge. It interfaces to numerical simulation to verify the design. The BLADES system only incorporated OPAMP circuits.

As for all the previous approaches, also the BLADES tool requires extensive preparation to create design plans.

2.3.1.4 Analog Module Generators (Layout)

ILAC implements a digitally oriented analog layout generation approach. An alternative is the implementation of a set of flexible analog module generators. The approach starts from a basic geometrical template (which is a full, parameterized layout), and completes it by correctly sizing the devices and the wires, as for instance [Kuhn 87]. More complex circuits are shown in [Been 93]. An analog layout language targeted to this type of module generators is BALLISTIC [Owen 95]. It is integrated in a commercial framework and handles OPAMP-level complexity layouts.

In fact module generators [Kuhn 87] are used in industrial practice nowadays [Lam 98, Lam 99]. The cost of maintaining templates [Owen 95] on the other hand, is only acceptable for highly reusable blocks. The advantage of this approach is not only its speed, but also its predictability. A number of different templates for the same circuit makes it possible to realize different aspect ratios and choose the best fit.

2.3.2 Second Generation

2.3.2.1 Sizing Synthesis: Plan-based versus Optimization-based

Early generation sizing tools all have one common problem: it is difficult and time-consuming to add knowledge or design plans to the synthesis system's library. This difficulty originates from the fact that starting from specifications and going directly to sizing, as shown in figure 2.4(a), is a hard problem.

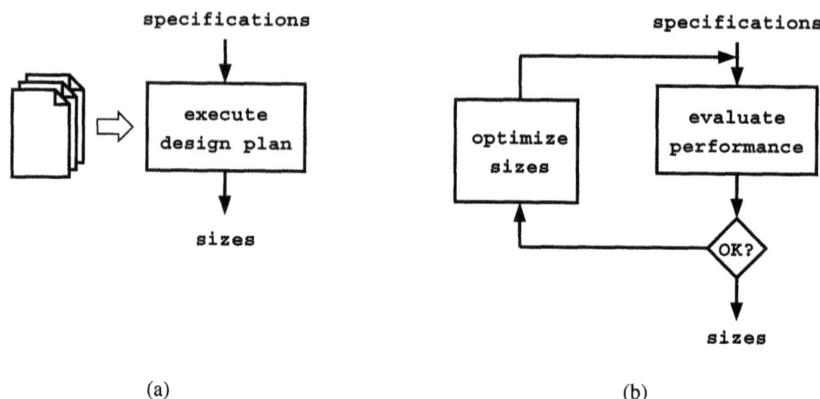

Figure 2.4: Plan-based sizing tools (a) versus optimization-based sizing tools (b) [Gie 00].

The second generation of experimental synthesis tools therefore rely on numerical optimization techniques to allow more flexibility and user control and reduce the setup time. Optimization techniques are used to solve for the degrees of freedom in the design such that the performance specifications are satisfied and user-defined design objectives (e.g. minimum power consumption) are minimized, see figure 2.4(b). Differences between the approaches in this category basically mount to the way how the circuit performance is evaluated at each iteration of the optimization loop.

A first group of methods uses analytic models that describe the basic performance relations in the circuit by a set of (explicit or implicit) symbolic equations. These methods are relatively fast but their accuracy is higher for rather linear (e.g. small-signal) characteristics. Examples of such systems include for instance at the level of basic analog blocks OPASYN [Koh 90], OPTIMAN [Gie 90, Gie 91c], STAIC [Harv 92] and ISAID [Tou 95, Mak 95], and at the level of Δ/Σ-converters SD-OPT [Med 95].

A second group of methods uses numerical simulation in the inner loop of the optimization. These methods have the full accuracy of a numerical device simulator (for instance SPICE), but are extremely slow (unless the optimization space considered is very restricted) and still require many design constraints to be incorporated into the optimization problem in order to guarantee a properly functioning circuit. Examples of such systems include for instance at the level of basic analog blocks FRIDGE [Med 94] and ASTRX/OBLX [Och 96]. The former uses plain-vanilla SPICE; the latter uses asymptotic waveform evaluation (AWE) to speed up the linear (small-signal) simulations but requires the designer to provide analytic formulas for all other characteristics.

2.3.2.2 Layout Generation: Device-level & Performance-driven

KOAN/ANAGRAMII [Cohn 91] is the successor of the ANAGRAM tools of the first generation. KOAN is an analog device-level placement tool that uses simulated annealing and a limited library of basic device generators. Complex structures, that required specialized module generators in first generation tools, are created on the fly by selectively merging devices by appropriately sharing of geometry. ANAGRAMII is a detailed area router that takes into account analog constraints: symmetry, shielding, crosstalk avoidance, ... Compared to the ILAC tool set KOAN/ANAGRAMII is a vast improvement, both in quality of results and maintainability.

In [Chou 90a, Chou 90b, Mala 96] the first analog performance-driven layout methodology has been proposed. The influence of layout parasitics on the performance of the circuit is modeled using sensitivities. The performance constraints of the circuit are then mapped on a set of constraints on layout parasitics. These parasitic constraints are used to drive the layout generation process. Application of this methodology to channel and area routing [Chou 90c, Mala 93], placement [Char 94a, Char 94b] and compaction [Felt 93] have been presented. KOAN/ANAGRAMIII uses a similar parasitic bounding strategy for routing [Bas 93].

2.3.2.3 Performance-driven Synthesis Methodology

In [Gie 91a, Gie 91c, Chang 92, Chang 96] the performance-driven approach has been extended to the complete synthesis flow. Not only layout, but also topology selection and sizing is steered by the performance constraints. Verification of the intermediate result is made against these performance specifications.

In [Chang 94, Neff 96] this design methodology has been applied to the design of interpolative current source D/A-converters and in [Chang 95a] to the design of Δ/Σ A/D-converter. Note that these works present the application of the methodology to certain circuits using amongst others the tools described in the previous section. They do not present an integrated environment that could allow automatic synthesis.

2.3.3 Most Recent Work

2.3.3.1 Sizing Synthesis: Equation-based & Simulation-based

The battle between equation-based and simulation-based approaches is still raging. Two recently reported tools are at the extreme of the divide.

At one end of the spectrum, there are the tools reported in [Kras 99, Phel 99, Phel 00]. These are simulation-based approaches. In MAELSTROM [Kras 99] a simulated annealing based evolutionary algorithm is applied to the sizing of OPAMP type circuits. The novelties of the presented approach are that: (1) the simulation environment is insulated from the optimizer, making the tool to a large degree simulator independent, (2) the exact same model used to verify the circuit, is used during optimization, removing redesigns caused by incorrect modeling and (3) the evolutionary algorithm is parallelized, reducing intractable total CPU times that would be in the order of days to an acceptable turn-around time (on 20 machines in parallel) of a few hours. The ANACONDA [Phel 99] tool uses the same encapsulation of the simulator and accurate model of the circuit in combination with a stochastic pattern search algorithm. In [Phel 00] the design of an ADSL front-end has been automated using ANACONDA [Phel 99] and compared with a manual (reference) design. The idea was to redesign the circuit, with the same specifications, potentially improving the design. As it turned out, the reference design could only marginally be improved. The automatic tool was run a few times, and almost all resulting designs were close to the reference design.

At the other end of the spectrum the tools reported in [Hers 98, Hers 99] are found. Here the idea is to apply an extremely fast optimization algorithm to the analog sizing problem. A Geometric Program (GP) [Duff 67] is an optimization problem of the following form: let $\mathbf{x}$ be a vector $(x_1, \ldots, x_n)$ of n real, positive variables and

$$\begin{aligned} \text{minimize} \quad & f_0(\mathbf{x}) \\ \text{subject to} \quad & f_i(\mathbf{x}) \leq 1 \quad i = 1, \ldots, m \\ & g_i(\mathbf{x}) = 1 \quad i = 1, \ldots, p \\ & x_i > 0 \quad i = 1, \ldots, n \end{aligned} \tag{2.1}$$

where $f_0, \ldots, f_m$ are posynomial functions and $g_1, \ldots, g_p$ are monomial functions. A function f is called a posynomial function of $\mathbf{x}$ if it has the form $f(x_1, \ldots, x_n) = \sum_{k=1}^{t} c_k x_1^{\alpha_{1k}} x_2^{\alpha_{2k}} \cdots x_n^{\alpha_{nk}}$ where $c_k > 0$ and $\alpha_{ij} \in \mathbb{R}$. When there is only one term in the sum, i.e., $t = 1$, f is a monomial function.

A geometric program is convex by definition, and the local optimum that is found using interior point methods is thus the global optimum. At this end of the spectrum almost no CPU time is required to size analog circuits (less than 60 seconds for a 15 transistor OTA). However, the modeling effort is high. Only equations can be used of the posynomial form as defined above. In [Hers 98] a MOS device model was presented, followed by applications of this optimization algorithm to linear circuits, as for instance OPAMPs with the GPCAD tool [Hers 98], and RF LC-based Voltage Controlled Oscillators (LC-VCOs) [Hers 99]. Note that in this case, due to the speed of the optimization algorithm, trade-off analysis becomes a feasible instrument for designing circuits. The most important drawback of the method is the limitation of the design equations to be of posynomial and/or monomial form.

As already mentioned, these recently reported research results are at the opposite ends of the spectrum. The first approach uses parallelism (i.e. using multiple machines in parallel) to keep the turn-around time of simulation-based approach within bounds. It reduces the tedious modeling work as much as possible, this to make the conversion to an optimization problem as easy as possible. The second method applies a fast, global optimization algorithm to a fine-tuned equation-based model of the circuit. The model has to meet the requirement as set forward in equation (2.1). This shifts the problem to modeling the circuit under design, and virtually eliminates any optimization difficulties.

As it stands now, neither the simulation-based, nor the equation-based approach is a definitive winner in this contest.

2.3.3.2 Layout Generation: Layout Representation & Direct Performance-driven

Recently new placement representation forms have been proposed. The placement presentation is the data structure which is used to hold the positions of the cells during placement. A slicing structure is a standard placement representation which finds its origin in digital standard cell placement. It is a hierarchical placement of in turn vertical and horizontal neighboring cells. The important disadvantage of the slicing structure is that it can only represent slice-able layouts. It can not represent every conceivable configuration of four or more cells.

That's why absolute placement representation has replaced the slicing structure in analog layout generation tools [Lam 99]. In the absolute placement representation all cells have absolute coordinates, and *any* configuration of cells is thus possible. The disadvantage of this approach is that the placement problem is burdened with a compaction problem that does not exist in slicing structures: The devices are placed anywhere in a rectangular box (playing field); the total area of the layout has to be made as small as possible by including an area term in the cost function or running a compactor after placement and routing.

Therefore new placement representations have been proposed. Sequence pair [Bala 99] representation and O-Trees [Pang 00] offer the advantage of the slicing structure: a relative placement which can easily be translated to an absolute, dense placement. At the same time they do not require that the layout has to be slice-able, thus extending the range of reachable layout configurations for four or more devices.

A last result of recent research is the introduction of *direct* performance-driven layout. Early performance-driven layout translated constraints on the performances to constraints on the layout parasitics before starting the layout generation process. In the LAYLA tool [Lam 98, Lam 99] the sensitivities of all the performances towards (layout) parasitics are derived before starting the layout tools, resulting in *direct* performance-driven layout generation. Note that LAYLA will be discussed further on in this work, since it has been integrated in the **AMGIE** system.

2.3.4 Conclusions

Most of the above tools cover only part of the entire analog design flow and therefore only partially fulfill the increasing need observed in industry today for an integrated synthesis environment that increases analog design productivity. For instance SD-OPT [Med 95] and FRIDGE [Med 94] can be used in combination to cover the higher-level respectively the lower-level design of Δ/Σ-converters, but no layout synthesis solution is provided. ASTRX/OBLX [Och 96] on the other hand has a companion analog layout synthesis tool KOAN/ANAGRAMII [Cohn 91] but no solution is offered for selecting a good topology from a library. In summary, all components of a viable synthesis environment exist, but no actual implementation has been realized and its functionality verified.

In this work a *fully integrated* analog synthesis environment, called **AMGIE**, is presented that implements a *hierarchical top-down refinement, bottom-up assembly performance-driven* design strategy for analog designs [Sans 94, Gie 95b, Reyn 96, VdPlas 01]. It covers the full design path from *specifications* over best *topology selection* and optimum *circuit sizing* down to automated *layout generation* followed by automatic *verification* and datasheet extraction. The system is also CMOS *process independent* and has an *open* library interface to add new circuit topologies into the library relatively easily. As every new circuit requires some amount of modeling, the approach is best suited for topologies that will be reused several times, i.e. topologies having a high reuse factor. For instance, in many companies always the same basic limited set of OPAMP structures is used for most applications. Hence their design could be entirely automated while guaranteeing a fully customized solution for every set of specifications and for every selected CMOS process. In this way also technology porting of a highly reusable cell library can be automated. On the other hand, some of the individual tools of the **AMGIE** system can also be used as point tools to leverage the design of the so-called "once-in-a-lifetime" circuits, as for instance is the case in domains like telecom and RF where the topologies tend to change with every new design.

In section 2.4 an overview will be given of the functionalities and capabilities of the **AMGIE** analog synthesis environment. Also the software architecture of the entire system will be described and the design controller (DC) which is the brains of the system. In the next chapter, chapter 3, the different design steps will then be discussed in detail. The corresponding design tools and their underlying algorithms will be explained. Small, easily understandable examples are used to demonstrate how the algorithms work. In chapter 4 the productiveness and efficiency of the system will be demonstrated by means of representative experimental results, including a fabricated design and measurement results. Conclusions will be formulated at the end of part I.

2.4 The AMGIE Synthesis System

In this section first the functionality of the **AMGIE** synthesis system [VdPlas 01] is described, including the supported design flow, followed by a description of the software architecture.

2.4.1 Functionality of the Analog Synthesis Environment

In the **AMGIE** system [VdPlas 01], the user first has to select the desired type of circuit that (s)he wants to synthesize (the so-called *functionblock*, e.g. an OPAMP) and then has to enter the desired specifications for this circuit (including the performance specifications, the optimization targets and a choice of the technology process). **AMGIE** then selects the most appropriate circuit schematic (*topology*) for these specifications from its library, optimally sizes this topology, verifies the sizing by detailed simulations, generates an optimal layout, verifies the result again with simulations after layout extraction, and generates a final datasheet.

For more complex circuits (e.g. data converters) these steps can be executed in an hierarchical way. According to the divide and conquer strategy, hierarchy is used when the circuit is too complex to be designed as one block, and therefore is decomposed in easier to design subblocks (like a comparator in the converter example). Hierarchy also results in more overall circuit schematics since every high-level topology can be realized with different lower-level subblock implementations. On the other hand the use of hierarchical split-up is complicated by the interactions between the different subblocks (e.g. there is a large interaction at the level of differential pairs and current mirrors in an OPAMP: DC bias, capacitive loading, ...). Therefore, our rule of practice is to introduce hierarchy only when the resulting subblocks can be designed separately much easier than the overall block as a whole; if not it is preferred to design the block (e.g. an OPAMP) *without* decomposition.

The **AMGIE** system can be run fully automatically in which case the designer accepts the solutions generated by the tools, or it can be used interactively in which case the designer is able to manually intervene and perform some changes to the generated solutions (e.g. select an alternative topology than the one proposed by the system). The system supports two different design styles: (1) *standard* cells, and (2) *custom* cells. Standard cells are cells which have been completely designed before within the **AMGIE** system or added to the **AMGIE** cell library by a silicon foundry, third party or the user himself or herself. In this way the system thus automatically supports the reuse of previous, possibly silicon-proven designs. Their major drawback however is that they are process-specific. The custom cells on the other hand are cells that still have all degrees of freedom (all design variables) free to customize the design and the layout in an optimal way to the requested specifications in the target technology process. These cells will be synthesized by following all steps in the complete design flow of the system. Custom cells can be more optimal than standard cells because they are fully tailored to the application, but they take longer to design (and they are not silicon proven). Note that every fully synthesized design is automatically stored as a standard cell in the system. So every custom cell may be accompanied by a number of fixed or standard cell implementations in the system's library, and the library will automatically grow along with the use of the system.

The supported design flow will now be explained in more detail.

2.4.1.1 Input to the AMGIE System

After starting **AMGIE**, the user first has to select the type of analog functionblock that he wants to design out of the list of types that are available in the **AMGIE** cell library. The corresponding specification template is then retrieved and the designer has to enter the following specifications required for his design in the specsheet editor (as shown in figure 2.5):

- the preferred design style (standard cell, custom cell — the default is in that order)
- the performance specifications for the selected functionblock type — the list of specifiable performances depends on the selected circuit type and the constraints on these specifications can be of equality or inequality (larger than or smaller than) type. The performance specifications are expressed in one of the following forms:
    1. $P \in [P_{lb}, P_{ub}]$: the performance value is constrained in an interval, possibly the upper or lower bound is $\pm\infty$. The interval can be open or closed (inequality constraint), or be a single value (equality constraint). The majority of the performance specifications belong to this category. An example of a performance value is for instance the gainbandwidth, that should be higher than or equal to 10MHz.
    2. $P \in [P_{lb}, P_{ub}]$ @ λ : the performance value is constrained in an interval at a certain parameter value. For instance the settling time should be smaller than 10ms for settling to within 0.1%. Both the settling time value and the settling accuracy are to be specified.
- the optimization targets and their relative weights in the cost function that control the sizing and optimization step. The designer indicates which performances are part of the cost function that is being minimized.
- operating constraints (such as power supply voltages, temperature range, etc.)
- the chosen technology process
- additional user options that control the **AMGIE** run, for instance:
    - choice of the optimization algorithm used in the sizing and optimization step
    - the level of detail with which the trace of the design run is displayed to the user in the session history.

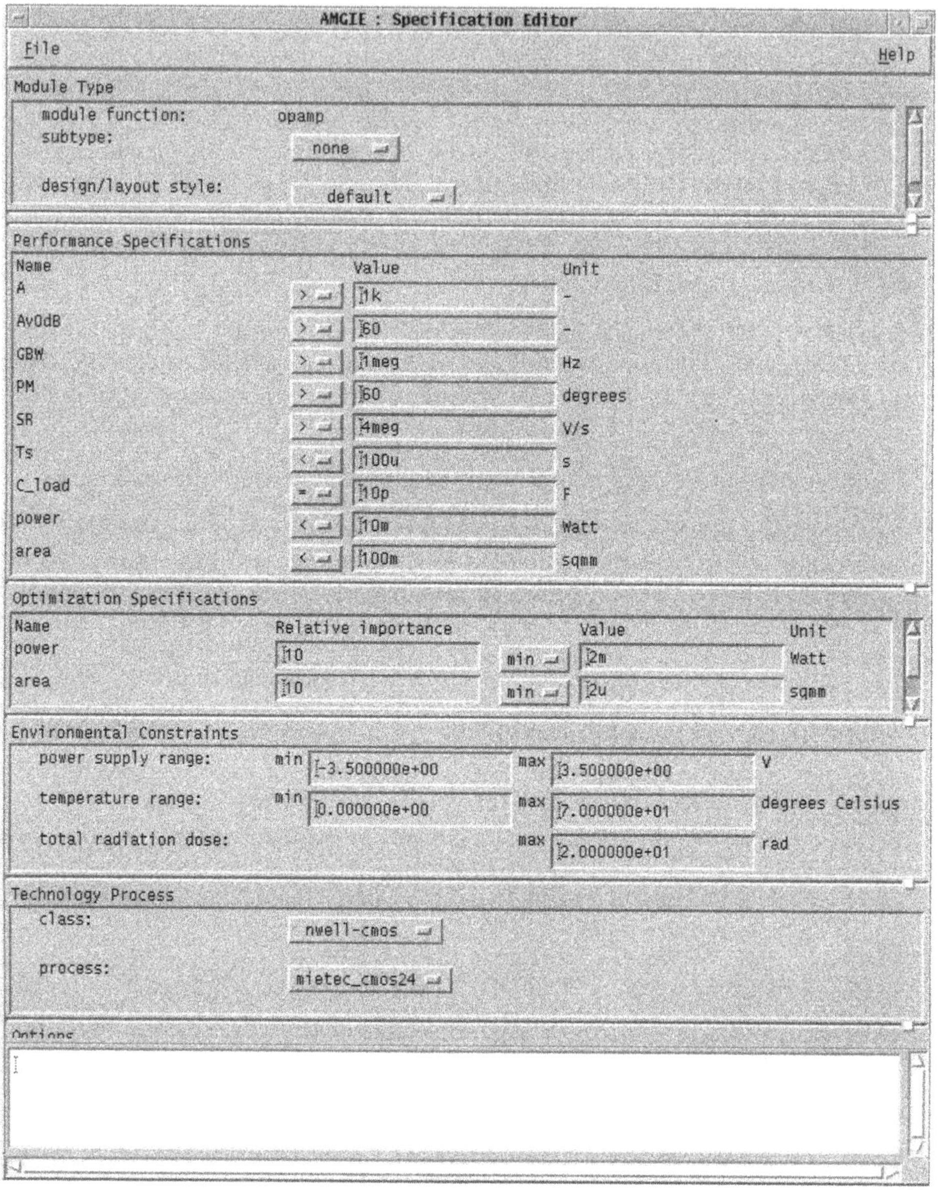

AMGIE : Specification Editor

File Help

Module Type

module function: opamp
subtype: none
design/layout style: default

Performance Specifications

Name		Value	Unit
A	>	1k	-
AvOdB	>	60	-
GBW	>	1meg	Hz
PM	>	60	degrees
SR	>	4meg	V/s
Ts	<	100u	s
C_load	=	10p	F
power	<	10m	Watt
area	<	100m	sqmm

Optimization Specifications

Name	Relative importance		Value	Unit
power	10	min	2m	Watt
area	10	min	2u	sqmm

Environmental Constraints

power supply range:	min	-3.500000e+00	max	3.500000e+00	V
temperature range:	min	0.000000e+00	max	7.000000e+01	degrees Celsius
total radiation dose:			max	2.000000e+01	rad

Technology Process

class: nwell-cmos
process: mietec_cmos24

Options

Figure 2.5: Snapshot of the **AMGIE** specification sheet editor.

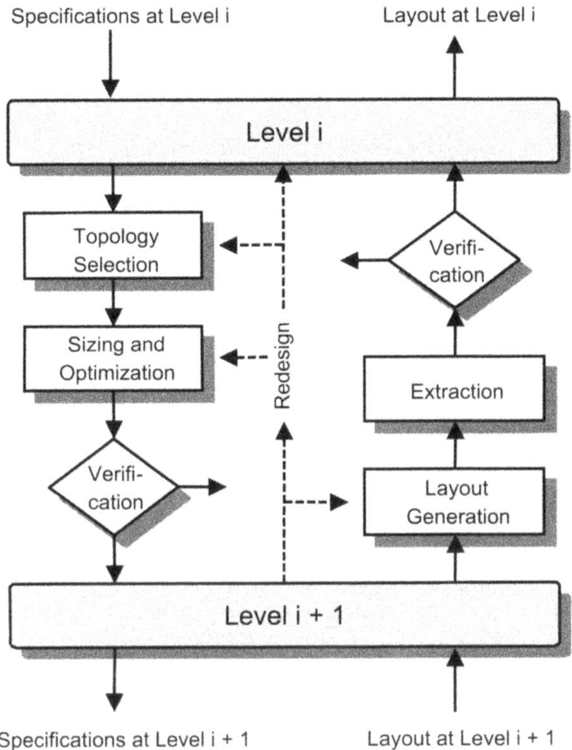

Figure 2.6: Hierarchical design flow implemented in the **AMGIE** synthesis system.

If the entered specification values are too stringent or unrealistic, the synthesis of course will fail. In order to anticipate such obvious problems, a specification value *checker* has been implemented that checks if the specification values entered by the user are within an allowed realistic range (specified in the library for the functionblock), and that warns the user immediately if the requested values are invalid or unrealistic while suggesting a reasonable default value. The user can also deactivate a performance specification parameter in case it is unimportant for his particular application.

This is basically all the input the **AMGIE** system expects from the user to start a synthesis run.

2.4.1.2 Design Flow and Hierarchy implemented in the AMGIE Synthesis System

The design strategy implemented in the **AMGIE** analog synthesis environment is a *performance-driven top-down refinement, bottom-up assembly* strategy, which consists of the following sequence of design steps. For each of these steps a separate software tool implements this step: either a new tool that has been developed or an existing commercial tool (especially for simulation and back-end tasks) that has been integrated in the system. Their details will be described in chapter 3. The design flow supported by the system is shown in figure 2.6 (for standard cells some of these steps are of course trivial):

1. starting from the input specifications entered by the user in the specsheet as specified in the previous section;
2. first the most promising topology for the functionblock is chosen from the cell library by the topology selection tool;
3. then this topology is optimally sized for the given requirements and optimization targets by the sizing and optimization tool;
4. the resulting design is then extensively simulated in the verification tool in order to verify that the design meets all performance specifications. If design failures or specification violations are noticed during this verification step, then previous design steps have to be changed and part of the design flow has to be iterated through backtracking (this is called redesign);
5. if the selected topology is defined in terms of non-primitive subblocks (e.g. an OPAMP within a filter), the system then first synthesizes these subblocks at this point in the design flow, by applying the complete design flow to every such subblock. When all non-primitive subblocks are synthesized, the design flow of the higher-level block continues;
6. an optimal layout is generated by the layout generation tool;
7. the circuit is then extracted from the layout (including all layout parasitics) and again extensively simulated in the verification tool and a datasheet is generated. In case of design errors or specification violations, the same redesign procedure as outlined in step 4 is followed. If not, the design is successfully completed and the synthesis run is finished when the cell has been stored as a standard cell.

Low-level circuits (such as OPAMPs) are handled in a flat way as fully expanded transistor-level circuit schematics in the above design flow (step 5 is then trivial). For circuits of a higher complexity level (e.g. A/D-converters) this is no longer possible, and the above design flow is executed in an hierarchical way. Sizing and optimization (step 3) is then rather *specification translation* which maps the specifications of the top-level cell to the individual specifications of each of the subcells (such as the comparator in the A/D-converter). The subcells are then synthesized separately (step 5), one by one, using the same design flow, and the resulting subblock layouts are returned up the hierarchy to assemble the layout of the top-level cell (bottom-up layout assembly in step 6). If needed, redesign iterations are carried out across the design hierarchy.

In such an hierarchical approach different alternative design strategies are possible. A first possibility is a depth-first approach in which all low-level cells are first fully synthesized top-down and bottom-up after which the top-level design flow is resumed (see figure 2.7(a)). The order in which the low-level cells are designed however will strongly determine the success

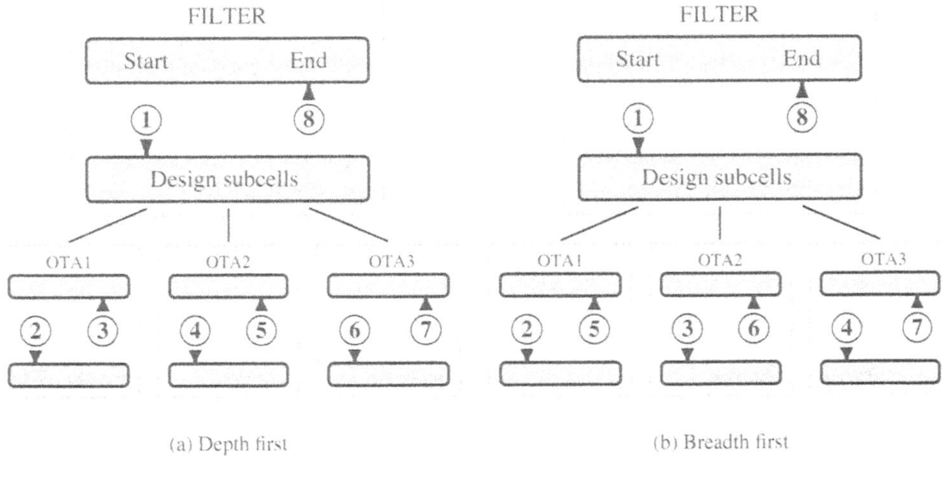

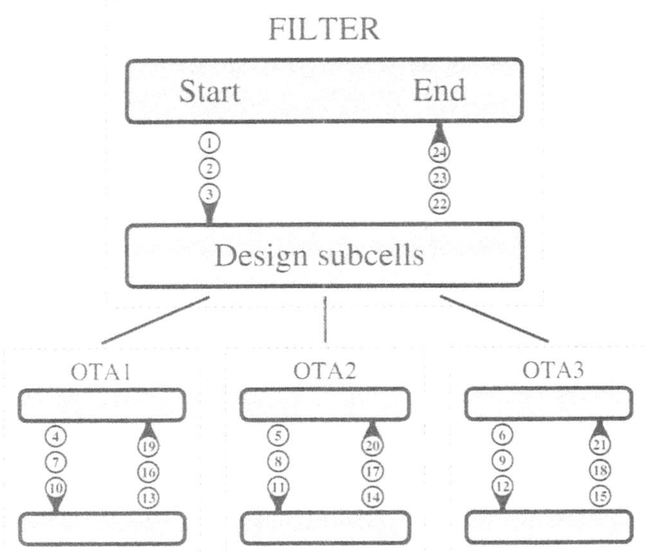

Figure 2.7: Different hierarchical design strategies (the numbers indicate the sequence of the steps executed).

rate of this approach. In general it is advisable to design the cells with the most demanding requirements first, since for these the chance of a design failure is the highest. To correct this failure the specifications will ultimately have to be relaxed, and other low-level cells will have to get stronger requirements to meet the same specifications at the top-level. It thus seems more appropriate to use a breadth-first strategy where only the top-down path (the topology selection and sizing steps) is executed for every low-level cell before any bottom-up path (the layout step) is started (see figure 2.7(b)). In this approach, an eventual design failure is detected quickly and causes less work to be wasted. The breadth-first approach can even further be refined to the level of the individual design steps (see figure 2.7(c)), where topology selection is performed first for every low-level cell, then sizing and optimization, etc. This approach is the most efficient (for detecting and correcting design failures) and therefore has been implemented in the **AMGIE** system.

The above design flow has been encoded in a software module called the Design Controller (DC). This module is the central "brain" of the **AMGIE** system and controls the execution of every synthesis run, according to the embedded design flow. The next step in the design flow can only be executed if the previous step has been terminated successfully. In this way the system can also guarantee full data consistency during the design, since no step can be executed before all required data have been correctly created before. Note however that the designer at any time can redo a previous step or — at his own responsibility — change the design after any step before proceeding. Part of the design flow is also the handling of redesign in the case of design failures. In the present **AMGIE** version, the Design Controller (DC) does not yet automatically impose the corrective action to be taken in case of redesign. As this largely depends on the actual design data, it would require sophisticated design expertise to be built in the design controller. Instead, the system includes a redesign wizard which is automatically invoked when a redesign action is needed and which proposes to the designer some context-specific alternative actions. The designer is then ultimately responsible for deciding on the actual backtracking action that has to be taken in order to correct the problem.

2.4.1.3 The Graphical User Interface

Although the **AMGIE** system can also be run in fully automatic batch mode, the system is most frequently operated interactively by an analog designer, who has the ultimate responsibility over the design. The designer supervises the design flow and design decisions, invokes the different subtools and views the status and data of the on-going design through the system's graphical user interface (shown in figure 2.8). All the individual subtools can run automatically and return their result to the user after completing their task, which makes batch mode runs possible. The designer can accept the solution suggested by each tool, and continues with the next step, or (s)he can change the solution manually in the appropriate editor, but at his/her own responsibility as no data consistency can be guaranteed anymore in this case.

The main graphical user interface (GUI) window of the **AMGIE** system is shown in figure 2.8. This is the *cockpit* of the system. This window is divided in the following panels:

1. *Hierarchical View Panel* at the top, which shows a graphical representation of the complete design hierarchy (top cell and the subcells down the hierarchy — multiple hierarchical levels are possible). From this panel the functionblock hierarchy can be navigated: switch to another functionblock, etc. Completely designed subblock nodes are

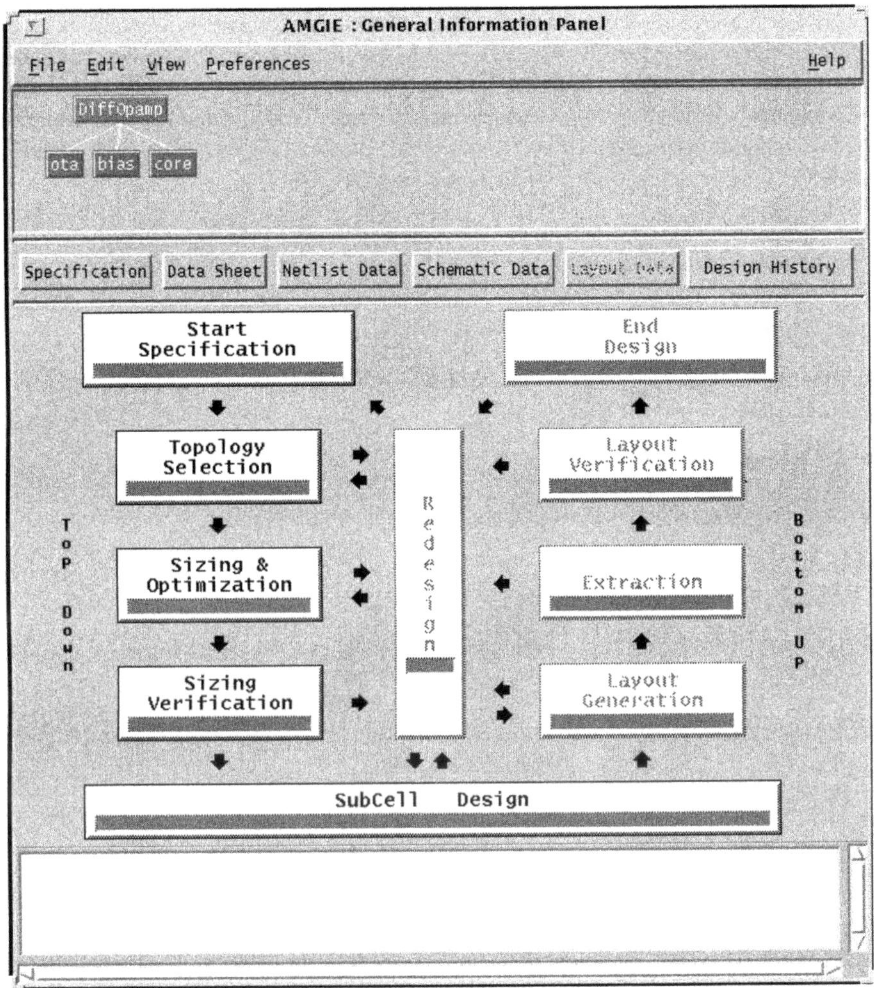

Figure 2.8: Graphical User Interface (GUI) of the **AMGIE** system.

colored green, yet to be completed subblock nodes are colored red, the current function-block under design is colored orange.

2. *Data View Panel* in the middle: this panel allows to open different pop-up editors that show the important design data (specifications, datasheet, netlist, schematic, layout, design history file) about the cell that is being designed at that moment. Each of these editors can be executed at any moment in the design flow, and the data are updated continuously with the progress in the design flow.

3. *Design Flow Panel* at the bottom, which allows the designer to execute the different tools in the order imposed by the design flow described above. The design flow panel is a graphical representation of the abstract design flow embedded in the Design Controller. It indicates through a *traffic light* coloring scheme (red — green) which design steps have already been executed successfully, and the next step can only be executed when the previous step has been terminated successfully.

4. a *message window* for warnings and messages at the very bottom and reporting the progress of the synthesis run.

2.4.1.4 Output of the AMGIE System

After running through the above design flow, the **AMGIE** system will return the following output to the user:

- the layout of the circuit
- the sized schematic (from which a netlist can be generated)
- the datasheet, which contains the simulated performance values obtained by the final design
- the design history, which is a file that contains the trace of the complete design session, for inspection purposes
- a design document that contains the specification values, intermediate results and a complete, detailed description of the final result
- an automatically created standard cell of the design, that can be reused in the system during later design runs.

All these data can be queried by the designer from within the main **AMGIE** GUI (see the middle panel in figure 2.8). For each type of information, a separate window pops up in the **AMGIE** GUI. This information is updated after each design step in the design flow, and is therefore continuously available for inspection by the designer during the synthesis run.

2.4.2 Software Architecture of the AMGIE System

The overall software architecture of the **AMGIE** system is shown in figure 2.9 and has been developed in a modular way. The system consists of a number of separate subtools, which are implemented as UNIX processes. The user interacts with the Design Controller (DC) by means of the Graphical User Interface. The individual subtools (such as the topology selection tool, the sizing and optimization tool, the verification tool with links to different simulators and the layout generation tool) are connected to the Design Controller and pass in this way design data between them. **AMGIE** stores data in a run-time database for the cell that is under design (*CUD* Database). Two libraries, the *technology library* and the *cell library*, store the design knowledge that is used by the design tools. The complete system has been integrated in a commercial EDA framework. The actual design database is implemented in this framework's

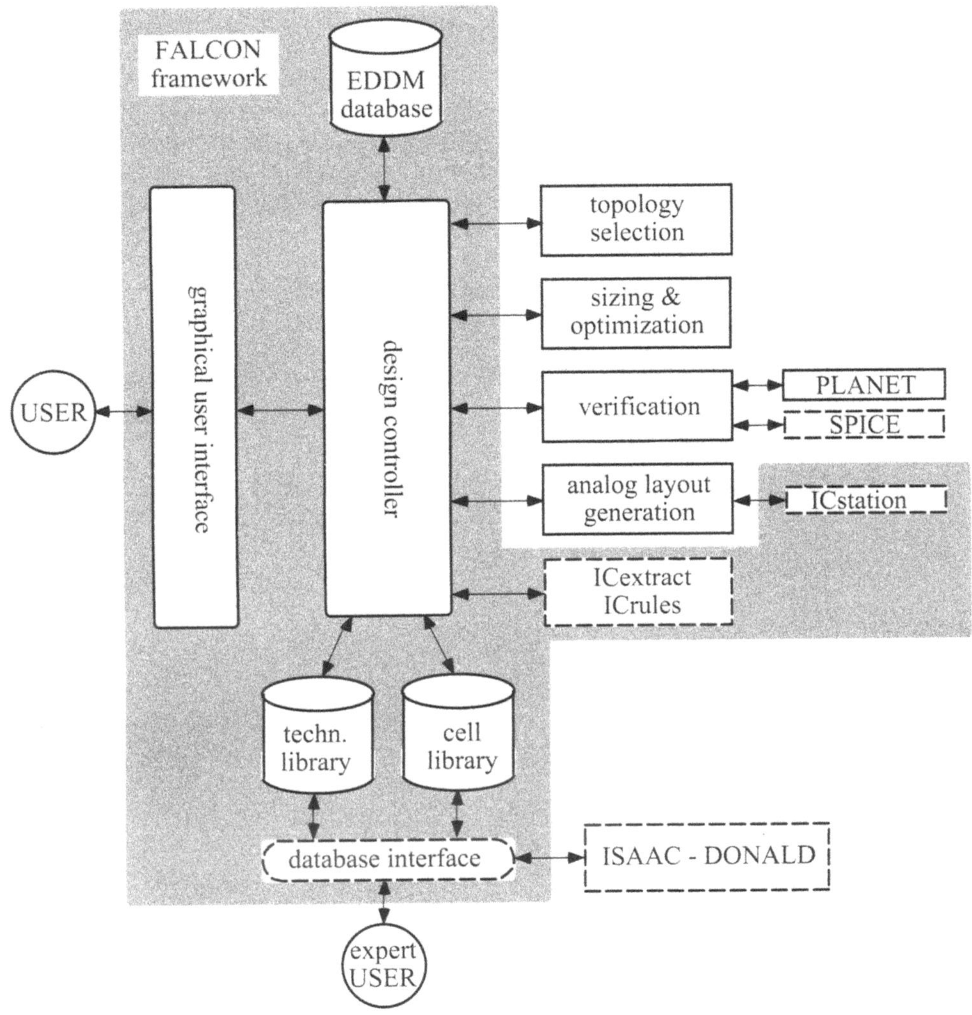

Figure 2.9: Software architecture of the **AMGIE** synthesis system.

database. The integration within a commercial framework also offered the advantage that existing commercial tools could be used for simulation, extraction, layout viewing, schematic capture and framework services. All data exchange occurs through a procedural interface, called *Data Representation Interface* (DRI). In this way the implementation details of the libraries and run-time database are hidden from the subtools and this modular design makes extension or modification of the libraries possible without changing the subtools. This should also make it possible to move to another EDA framework with a relatively small effort, or to extend **AMGIE** relatively easily with new software modules.

The **AMGIE** system needs 2 libraries for its operation:

1. cell library: this library contains all information about the analog cells needed for topology selection, sizing and optimization, verification and layout generation. The **AMGIE** system can only design circuits for which the corresponding data are included in the cell library. In order to allow the designer to trade off short design time for flexibility and optimized performance depending on his/her particular application, the cell library contains both standard and custom cells.

2. technology library: this library contains all technology process specific information that is needed by the different tools in the system.

Two user-cases of the **AMGIE** system can be distinguished:

1. the typical **AMGIE** user. This can be a novice analog designer, a system-level or digital designer. This designer is on average not capable of *manually* designing an analog circuit to a specified performance. He/she uses the **AMGIE** system through the interface shown in figure 2.8, and relies on the knowledge stored in the libraries. He/she is in full control of the design process through the user interface and leaves the point tools of the **AMGIE** system solve all design problems (topology selection, sizing, verification and layout generation). An experienced analog designer can also use the **AMGIE** system in this mode: (s)he wants a low-challenge analog design solved quickly in this case.

2. the library developer or expert user. The **AMGIE** system relies on libraries for its operation. Library developers provide this information. This category of users has an interface to the libraries (cell and technology) where they can add, modify and remove device, topology and functionblock data. A library developer is a highly trained person: ideally (s)he is an experienced analog designer, who has an extensive understanding of the **AMGIE** system and its operation. This set of skills is however hard to develop. In practice a number of library developers work in parallel, all being experts at a specific part of the developer's job: some derive sizing models, see section 3.3, others provide template files for verification, see section 3.5, etc. The library developer uses the standard **AMGIE** user interface of figure 2.8 in *library mode* and command-line user interfaces to the libraries (bottom of figure 2.9).

Design Process and Design Data Management

The Design Controller (DC) is at the heart of the **AMGIE** system, as shown in figure 2.9. It manages the design process and design data [VdPlas 94]. The design controller implementation is centered around a state transition model of the design process. A Petri model of the design process is shown in figure 2.10. Note that the breadth-first strategy as explained in section 2.4.1.2 is not visible on this graph. The shown graph represents the *forward* design flow at one level of the hierarchy (i.e. without redesign steps). The complete graph with inclusion of all redesign paths would be too complicated to show. What is modeled in this graph is the state of the system, represented by the circles, and the processes being executed going from one state to the next. For instance, the specification state is the start of a new design. From

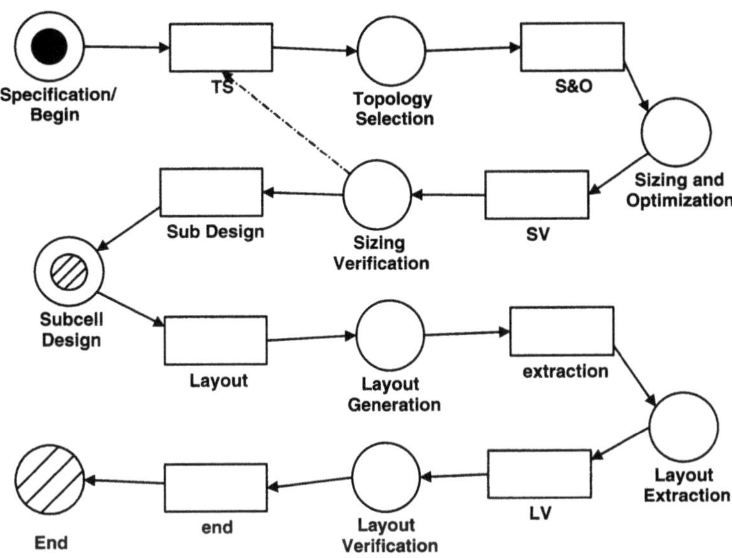

Figure 2.10: Petri net of the design controller (one hierarchical level — forward path only, redesign has not been included in the figure).

there Topology Selection is run and one ends up in the topology selection state. The next logical step is running sizing and optimization, reaching the sizing and optimization state, and so on. A dashed transition line has been added, from Sizing Verification state back to the Topology Selection process. Following this transition would equate to rechoosing another topology after sizing and verification. This is possible but not part of the forward design flow and it is very likely a manual intervention from a user. In the design controller the valid transitions are coded, as well as the automatic (forward) transitions. The latter allow an automatic synthesis run of the tool. This concludes the *design process management features* built into the design controller. But the design controller does more than this. It also manages all design data. In figure 2.11 the design data management of the design controller is shown when a point tool is run, for instance to choose a topology. First of all, the cell library, technology library and the database of the cell under design (CUD) are accessed by the design controller and all appropriate design data is retrieved. This data is passed on to the design point tool. The tool is run and its return value is checked. If the tool returned success, which means it didn't experience any problems finding a valid solution, the resulting design data is stored in the CUD database. In this way all the tools have been interfaced to the three main databases of the **AMGIE** system. In total more than 50 design data types have been defined. The most important of these data types have corresponding editors and/or viewers that can be called from the main GUI window, figure 2.8. An example of such an editor is the specification sheet editor that is shown in figure 2.5. Other examples are the schematic editor, layout editor, netlist editor, datasheet editor, design history browser, etc. For further snapshots of these editors/viewers, the reader is referred to the **AMGIE** user manual [VdPlas 96a].

The modular implementation approach that has been chosen, makes it possible to replace

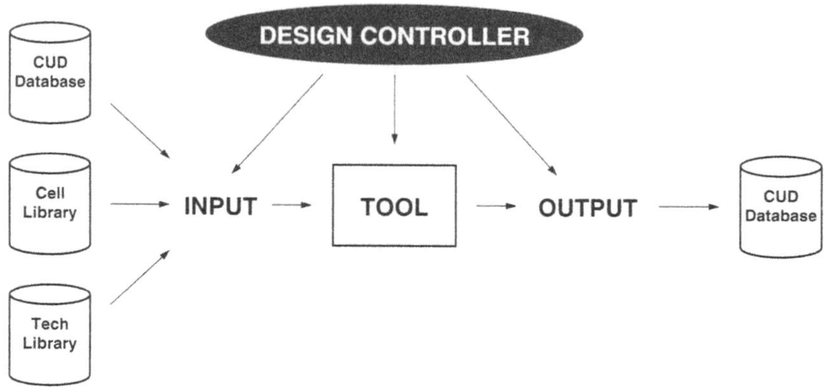

Figure 2.11: The Design Controller (DC) retrieves the input, runs the tool and stores the results.

existing point tools with compatible, alternative implementations (which could even be manual). The strength of the **AMGIE** synthesis system is that for all design steps *automated* solutions have been implemented. These design tools will be presented in the next chapter.

2.5 Summary

In this chapter, first the terminology has been defined that will be used throughout this work. A definition has been given for *analog synthesis*, which is the main topic of this text. Next an overview has been given of the research that has been carried out over the years in this area. Three generations of synthesis tools and systems have been identified and their advantages and disadvantages summarized. The major limitations of the approaches proposed up till now are: (1) that they do not offer an integrated environment, (2) that they do not cover the complete design flow, and (3) that they are not easily extendible with new circuits, ideas, etc.

The **AMGIE** analog synthesis system [VdPlas 01] was introduced next. It aims to solve the major limitations of the earlier tools: it is an *integrated environment*, that covers the *complete design flow* from specification down to layout. It implements a top-down, bottom-up, performance-driven design methodology. Complex circuits are decomposed using a functional abstraction, both depth-first and breadth-first design flows are possible. It uses two libraries: a cell library and a technology library. Its objective is to increase the productivity of both novice and experienced designers by automating the design of analog integrated circuits. The **AMGIE** synthesis system has a *modular software architecture*, defines clear interfaces for design data and management, and can more easily be extended than its predecessors.

This concludes the architectural overview of the **AMGIE** system. In the next chapter the implementation of the **AMGIE** synthesis system will be described. The point tools integrated in the **AMGIE** synthesis system will be discussed, their underlying algorithms and techniques will be explained using illustrative examples. In chapter 4 experimental results obtained with the **AMGIE** system will be presented, including an actually fabricated and measured design.

Chapter 3

Detailed Description of the AMGIE Analog Synthesis System

In the previous chapter a global overview of the **AMGIE** analog synthesis environment was given. The design management features of the design controller and the overall interfaces were described, making it possible to provide a completely integrated solution to the analog synthesis problem. The actual design tasks have already been defined but no implementation was supplied. In this chapter the core steps in the analog design flow and the technical and algorithmic details of the corresponding design tools will be described.

But first two remarks are formulated: (1) on the hierarchy model of the **AMGIE** analog synthesis system and the relation to its point tools and (2) on the performance-driven approach (represented by the functionblock's specifications) as seen by the point tools.

The sections thereafter describe the following design tools in detail:

- Topology Selection tool, section 3.2
- Sizing and Optimization tool, section 3.3
- Layout Generation tool, section 3.4
- Verification tool, section 3.5
- Redesign wizard, section 3.6

In these design task sections small and illustrative examples are provided, primarily to explain how the algorithms work. In chapter 4 full examples will be presented, proving the capabilities and showing the limitations of the **AMGIE** analog synthesis system.

3.1 Specifications and Hierarchy

As already explained in section 2.4 **AMGIE** uses a functional decomposition of circuits. This hierarchy leads to the definition of functionblocks in the cell library. Examples of typical functionblocks are: OPAMP, OTA, COMPARATOR, SWITCAP_BIQUAD, CSA-PSA, A/D-CONVERTER, D/A-CONVERTER, …

These functionblocks define an interface and a parameterized behavior. These behavioral parameters are the functionblock's specifications. Every point tool of the system uses the values of the specification parameters to select its design decisions. Since the functionblock decomposition is rather coarse (although completely under control of the library developer), it is often appropriate that individual point tools use a more refined decomposition of the circuit. All the design point tools (Topology Selection, Sizing and Optimization, Layout Tool and Verification) have the opportunity to exploit a further refinement of the hierarchy for a functionblock. This refinement can however only be done in terms of structural, geometrical or other decomposition techniques, since at this level no functionblocks have been defined. The sizing tool for example can introduce another level of structural hierarchy between OPAMPs and devices, for instance current mirrors and differential pairs. The layout tools can do the layout generation of a block in terms of subblocks, solving multiple placement and routing problems in one global optimization loop, see for an example of this in section 4.3.5 on page 102.

Take note however that the design is only verified at the functional hierarchy nodes. Extra hierarchical decomposition inside the point tools does have to be done with appropriate care in order not to violate this performance-driven design paradigm.

Stated in this way, the selection of the functional decomposition of the circuits in the cell library combined with the potentially further fine-grained decompositions in the point tools is the most important decision a cell library developer has to take. A successful library exploits this hierarchy in the most optimal manner. It is very much possible that no optimum exists for all applications, which leads to a set of cell libraries, each targeted towards a specific application domain. In the remainder of the chapter the functionblock hierarchy of a cell library is not further discussed: it is assumed that a choice has been made by the cell library developer.

By now it must be clear that the performance specifications play a crucial role in the **AMGIE** analog synthesis system. These are initially supplied by the user for the top-level functionblock; the sizing and optimization point tool derives these values for all subblocks. In both cases, they fully drive the design algorithms. Consider a specification P, which has to lie in a *bounded*[1] interval $P_{requested}$, as is shown in figure 3.1. In figure 3.1(a), the bounded interval is shown, and extra margins have been introduced; when a design is first attempted no actual layout degradation is available, nor an idea of the spread (tolerance) of the specification after sizing. Estimated margins are thus subtracted from the interval: $\Delta P_{est}^{lay\pm}$ and $\Delta P_{est}^{tol\pm}$ leading to an acceptable nominal specification interval P_{acc}^{nom}. This interval is used to select topology candidates. Since all topologies are modeled using nominal specifications, any candidate providing specifications within this nominal specification interval is valid, this is shown in figure 3.1(a). The sizing and optimization tool then uses the P_{acc}^{tol} interval to size the circuit, as shown in figure 3.1(b). It uses estimates internally to account for the technology variations or uses a direct yield method [Debyser 98a, Debyser 98b] to include the (manufacturing) tolerances. After verification, the nominal performance and specification variability (a normal distribution is assumed) is extracted. This is shown in figure 3.1(c). The available layout margins can now exactly be calculated: $\Delta P_{acc}^{lay\pm}$. These can all be consumed by the layout tool to provide an acceptable design. After layout extraction and verification the actual performance is known, as shown in figure 3.1(d). To account for estimation errors, the margins are typically overestimated, resulting in a specification value which is well within bounds, leading to the unused specification margin of $P_{unused}^{\pm}$, shown in figure 3.1(d).

[1] most specifications are of the format $P \lesseqgtr$ value, where one of the bounds is $\pm\infty$.

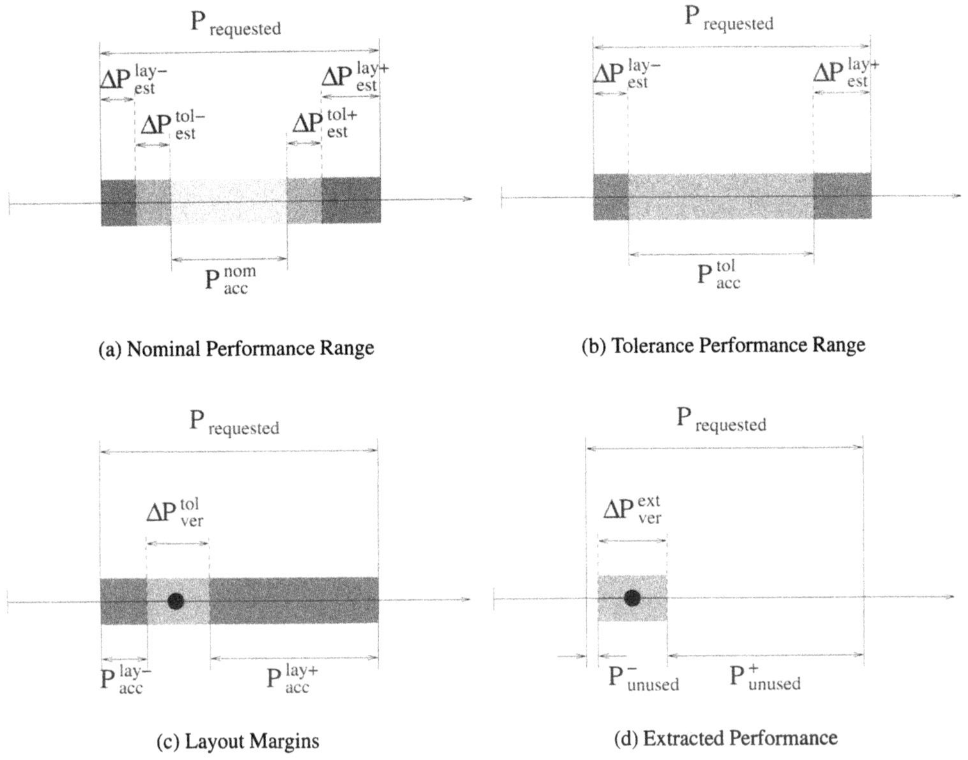

Figure 3.1: Specification margins and ranges.

The estimated margins ($\Delta P_{est}^{lay\pm}$ and $\Delta P_{est}^{tol\pm}$) are calculated as follows:

$$\Delta P_{est}^{lay\pm} = \frac{f_P^{lay\pm}}{100} P_{lowerbound,upperbound} + \Delta P_{fixed}^{lay\pm} \tag{3.1}$$

$$\Delta P_{est}^{tol\pm} = \frac{f_P^{tol\pm}}{100} P_{lowerbound,upperbound} + \Delta P_{fixed}^{tol\pm} \tag{3.2}$$

where $f_P^{lay\pm}$, $f_P^{tol\pm}$ (expressed as a percentage) and $\Delta P_{fixed}^{lay\pm}$, $\Delta P_{fixed}^{tol\pm}$ have default values (that can be zero) dependent on the specification at hand. These default values can be overridden by the user. For small, closed intervals, i.e. specifications that have a lower- and upperbound close together, the design will be infeasible if these margins are strongly overestimated; there is not enough specification slack for handling the technology variations. In this case the margins of the infeasible narrow specifications must be lowered, until the circuit becomes feasible. It must be noted that most specifications have *open-ended* intervals (the required specification range is of the form $P > P_{lowerbound}$ or $P < P_{upperbound}$), and an over-specified margin does not lead to an infeasible design. By overestimating the performance margins a sub-optimal result is found. The result can be improved much in the same way as the infeasibility of a design can

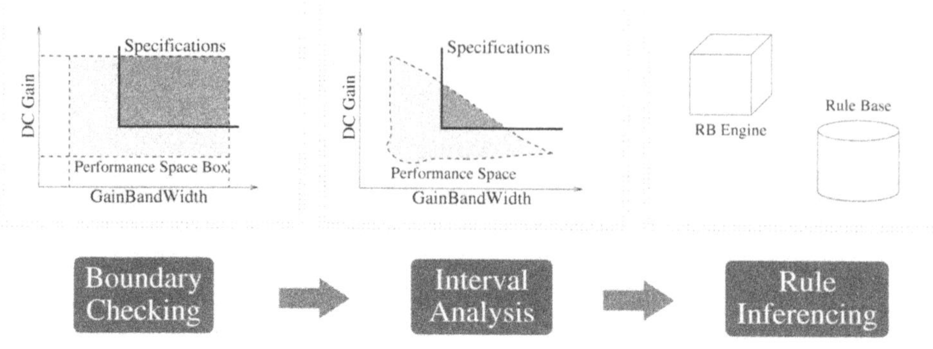

Figure 3.2: Filter sequence implemented in the Topology Selection (TS) tool; the darker grey area indicates the overlap between specifications and performance space or its bounding box.

be resolved. In general design failures caused by infeasible margins occur rarely.

These specification values and margins are stored in the design management system. The individual design point tools access their set of specification values. The next sections are dedicated to these design point tools, starting with Topology Selection.

3.2 Topology Selection Tool

The topology selection (TS) tool selects from all topologies in the **AMGIE** cell library those that are able to satisfy the specifications of the requested functionblock as determined in the specification sheet and ranks them in order of preference.

The topology selection tool actually works by eliminating inappropriate topologies from all possible candidates stored in the library and by ranking the remaining ones (see figure 3.2).

Elimination of a circuit topology can be because the topology does not have the correct functionality, does not fit to the selected process, or is incapable to meet the required specifications.

The latter elimination is being carried out by applying a sequence of three consecutive filters on the list of candidate topologies [Ves 95, Ves 97, VdPlas 01]: first a boundary checking filter is applied, then an interval analysis based filter and finally a rule inferencing based ranking filter.

The resulting list is presented in order of preference to the user through a graphical user interface. The user can accept the proposed topology, or force the **AMGIE** analog synthesis system to choose any other topology from the list. The three filters are now discussed.

3.2.1 Boundary Checking Filter

The first two filters use quantitative information about the feasible nominal performance space of a topology which is stored in the cell library. This means that it is calculated based on the stored models, what the achievable performances of each topology in the selected technology process are, given the acceptable ranges in biasing values and device sizes, and that it is checked whether the specified performances are included in this performance space or not.

Since the calculation of the actual performance space is a time-consuming process, this step is split in two consecutive filters. The first filter only calculates the multidimensional boundary box of the feasible performance space and checks whether this box overlaps with the space determined by the input specifications. This is called boundary checking (BC) and is the first filter in figure 3.2.

If we denote the performance specification for performance j as $P_j \in [P_{lb_j}, P_{ub_j}]$, and its feasible range for topology k in a given technology process as $P_j \in [\psi_{lb_j^k}, \psi_{ub_j^k}]$, then topology k is an acceptable topology for these specifications in that process if:

$$\forall j : [P_{lb_j}, P_{ub_j}] \cap [\psi_{lb_j^k}, \psi_{ub_j^k}] \neq \emptyset \tag{3.3}$$

The feasible performance interval values are calculated from the declarative model that characterizes every circuit in the library (see next subsection). Since the boundary checking filter essentially considers each performance parameter independently of all the others, boundary checking is simple and fast, and can already eliminate most of the unfit topologies from the library.

The disadvantage however is that no interdependencies between different performances are taken into account, and therefore that some topologies may pass the boundary checking filter but cannot meet the combined set of specifications in the end.

Eliminating those topologies is exactly the task of the second filter as will be discussed in section 3.2.2. Some heuristics based on the relative position of the specification values within the feasible performance intervals or on the maximum size of the intervals' intersection can be applied to perform already an initial ranking of the surviving topologies. In our case the ranking is based on the ranking value rv_k which for a topology k is calculated according to:

$$rv_k = \sum_{i=1}^{N} \frac{||parameter.\max_i| - |parameter.\min_i||}{||parameter.\max_i| + |parameter.\min_i||} \tag{3.4}$$

where $parameter.\max_i$ and $parameter.\min_i$ are the maximum and minimum values of the overlap region for performance i.

3.2.1.1 Example

Figure 3.3(a) shows a comparison of four topologies ($\mathbf{T_1}$ till $\mathbf{T_4}$) based on the feasible interval for one performance parameter i with a specification range P_i. The selection process rejects $\mathbf{T_2}$ whose feasible interval does not overlap with P_i, and ranks the remaining topologies as $\mathbf{T_3}$, $\mathbf{T_1}$, $\mathbf{T_4}$ depending on the size of the intersection region. Figure 3.3(b) depicts another comparison of four topologies, this time based on feasible ranges for two performance parameters P_1 and P_2. $\mathbf{T_1}$ and $\mathbf{T_4}$ are rejected and the ranking of the remaining topologies is $\mathbf{T_3}$, $\mathbf{T_2}$.

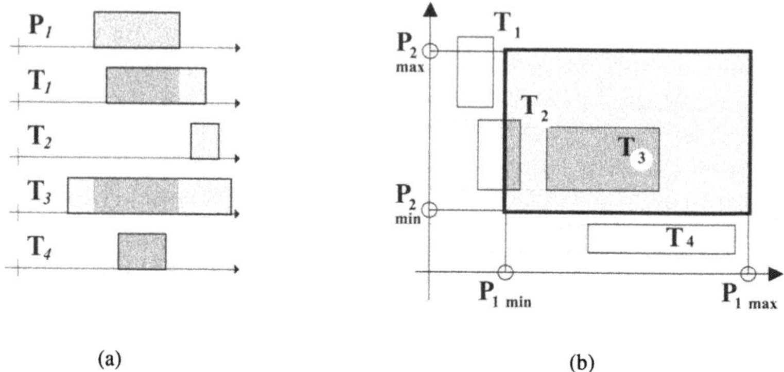

Figure 3.3: Boundary checking illustrated for (a) one and (b) two performance characteristics.

3.2.2 Interval Analysis Filter

The second filter (see figure 3.2) takes the interdependencies between the different performances into account in order to calculate the complete feasible performance space more accurately, and to eliminate more inappropriate topologies that have passed the first filter. This means solving all (in)equalities simultaneously for the performance variables bounded by the required nominal specifications.

In order to do so, techniques from interval analysis are used in combination with Chernykov's algorithm [Tscher 71, Leen 90] that can solve all systems of nonlinear equations, including inequalities, using a piecewise-linear (PWL) approximation for all nonlinear functions [Ves 95, Ves 97]. This system of equations is derived from the declarative model (see next subsection) that is stored with every topology in the library.

Topology selection now consists of checking if the calculated solution space constrained by the specifications is empty or not. If not, the topology is accepted; otherwise it is rejected. The drawback of the technique is its exponential computational complexity behavior with the size of the problem. Therefore only the most important specifications (as determined by the library developer introducing the topology in the library) are taken into account in this filter. This makes the CPU time still acceptable in practice. Note also that this filter is only applied to the topologies that survived the boundary checking filter. For a more detailed description of the boundary checking and interval analysis filter and how the models stored in the cell library can be derived starting from the declarative model, the reader is referred to [Ves 97].

3.2.2.1 Example

The improvement that this filter brings over boundary checking is depicted in the examples of figures 3.4(a) and 3.4(b). Figure 3.4 differs from figure 3.3(b) in that the interdependency (functions f_1 and f_2) between the performance parameters P_1 and P_2 has been taken into account. For the topology $\mathbf{T_3}$ and for two performance parameters P_1 and P_2, figure 3.4(b) shows the user-specified specification intervals (1), the initial boundary intervals (2) as stored

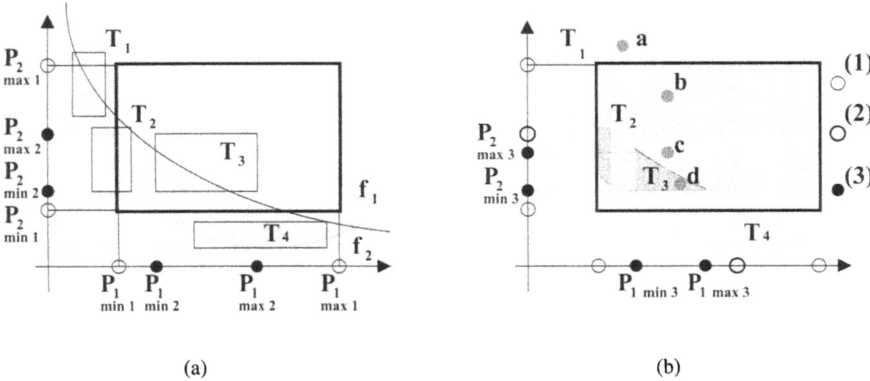

Figure 3.4: Feasibility check with the relations between two parameters (a) and the result of the combination of both filters (b).

in the cell library, together with the remaining solution space (3) for those parameters after a calculation took place taking into account the relationship between P_1 and P_2. Point *d* for example belongs to the solution space of the topology $\mathbf{T_3}$ for the given specifications, while point *c* is outside of it, in contrast with simple boundary checking that would accept both *c* and *d*.

3.2.3 Rule-based Ranking Filter

The last filter that — if desired — can be applied to (re)rank the remaining list of candidate topologies is a heuristic rule-based filter approach, where an inference engine executes a number of rules stored in a database, to decide on the final ranking of the remaining topologies. The rules can encode both general heuristics as well as designer-specific preferences. They are implemented in *if–then* form. An example of such a rule (based on cell attributes) is:

$$\textbf{IF} \quad \{nr\_integrator.cell_A < nr\_integrator.cell_B\} \quad \textbf{THEN} \quad cell_A \ \text{before} \ cell_B; \tag{3.5}$$

3.3 Sizing and Optimization Tool

After topology selection an unsized schematic is available. The next step in the design flow is sizing and optimization (S&O) where — for the cells at the device level — the optimal device sizes and biasing will be determined for the selected topology to meet the performance specifications in the target technology process while minimizing some cost function (e.g. power consumption). At higher levels in the design hierarchy the tool searches for the optimum subblock parameters. Note that hierarchy is used only when a decomposition in more or less non-interacting subblocks is possible. For example, in our approach an OPAMP is sized as one block and is not further decomposed into subblocks like differential pairs, current mirrors, etc. because it is impossible to easily distribute specifications such as power-supply rejection ratio (PSRR) or settling time over the different subblocks.

The most difficult problem in circuit sizing is to solve for the degrees of freedom in the design, while managing the many conflicting performance trade-offs. The approach taken for the sizing in the **AMGIE** analog synthesis system is *improved equation-based circuit optimization*. The use of optimization provides flexibility and reduced setup time; the use of equations provides speed of execution. Table 3.1 gives an overview of different methods that have been used to perform the circuit sizing [Carl 96, Gie 00] and their advantages and disadvantages. The earliest methods were knowledge-based, and tools like IDAC [Degra 87] and OASYS [Harj 89] used explicitly derived procedural sizing plans to directly calculate the circuit sizes from the specifications. This approach is extremely fast for sizing circuits. It has many disadvantages when compared to optimization based approaches, as shown in Table 3.1: the time required to formalize and encode the design plan for every circuit is larger than with any other method. The overall obtained accuracy is rather poor: typically level 1 SPICE models are used to model the devices, the equations modeling the performance specifications have been simplified, and technology information has to be hardcoded in the plans. The time needed to derive and craft a plan is long and the flexibility in changing the plan to a new specification target set is low.

	procedural sizing plans	**equation-based optimization**	**simulation-based optimization**	**AMGIE approach**
speed (CPU time)	+++	++	−−	+
device model accuracy	−−	−	++	++
specification model acc.	−−	++	+++	++
technology independence	−	−	+	++
off-line setup time	−−−	−−	++	+

Table 3.1: Characteristics of analog circuit sizing approaches.

Therefore later approaches adopted an optimization-based approach where the design problem was recast as a constrained optimization problem, which offers maximum flexibility and reduces the preparation time at the cost of larger on-line run times. The degrees of freedom in the design are in this case not explicitly eliminated by heuristics but solved for at run-time by the optimization algorithm. There are still two subcategories in this approach depending on the way how the circuit performance is evaluated at every iteration of the optimization. The first subcategory uses (simplified) equations to characterize the circuit performance (OASYS [Harj 89], OPTIMAN [Gie 90], STAIC [Harv 92] and GPCAD [Hers 98]). The evaluation of these equations is relatively fast, thereby limiting the on-line CPU time overhead of optimization-based approaches, but the drawback is that the equations themselves still have to be derived and many show a simplification error. The second subcategory calls a numerical simulator at every iteration of the optimization to calculate the circuit performance (FRIDGE [Med 94], ASTRX/OBLX [Och 96], MAELSTROM [Kras 99], ANA-

CONDA [Phel 99] or [Schwe 99]). These approaches can reach full SPICE-level accuracy for all simulated characteristics, but the run times are long (hours or more). This is especially the case if the design space is not a priori restricted to a small number of optimization variables. Note also that the setup time in these cases is not zero either, since the design problem still has to be formulated with the correct constraints (e.g. stability constraints) in order to obtain decent design solutions.

The approach taken for circuit sizing in the **AMGIE** analog synthesis system is an *improved equation-based approach.* This approach alleviates many of the drawbacks of the traditional equation-based approaches, by using techniques of computer-automated symbolic analysis [Gie 89, Wamb 95, Fern 98, Gie 00] for declarative model derivation and constraint satisfaction for sizing model generation [Swi 90, Swi 91, Swi 95] on the one hand, and encapsulated device models to obtain high accuracy on the other hand [Debyser 00, VdPlas 01]. Also, an operating-point driven formulation of the design problem is used to speed up the evaluations [Leyn 98, VdPlas 01]. This is shown in figure 3.5. On the left of figure 3.5 (Off-line setup) the sizing model generation methodology is shown, implementing the *improved equation-based approach.* On the right of figure 3.5 (Synthesis run) the sizing and optimization as run by the typical **AMGIE** user is shown. The sizing model stored in the cell library is combined with the performance specifications and technology data of the cell under design and the selected optimization algorithm. The result of the optimization is a sized circuit (figure 3.5).

This will now be explained in more detail in the next subsections. In the first subsection the sizing model generation methodology will be explained. The optimization setup will be discussed in subsection 3.3.2. A practical example will illustrate the capabilities of the implemented sizing and optimization tool in subsection 3.3.3.

3.3.1 Sizing Model Generation

The general flow for generating a sizing model is shown in figure 3.5 on the left (off-line setup) [VdPlas 01]. The circuit behavior is first characterized by a declarative model that contains all the equations (DC, AC, transient, ...) that fully describe the relationships between the circuit behavior and the circuit parameters. These equations are declarative, i.e. they only specify relationships that must hold simultaneously between different variables, they don't describe a direction nor sequence of solution; they are *not* assignments but simply declarations of constraints between variables. DC equations (Kirchoff laws) are derived automatically from the circuit topology; AC equations are derived by means of symbolic analysis techniques like with the ISAAC [Gie 89] or SYMBA [Wamb 95] tools; transient and other equations to date still have to be provided by the designer unless they are simulated for.

In this way most of a declarative model can be generated automatically, i.e. over 90 to 95% of the equations. The resulting model however is still declarative and therefore not yet suited for computer execution. The equation manipulation tool DONALD [Swi 90, Swi 91, Swi 95] is therefore used to automatically determine the degrees of freedom in the design, then to choose a set of independent input variables (equal to the number of degrees of freedom), and then to turn the undirected declarative model into a directed sequential computational plan, which indicates how (by means of which equations, in which direction and in which sequence) all the dependent variables are to be calculated from the values of the independent ones.

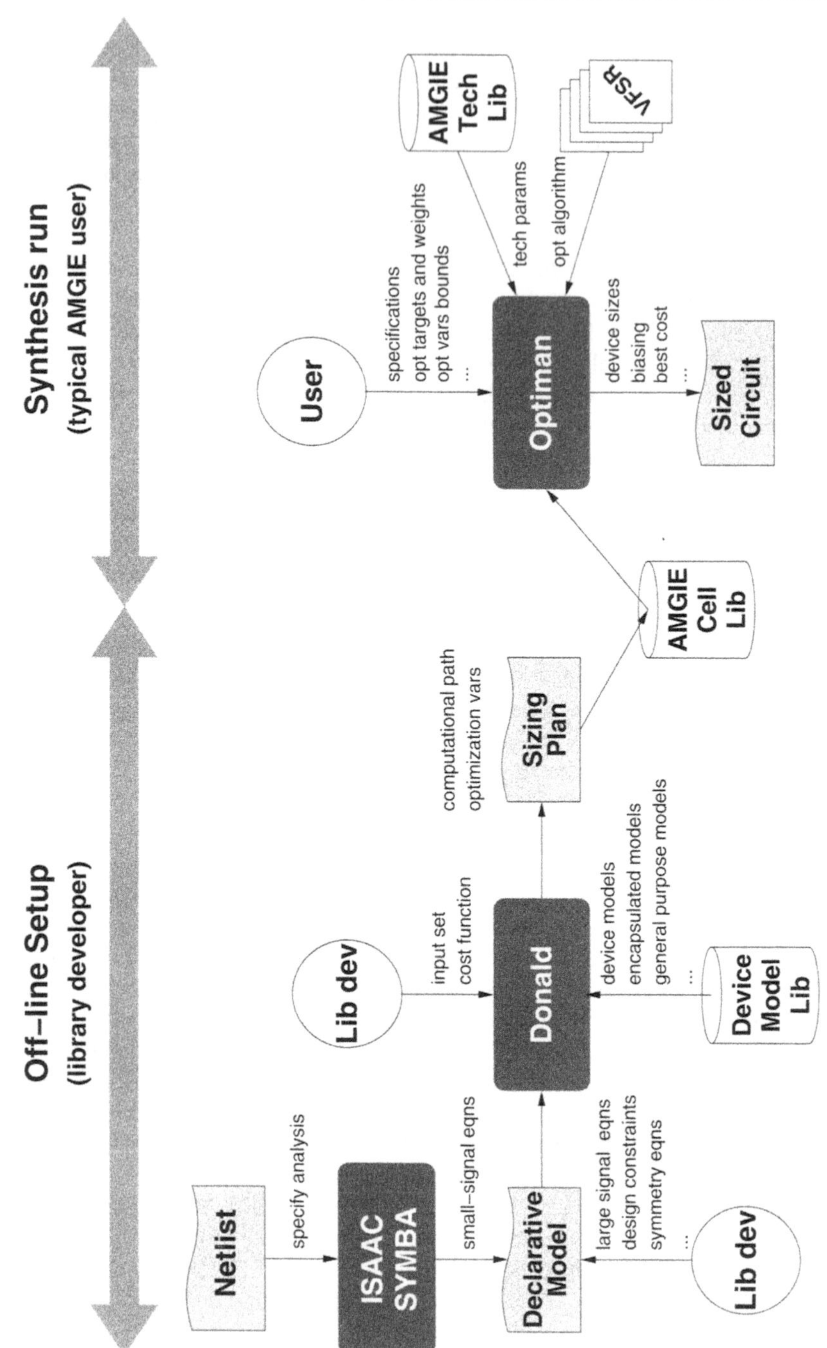

Figure 3.5: Sizing model generation procedure and application.

DONALD uses techniques of constraint satisfaction to determine the ordering of the computational plan, and has a built-in algorithm to find a computational plan that is free of equation clusters if possible. The computation or design plan is then written out in C code, compiled and stored in the **AMGIE** cell library, ready to be used for circuit sizing and optimization by the **OPTIMAN** tool during an actual **AMGIE** synthesis run.

All this model generation is done off-line in a process independent way and thanks to the supporting tools drastically reduces the setup time needed to include a new topology in the **AMGIE** analog synthesis system. With this approach setup times of less than 8 hours have been achieved for moderate-complexity circuits [Gie 95c, Gie 95a], i.e. circuits consisting of approximately 10 to 20 devices; for a discussion of this experiment see also section 4 in the next chapter. Considering that the whole flow of figure 3.5 can be executed in less than 20 minutes (on a typical SUN Ultra-1/170 workstation) for these moderate-complexity circuits, the proposed environment allows quick sizing model development (i.e. debugging). This is not true for any other reported previous approach (equation-based or simulation-based), since either the setup time (off-line) in those approaches is much higher or the optimization time (run-time) is much larger. Reported times for those approaches are an order of magnitude larger, in the order of hours.

In the next subsections the important contributions of the proposed method are explained in more detail: the operating-point driven formulation in subsection 3.3.1.1, the device model and technology parameters in subsection 3.3.1.2, a simplified example illustrating the proposed declarative modeling in subsection 3.3.1.3 and the use of estimators in subsection 3.3.1.4.

3.3.1.1 Operating-point Driven Formulation

The choice of the independent input variables in the computational plan (shown in figure 3.5), which of course are also the optimization variables in the circuit optimization, is an important factor in the performance of the sizing tool. As shown in [Leyn 98, VdPlas 01], the choice of variables directly controlling the operating-point of all MOS devices is to be preferred over all other input sets.

In our approach the voltages at all nodes and currents in all branches are therefore specified as input variables, of course taking into account the physical dependencies resulting from the Kirchoff laws to obtain independent variables only. As a result of this choice, the time-consuming DC operating-point calculations can be avoided as all devices in the circuit can be solved independently, and DC operating-point convergence problems often encountered in numerical simulations are completely avoided.

Solving a device in our case requires calculating the value of W for which:

$$I_{ds} = f_I(V_{gs}, V_{ds}, V_{bs}, W, L, \Theta, T) \tag{3.6}$$

in which I_{ds} is the drain current, V_{gs}, V_{ds}, V_{bs} are the operating-point voltages applied to the transistor, W and L are the width and length of the transistor, Θ is the device model's parameter set and T is the temperature of the device.

Some simple device models, like SPICE MOS level 1, allow an explicit solution of this equation:

$$W = f_W(I_{ds}, V_{gs}, V_{ds}, V_{bs}, L, \Theta, T) \tag{3.7}$$

For deep submicron technologies more advanced device models must be used, such as *BSIM3v3*, *MOS level 9* or the *EKV* model [Foty 96]. In this case the device equation must be iterated according to equation 3.6, for instance using a bisection method, which converges always since the function f_I typically is monotone. In our approach these device models are therefore integrated as encapsulated functions in the sizing tool and are *not* hard-coded in the design plans. This also means that our approach may use simplified small-signal expressions, but has the full accuracy of SPICE for the device modeling.

3.3.1.2 Device Model and Technology Parameters

The whole sizing approach is technology process independent through the use of a technology meta-model, i.e. all technology parameters are represented as variables in the equations used in the sizing model. Their actual values during sizing are read in from the technology file in the technology library corresponding to the technology process that was selected by the user at the start-up of a synthesis session.

Parameter set	**Examples**
Spice Model Parameters	LEVEL, VT0, TOX, UO, UCRIT, UEXP, XJ, CGSO, CGDO, RSH, ...
Geometric Model Parameters	GCM, DIFFUSION_WIDTH, GATE_STRAP, MINIMAL_AREA, ...
Mismatch Model Parameters	AVT, AB, SVT, SB, ...
Technology Info Parameters	LMIN, WMIN, LGRID, WGRID, LMAX, WMAX, WELL, ROUTING_SPACE, MIN_WIDTH, MAX_CURRENT, ...

Table 3.2: Meta-model technology parameters and categories.

The parameters of the technology meta-model for a MOS transistor are summarized in Table 3.2. Four categories of parameters have been identified:

1. The *SPICE device model* parameters: these are the well known parameters used for simulation of circuits in any SPICE-like simulator. They are used to determine the operating current and terminal voltages and small-signal parameters of each device.

2. The *mismatch model* parameters: these model the statistical intra-die differences between nominally identical devices, which heavily influence characteristics such as offset voltage or power-supply rejection ratio (PSRR). These mismatches are modeled using the model of [Laksh 86, Pel 89]:

$$\sigma^2(\Delta V_T) = \frac{A_{V_T}^2}{WL} + S_{V_T}^2 D^2 \tag{3.8}$$

$$\sigma^2(\frac{\Delta\beta}{\beta}) = \frac{A_\beta^2}{WL} + S_\beta^2 D^2 \tag{3.9}$$

They mainly depend on the active area WL of the devices; their distance D is not known during sizing. During layout generation afterwards the active area is fixed and only the distance term can be varied to improve the layout. The parameters A_{V_T}, A_β, S_{V_T} and S_β depend on the selected technology process and device type.

3. The *geometric model* parameters: these define the layout implementation of the device. Since in general there are multiple ways of laying out a given sized device (e.g. the normal and the fingered variants of a MOS transistor), the Geometry Calculation Method (GCM) parameter is used to indicate the correct layout variant. This GCM parameter triggers the proper set of equations to calculate or estimate the geometric dimensions of every device from its device sizes in the selected technology. For example, in the case of a fingered transistor the source and drain areas are shared, resulting in smaller overall source and drain area and junction capacitance. The GCM parameter determines which MOS variant and therefore which drain/source area function is used. For example, the total area occupied by a simple MOS transistor (GCM=1) is given by:

$$area_{est} = \sqrt{(area_{MOS} + area_{routing})^2 + MINIMAL\_AREA^2} \tag{3.10}$$

where the core MOS area and the routing space are estimated as:

$$\begin{aligned}
area_{MOS} &= area_{active} + area_{gate_strap} + area_{source_drain} && (3.11)\\
area_{active} &= W \times L && (3.12)\\
area_{gate_strap} &= \sqrt{area_{active} + area_{source_drain}} \times GATE_STRAP && (3.13)\\
area_{source_drain} &= W \times DIFFUSION_WIDTH/2 && (3.14)\\
area_{routing} &= 4 \times (\sqrt{area_{MOS}} + ROUTING_SPACE) \times ROUTING_SPACE && (3.15)
\end{aligned}$$

where $MINIMAL\_AREA$, $ROUTING\_SPACE$, $DIFFUSION\_WIDTH$, $GATE\_STRAP$, etc. are technology dependent constants.
The resulting estimated area as a function of the width and length is shown in figure 3.6. Also other device geometry parameters like *ps*, *pd*, *nrs*, *nrd* are derived in this way. These are essential to estimate during circuit sizing parasitics of the devices like the bulk capacitances, extrinsic drain/source resistances, etc.

4. The *technology info model* parameters: these define extra technology-specific information used to characterize the devices. For example, the width and length of MOS transistors are constrained between a minimal and possibly maximal value, and they need to be snapped to grid. These technology constants are implemented through the process-specific parameters *LMIN*, *WMIN*, *LGRID*, *WGRID*, *LMAX* and *WMAX*. By specifying the length and width of the MOS transistors as a ratio to their minimal value according to:

$$W = WMIN \times 10^{logW}, \qquad logW = \log_{10}(\frac{W}{WMIN}) \tag{3.16}$$

$$L = LMIN \times 10^{logL}, \qquad logL = \log_{10}(\frac{L}{LMIN}) \tag{3.17}$$

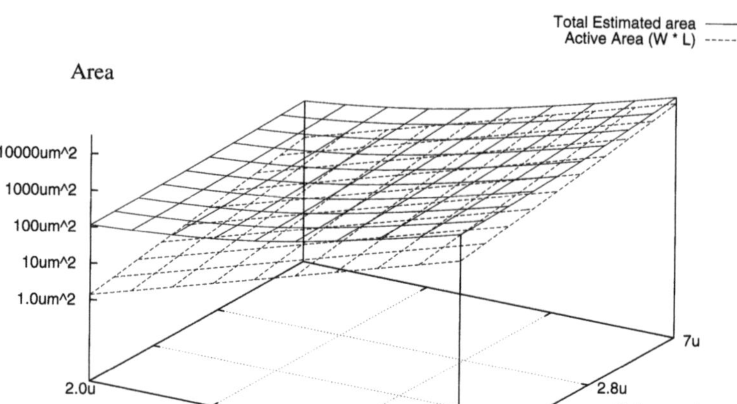

Figure 3.6: The estimated area of a MOS transistor (including routing space) as a function of its W and L compared to its active area ($W * L$).

and by using the $logW$ and $logL$ design model variables instead of the process-dependent W and L, an important technology dependence can be removed from the design plans. Additional technology parameters include for instance the availability of a floating well (in which the transistor is created), the minimal width of interconnections, maximal currents through minimal-width metal lines, ...

3.3.1.3 Example

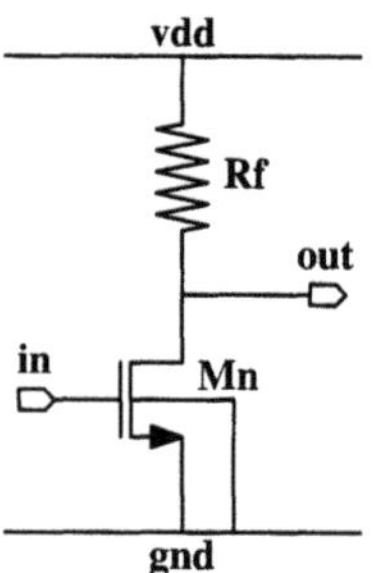

Figure 3.7: One-transistor amplifier circuit.

The approach is now illustrated for a simplified example to demonstrate the concepts. Figure 3.8 shows part (the DC part) of the declarative model that corresponds to a common-source

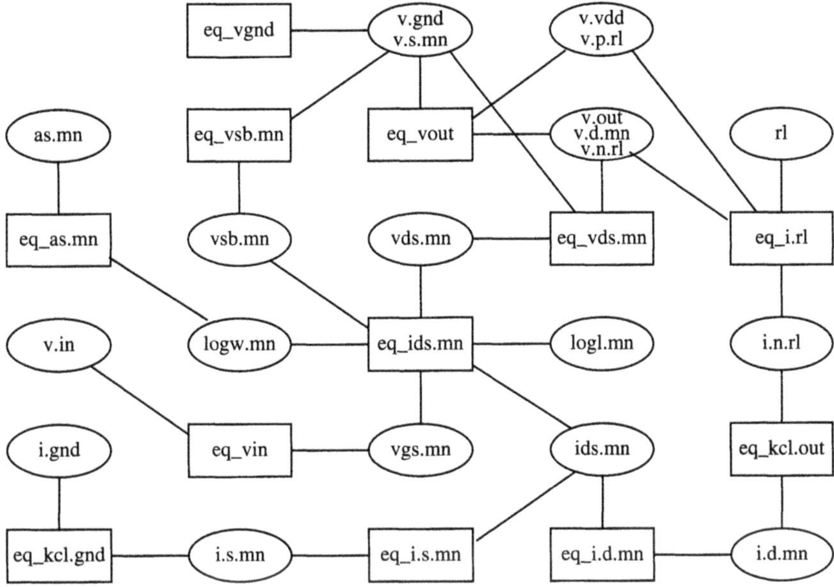

Figure 3.8: Undirected bipartite graph of the one-transistor amplifier circuit.

single-transistor amplifier with resistive load as shown in figure 3.7. The model is represented as a bipartite graph containing two different types of vertices: ovals for the variables, rectangles for the constraining equations. Note that the graph is undirected.

The declarative equations are:

$$\text{eq\_vgnd}: \quad \text{v.gnd} = 0 \tag{3.18}$$

$$\text{eq\_vout}: \quad \text{v.out} = \frac{\text{v.dd} - \text{v.gnd}}{2} \tag{3.19}$$

$$\text{eq\_vin}: \quad \text{v.in} = \text{vgs.mn} \tag{3.20}$$

$$\text{eq\_vsb.mn}: \quad \text{vsb.mn} = \text{v.s.mn} - \text{v.b.mn} \tag{3.21}$$

$$\text{eq\_vds.mn}: \quad \text{vds.mn} = \text{v.d.mn} - \text{v.s.mn} \tag{3.22}$$

$$\text{eq\_ids.mn}: \quad \text{ids.mn} = f_I(\text{logw.mn}, \text{logl.mn}, \text{vgs.mn}, \text{vds.mn}, \text{vsb.mn}) \tag{3.23}$$

$$\text{eq\_as.mn}: \quad \text{as.mn} = f_{as}(\text{logw.mn}) \tag{3.24}$$

$$\text{eq\_i.rl}: \quad \text{i.rl} = \frac{\text{v.p.rl} - \text{v.n.rl}}{\text{rl}} \tag{3.25}$$

$$\text{eq\_kcl.out}: \quad \text{i.d.mn} + \text{i.n.rl} = 0 \tag{3.26}$$

$$\text{eq\_i.d.mn}: \quad \text{i.d.mn} = \text{ids.mn} \tag{3.27}$$

$$\text{eq\_i.s.mn}: \quad \text{i.d.mn} = -\text{ids.mn} \tag{3.28}$$

$$\text{eq\_kcl.gnd}: \quad \text{i.s.mn} = \text{i.gnd} \tag{3.29}$$

In total there are 16 variables constrained by 12 *independent* equations. Hence, there are 4

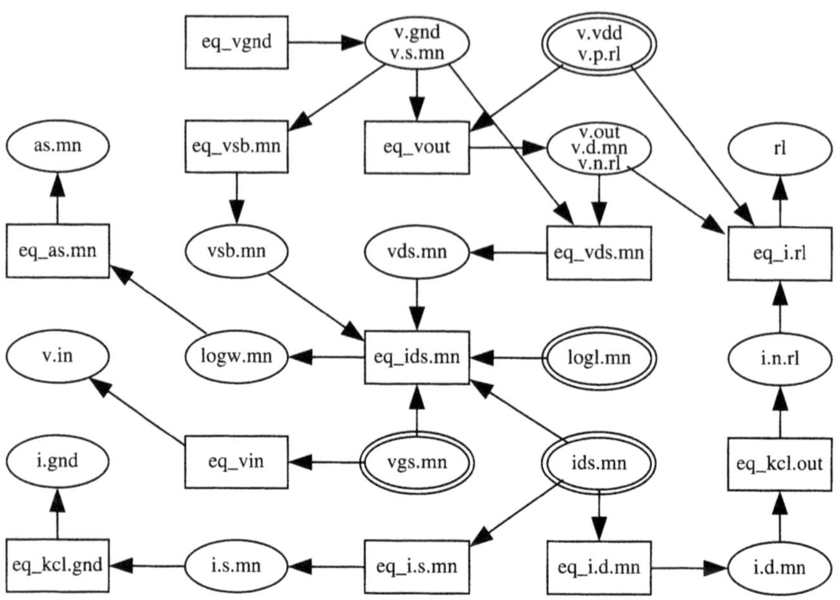

Figure 3.9: Directed bipartite graph of the one-transistor amplifier circuit.

degrees of freedom in this (simplified) example. (In reality there are more equations capturing also the AC and transient behavior of the circuit). However, only equality constraints eliminate degrees of freedom; inequality constraints don't. This means that 4 independent variables can be selected as input variables. Note that many combinations are possible: C_4^{16}.

If we choose for instance the variables {v.vdd, vgs.mn, ids.mn, logl.mn} as input set, then the originally undirected bipartite graph can be directed using constraint propagation techniques, resulting in an directed (matched) bipartite graph as shown in figure 3.9. In this graph the direction and order in which the equations have to be solved is indicated. In this way the values of the remaining 12 dependent variables (single line ovals) can be calculated out of the values of the independent variables (double line ovals). This information is then written out in C code as a procedural computational plan and subsequently compiled and stored in the sizing model library, allowing fast evaluation of the sizing model in an optimization loop. During optimization the optimization algorithm will then vary the independent variables to find the optimum design solution that satisfies all (specification) constraints.

Of course in a real sizing model, the device model of the previous paragraph is included (implementing f_I and f_{as}) and values are calculated for all small-signal parameters of the device based on the geometry model. These are then subsequently used to calculate performance specifications.

3.3.1.4 Hierarchical Circuits: Power and Area Estimators

When sizing hierarchical blocks, the performance specifications of the subblocks have to be determined by the specification translation tool using optimization. To associate a cost with a set of proposed subblock specifications estimators are used. They link the subblock's performance with its *feasibility*, *power* consumption and *area*:

$$feasibility_k = f_{FB}(\mathbf{S}_k) \tag{3.30}$$

$$power_k = g_{FB}(\mathbf{S}_k) \tag{3.31}$$

$$area_k = h_{FB}(\mathbf{S}_k) \tag{3.32}$$

in which $\mathbf{S}_k$ is a vector representing the specifications of subblock k. $feasibility_k$ is a boolean range function, returning either *true* or *false*, indicating the feasibility of the specification values supplied ($\mathbf{S}_k$). In some instances the $feasibility_k$ estimator is left out; its functionality is then implemented by returning values close to ∞ for $power_k$ and/or $area_k$ when infeasible specification sets are requested. In case of feasible specifications, $power_k$ and $area_k$ return estimates of the power consumption and area.

These estimators can be implemented with (1) manually derived equations (an example for an analog sensor interface is presented in [Vdbus 98a]), (2) by fitting to (automatically generated) design points [Harj 96, VdPlas 97], or (3) by empirically derived formulas, as for A/D-converters in [Lau 99] or (4) by combinging high-level design with lower-level estimators (the so-called meet in the middle approach), as done for filters in [Lau 00].

Using optimization the top-level block parameters are then translated to *optimal* subblock specifications. With high-quality estimators an optimal trade-off in terms of power and area of the overall system can be achieved in this process.

3.3.2 Circuit Optimization Setup

Once the design plan is available in the library, the **OPTIMAN** program [Gie 95a, Gie 95c, VdPlas 01] can then perform the actual circuit sizing and optimization as part of an **AMGIE** synthesis run, as shown in figure 3.5 on the right. The compiled sizing model of the selected circuit schematic is retrieved from the cell library and linked to an optimization algorithm to tune the circuit towards the user-defined specifications while optimizing some user-defined design target, e.g. minimum power consumption.

The **OPTIMAN** tool is modular: the same optimization problem can be solved with several different optimization algorithms. The user selects in the **AMGIE** analog synthesis system the optimization algorithm as one of the options to be chosen in the specification sheet window. At this moment both global optimization algorithms like Very Fast Simulated Re-annealing [Ingb 89] (VFSR), as well as local optimization algorithms like Hooke–Jeeves [Hooke 61], minimax [Leyn 97a] or Sequential Quadratic Programming (SQP) [Fle 93, Spel 98] can be chosen. The range of all optimization variables as well as a default initial solution is provided for every schematic in the cell library, but can also be modified by the user. After the sizing optimization in the **AMGIE** analog synthesis system the resulting optimal device sizes are automatically back-annotated onto the schematic of the cell under design in the system's database.

The used formulation of the analog circuit sizing as an optimization problem is as follows:

$$\begin{aligned} &\text{find } \mathbf{x} \in D \text{ such that } f(\mathbf{x}) \text{ is minimal} \\ &\text{while: } g_i(\mathbf{x}) \leq 0 \quad \text{for } i = 1 \ldots n, \\ &\qquad h_j(\mathbf{x}) = 0 \quad \text{for } j = 1 \ldots m \end{aligned} \tag{3.33}$$

The optimization variables $\mathbf{x}$ are the independent input variables of the stored design plan of the selected schematic. For optimization algorithms that cannot handle the constraints directly, like for instance VFSR, penalty functions are added to the optimization target. The cost function used during optimization is then as follows:

$$\Phi(\mathbf{x}) = f(\mathbf{x}) + \beta u(G(\mathbf{x})) + \gamma u(H(\mathbf{x})) \tag{3.34}$$

$$\text{with } u(G(\mathbf{x})) = \sum_{i=1}^{n} u(g_i(\mathbf{x})) \text{ and } u(H(\mathbf{x})) = \sum_{j=1}^{m} u(h_j(\mathbf{x}))$$

where the penalty terms $u()$ have been added to handle the equality and inequality constraints; β and γ are scaling factors. Different choices of penalty functions are possible, such as (for $g_j(\mathbf{x})$):

$$u(g_j(\mathbf{x})) = w_j g_j^2(\mathbf{x}), \qquad g_j(\mathbf{x}) \geq 0 \tag{3.35}$$

$$= 0, \qquad g_j(\mathbf{x}) < 0 \tag{3.36}$$

or,

$$u(g_j(\mathbf{x})) = w_j \ln(1 + \frac{g_j(\mathbf{x})}{g_{j0}}), \quad g_j(\mathbf{x}) \geq 0 \tag{3.37}$$

$$= 0, \qquad g_j(\mathbf{x}) < 0 \tag{3.38}$$

For optimization algorithms that can handle constraints directly like SQP, of course no penalty terms are added to the cost function.

Originally only the nominal performance could be optimized. Recently, however, the approach was extended to include the impact of process parameter and operating parameter variations on the circuit performance, allowing to simultaneously optimize the circuit performance and the design yield and robustness [Debyser 98a, Debyser 98b]. The method proposed in [Debyser 98a, Debyser 98b] uses the operating-point driven approach to nominally size the circuit (which is compatible with the presented approach). The sizing model is then extended with a SPICE-like, non-operating-point driven sizing model. This normally results in the creation of large clusters of equations, causing convergence problems well known by simulator users (DC convergence of numerical simulators). However, since the circuit has been sized starting from the operating point, the voltages and currents are known, and the clusters don't have to be solved, the voltage and current values are simply filled in. The method then proceeds with calculating the sensitivities (first order derivatives) of the performance specifications (P_j) to the independent technology parameters (Θ_i) that were derived with principal components analysis (PCA) [Chen 93, Aftab 94]. These sensitivities are then used to calculate the specification variance $var\{\mathrm{P}_j\}$:

$$var\{\mathrm{P}_j\} = \sigma^2_{\mathrm{P}_j} \approx \sum_{i=1}^{n} (S^{\mathrm{P}_j}_{\Theta_i})^2 \sigma^2_{\Theta_i} \tag{3.39}$$

where $S^{\mathrm{P}_j}_{\Theta_i}$ is the sensitivity of the performance specification to the technology variable. The yield is then optimized by minimizing the capability indices of [Aftab 94]; the capability *potential* index C_p and the capability *performance* index C_{pk} for a performance specification P_j:

$$C^{\mathrm{P}_j}_p = \frac{\mathrm{P}^{\mathrm{tol}+}_{\mathrm{est},j} - \mathrm{P}^{\mathrm{tol}-}_{\mathrm{est},j}}{6\sigma_{\mathrm{P}_j}} \tag{3.40}$$

$$C^{\mathrm{P}_j}_{pk} = \min\{\frac{\mathrm{P}^{\mathrm{tol}+}_{\mathrm{est},j} - \mathrm{P}^{\mathrm{nom}}_j}{3\sigma_{\mathrm{P}_j}}, \frac{\mathrm{P}^{\mathrm{nom}}_j - \mathrm{P}^{\mathrm{tol}-}_{\mathrm{est},j}}{3\sigma_{\mathrm{P}_j}}\} \tag{3.41}$$

where $\mathrm{P}^{\mathrm{nom}}_j$ is the nominal value of performance specification P_j. A combination of the C_p, C_{pk} indices for all performance specifications is then included in the cost function [Debyser 98a, Debyser 98b], resulting in a yield optimization of the circuit under design.

The developed sizing approach results in a fast sizing process. CPU times between a few minutes (for low-complexity circuits of approximately 15 MOS transistors) to one hour (for complex circuits of approximately 100 MOS transistors) are obtained on a standard SUN Ultra-1/170 workstation, while at the same time achieving high accuracy.

To enable the user to follow and possibly interact with the optimization process, an interactive graphical viewer has been developed. This viewer, shown in figure 3.10, gives the user a view on the evolution of the value of the optimization variables (top left window in the figure), of selected variables (two windows middle right, schematic top right), of the circuit performances and of the cost function throughout the optimization (top right window) and constraints (bottom left). All values are continuously updated throughout the progress of the optimization run, and a coloring scheme (red/orange/green) indicates whether the specifications are satisfied or not. The user can intervene by changing for instance the upper or lower bound of a certain variable and then continue the optimization. The user can also deduce what the most constraining specifications in the design are. In this way, the viewer is also used to debug design plans during the initial setup phase.

3.3.3 Practical Example

Let us now consider the practical example of a symmetrical OTA with class-AB output buffer that is depicted in 3.11. The specification set has been limited to the following specs: low-frequency gain (A_{v0}), gainbandwidth (GBW), slew rate (*SR*), phase margin (*PM*), total offset voltage (V_{off}, this is the sum of the absolute value of the systematic offset and three times the standard deviation of the random offset voltage) and capacitive load (C_{load}). The *power* consumption and *area* are to be *minimized*. The specification values used for optimization are summarized in Table 3.3.

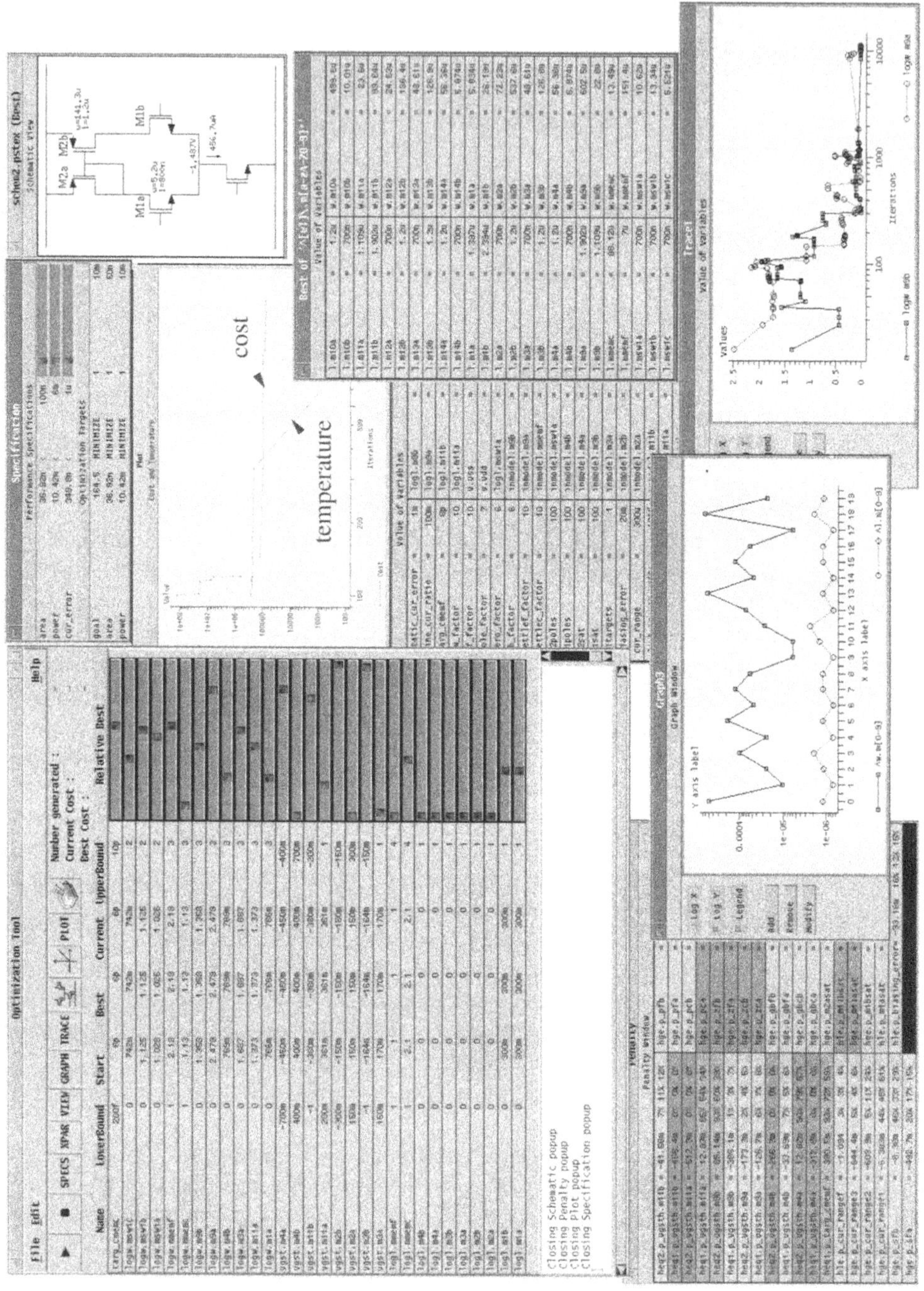

Figure 3.10: Snapshot of the viewer of the sizing optimization process.

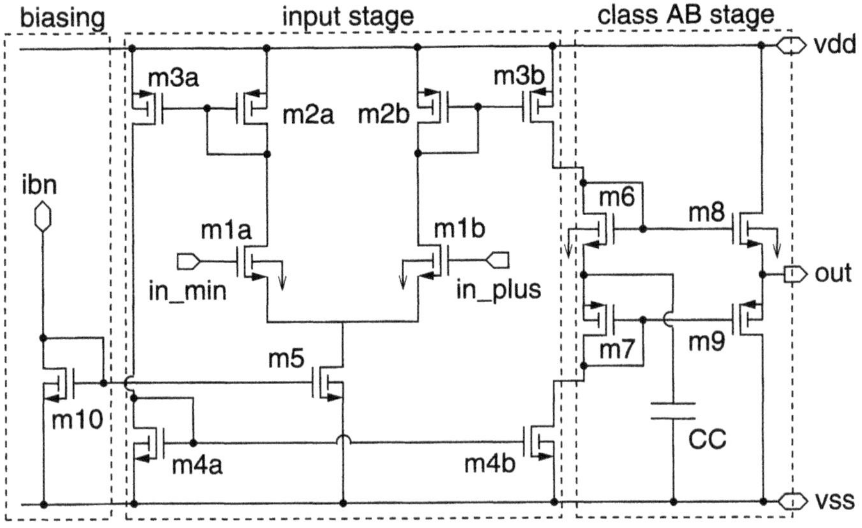

Figure 3.11: Schematic of the symmetrical OTA with class-AB output stage.

Specification	Symbol		Value	Unit
Low-frequency gain	A_{v0}	>	1000	–
Phase margin	PM	>	65	°
Total offset voltage	V_{off}	<	3	mV
Slew rate	SR	>	1	V/μs
Gainbandwidth	GBW	>	1	MHz
Load capacitance	C_{load}	=	100	pF
Technology	Θ	=	2P2M 0.7μm CMOS	–
Power consumption	*power*	MIN	1	mW
Area	*area*	MIN	0.05	mm^2

Table 3.3: Synthesis specifications of the symmetrical OTA with class-AB output stage.

Using DONALD and ISAAC and adhering to the principles proposed previously in this section, a fast computational plan (sizing model) has been created. It uses the encapsulated device models, the DC operating-point driven formulation and analytical equations linking the specifications to the device parameters. In addition to these equations design constraints have been added that generate a penalty when transistors leave preferred operating-point regions (overdrive voltage limits, saturation limits, ... [Leyn 97b, Leyn 98, VdPlas 01]). The thus generated sizing model has then been used to perform optimizations.

Since at first no *good* design point is known (to start up the optimization), the global optimization algorithm (VFSR) is employed (which takes a random starting point). In figure 3.12(a) both the temperature and best cost achieved during a typical optimization run is

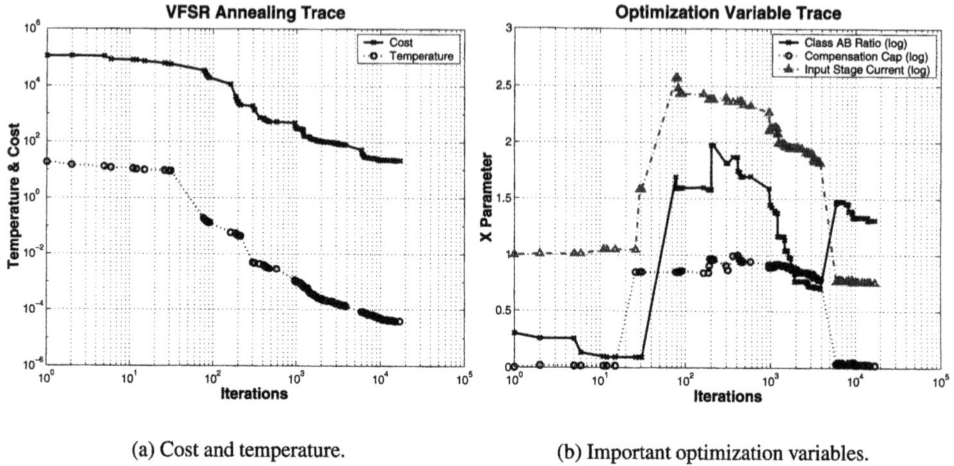

(a) Cost and temperature.

(b) Important optimization variables.

Figure 3.12: Trace of the VFSR optimization.

shown. The corresponding trace of the most important optimization (independent) variables is shown in figure 3.12(b).

It can be clearly seen that after a short period of random exploration the annealing algorithm finds a design point that conforms to the constraints (specifications, extra design constraints), and that subsequently the power and area target are minimized. However in the latter optimization stage, large changes in the optimization variables are still possible. As can be seen on figure 3.12(b) at about iteration 5000 the three most important design variables change simultaneously. The input stage current drops in value, the compensation capacitance is decreased correspondingly and the class-AB ratio (i.e. driver to output stage) is increased. In fact the optimization algorithm has found that decreasing the input stage current and compensation capacitance and at the same time keeping the output stage current constant is advantageous to reduce the overall power consumption, while still fulfilling all specifications.

Since we now have a good design point we can calculate the power–area trade-off curve (Pareto) using the local optimization algorithm SQP. While maintaining the specification set of Table 3.3, the power and area weights are modified to look for alternative designs. In figure 3.13 the resulting power/area Pareto points have been plotted, for the original specification set and two modified sets (low-frequency gain and total offset voltage). As can be seen from figure 3.13, the power–area trade-off curve is decreased to a flat region. This is explained by the fact that a power minimum does allow large transistors to be used, while an area minimum shrinks all transistors to their minimal sizes and thus allows only *one* power point. Furthermore, relaxing the low frequency gain and total offset voltage specifications influences the lowest possible area, but not the power. This is because power is predominantly determined by GBW and C_{load}. In addition, relaxing the specifications increases the extent of the trade-off curve considerably.

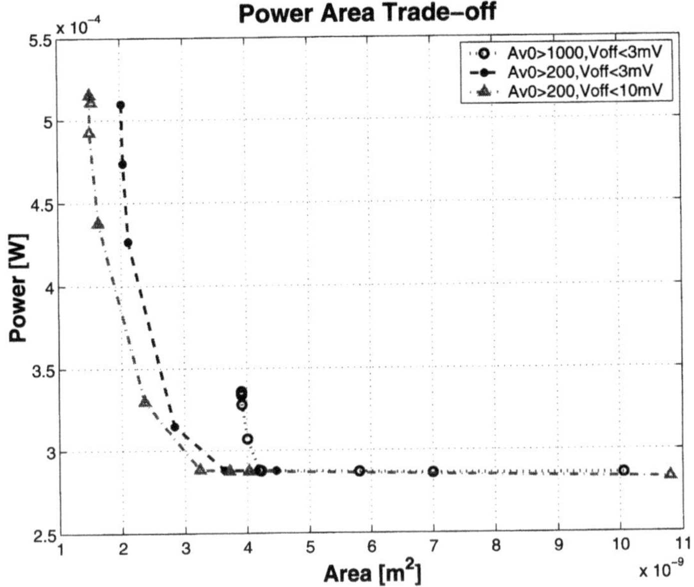

Figure 3.13: Power–area tradeoff of the symmetrical OTA with class-AB buffer stage.

3.4 Layout Generation Tool

After sizing, the circuit performance is verified (see next section). If this verification is passed successfully, a fully customized layout of the circuit is automatically generated by the LAYLA tool [Lam 99]. This tool implements a direct performance-driven macro-cell place & route methodology [Mala 96, Lam 99], shown in figure 3.14. The placement and route steps are preceded by a sensitivity extraction. The placement uses built-in and external module generators to create alternative variants for the macro cells. The routing then connects the placed macro cells. The performance degradation due to layout-induced effects is quantified for every layout iteration solution, and the placement and routing routines are driven in such a way that this performance degradation $\Delta \mathrm{P}_j$ for every performance P_j does not exceed the acceptable layout performance margins $\Delta \mathrm{P}^{\mathrm{lay}-}_{\mathrm{acc},j}$ and $\Delta \mathrm{P}^{\mathrm{lay}+}_{\mathrm{acc},j}$ in the final layout solution:

$$\Delta \mathrm{P}^{\mathrm{lay}-}_{\mathrm{acc},j} \leq \Delta \mathrm{P}_j \leq \Delta \mathrm{P}^{\mathrm{lay}+}_{\mathrm{acc},j} \tag{3.42}$$

where the acceptable layout performance margins $\Delta \mathrm{P}^{\mathrm{lay}\pm}_{\mathrm{acc},j}$ have been defined in section 3.1 and on figure 3.1(c).

The performance degradation is calculated using a first-order linear approximation using the sensitivities of the performances to the different layout parasitics:

$$\Delta \mathrm{P}_j = \sum_i S^{\mathrm{P}_j}_{y_i} y_i \tag{3.43}$$

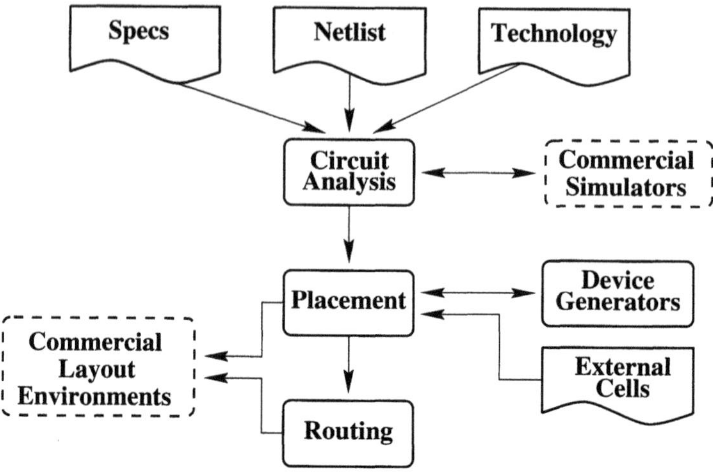

Figure 3.14: The macro-cell place and route methodology used in LAYLA [Lam 99].

resulting in:

$$\Delta \mathrm{P}^{\mathrm{lay}-}_{\mathrm{acc},j} \leq \Delta \mathrm{P}_j = \sum_i S^{\mathrm{P}_j}_{y_i} y_i \leq \Delta \mathrm{P}^{\mathrm{lay}+}_{\mathrm{acc},j} \tag{3.44}$$

The values of the layout parasitics y_i are extracted (calculated and/or estimated) for every intermediate layout solution. The sensitivities $S^{\mathrm{P}_j}_{y_i}$ are obtained from numerical simulations that are performed only once at the beginning of the layout generation process (the verification tool that will be described in the next section can be used to derive these sensitivities).

In addition to performance constraints, additional geometrical constraints can be enforced by the cell library developer or the user, such as symmetry constraints both for devices and for nets; devices can be grouped in arrays; also the orientation of devices can be fixed; buses and pins can be constrained to be placed on a specific side of the circuit layout, etc.

The layout generation is split up in two parts: first placement, followed by routing. The placement algorithm [Lam 95] uses simulated annealing to place the devices. Symmetry constraints are enforced in the move set. Other constraints are enforced through the performance-driven mechanism: any violation of the performance margins for a layout solution according to equation (3.44) is penalized via an extra penalty term that is added to the cost function. A first effect included in this way is the performance degradation caused by (estimated) interconnect parasitics (capacitances associated with every wire and resistances associated with every wire segment in the layout) according to:

$$C_{par} = C_{junction} + C_{wire} \tag{3.45}$$

$$R_{par,i} = \rho_{wire} \frac{L_{wire,i}/n_p}{W_{wire,\,i}} \tag{3.46}$$

Resulting for equation (3.43) in:

$$\Delta P_j = \sum_{k=1}^{m} \left(S^{P_j}_{C_{par,k}} C_{par,k} + \sum_{i=1}^{n_k} S^{P_j}_{R_{par,ki}} R_{par,ki} \right) \tag{3.47}$$

The inclusion of junction capacitances in the above formula favors on-the-fly device merges at the diffusion level.

A second effect included is the matching of devices. Matching devices are handled simultaneously in the move set (same orientation and variant of the devices), but as it is not possible to put all matching devices exactly next to each other while also satisfying all other constraints, their distance is determined by the performance-driven mechanism according to the impact of their mismatch on the performance:

$$\sigma^2(\Delta V_T) = \frac{A^2_{V_T}}{WL} + S^2_{V_T} D^2 \tag{3.48}$$

$$\sigma^2(\frac{\Delta\beta}{\beta}) = \frac{A^2_{\beta}}{WL} + S^2_{\beta} D^2 \tag{3.49}$$

Using pre-derived sensitivity information the performance degradation of performance P_j is then estimated as follows:

$$\Delta P_j = \sum_{k=1}^{m} \left(3|S^{P_j}_{\Delta V_T k}|\sigma(\Delta V_T)_k + 3|S^{P_j}_{\Delta\beta k}|\sigma(\frac{\Delta\beta}{\beta})_k \right) \tag{3.50}$$

where $S^{P_j}_{\Delta V_T k}$ and $S^{P_j}_{\Delta\beta k}$ are the sensitivities of performance P_j with respect to small changes in ΔV_T and $\frac{\Delta\beta}{\beta}$ of matching transistor pair k. The sum is taken over all m pairs of matching devices. Equation (3.50) can be rewritten as:

$$\Delta P_j = \Delta P_{j,area} + \Delta P_{j,distance} \tag{3.51}$$

Since the active transistor area ($W * L$) is not altered during layout generation (it has been determined during sizing), the first term of (3.51) is constant during placement. The performance degradation due to the distance is however determined by placement. This term can be computed as follows:

$$\Delta P_{j,distance} = \sum_{k=1}^{m} S^{P_j}_{D_k} D_k \tag{3.52}$$

in which D_k is the distance between devices of the matching pair k and $S^{P_j}_{D_k}$ is the sensitivity of performance P_j to small variations in distance D_k.

Other effects have been included following the same mechanism, for example thermal effects due to self-heating of the circuit [Lam 96b].

The resulting placement is then interconnected by a performance-driven router [Lam 96a, Lam 99]. The performance degradation caused by the actual routing parasitics is quantified and constrained in the same way as during placement by including any excess performance degradation in the cost function of the line expansion algorithm. In addition, as a post operation, the router can also trade off any remaining slacks on the performance degradation for an improved yield with respect to local catastrophic defects (pinholes and spot defects). By ripping up and re-routing nets according to the modified cost function, the layout can be made less sensitive to these defects, always without exceeding the original performance degradation margins. In this way a fully customized circuit layout is obtained that satisfies all specifications and has a high robustness; an example will be shown in section 3.4.1 below.

The final layout is then checked for layout rule violations (DRC) and compared with the schematic (LVS) by the Extraction Tool (ET). If these checks don't return any errors, the actual parasitic elements of the circuit are extracted from the mask layout and back-annotated on the schematic to allow a detailed verification of the circuit performance.

3.4.1 Practical Example

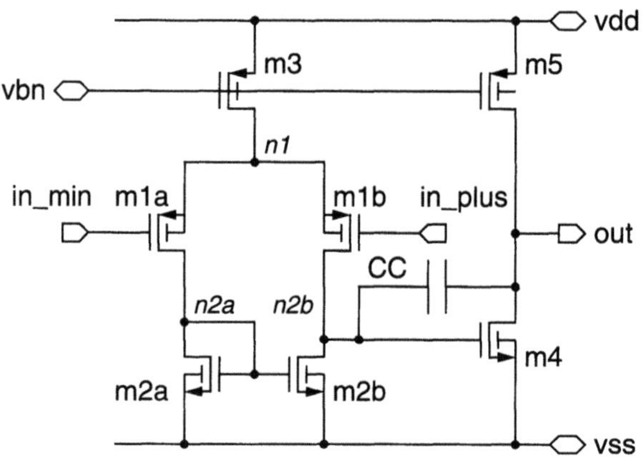

Figure 3.15: Schematic of the Miller-compensated OTA.

Net	$S^{PM}_{cap_{net}}$ (°/F)	ΔPM_{placed} (°)	ΔPM_{routed} (°)	$S^{GBW}_{cap_{net}}$ (Hz/F)	ΔGBW_{placed} (Hz)	ΔGBW_{routed} (Hz)
n1	-1e10	-0.00009	1e-4	–	–	–
n2a	-8.1e12	-0.12	-0.13	-6.9e17	-10300	-11000
n2b	-6.8e12	-0.24	-0.20	-1.6e18	-55400	-45800
out	-2e12	-0.063	-0.09	-4.2e17	-13200	-11020
vbn	7e10	0.0007	0.0012	-1e16	-104	-184
Sum	–	-0.428	-0.421	–	-79100	-76200

Table 3.4: Sensitivity and performance degradation of the Miller-compensated OTA after placement and routing (internal nodes only); *PM* is 60.7°, *GBW* is 30MHz.

In figure 3.15 the schematic of a Miller-compensated OTA is shown. With the discussed performance-driven macro-cell place and route approach the layout of figure 3.16 has been

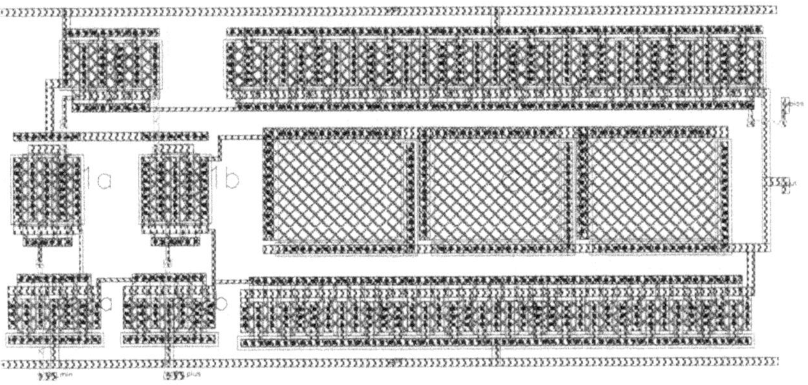

Figure 3.16: Performance-driven layout of the Miller-compensated OTA.

Performance	Requested	Nominal	$\Delta Perf_{placed}$	$\Delta Perf_{routed}$	Extracted	Unit
Phase margin	> 60	61.2	-0.428	-0.421	60.7	°
Gainbandwidth	> 30meg	30.28meg	-79100	-76200	30.2meg	Hz

Table 3.5: Performance of the Miller-compensated OTA.

generated. In this (limited-complexity) example, two performance specifications have been taken into account: the phase margin (*PM*) and the gainbandwidth (*GBW*). In Table 3.4 the sensitivities of these specifications with respect to the internal node capacitances are summarized, as are the estimated degradations of the placement and routing phase. The final performance degradation remains within the requested values, as shown in Table 3.5.

3.5 Verification Tool

Detailed verification of the circuit performance is performed twice in the design flow: a first time in the top-down path to verify the circuit sizing without the layout-induced degrading effects, and the second time in the bottom-up path after layout extraction to verify the circuit with inclusion of the actual layout-induced degrading effects. Verification implies a number of checks to be performed on the circuit as well as the execution of a simulation script to simulate and extract all actual performance values obtained by the design. For this a link to existing numerical simulators is provided; the actual simulator used can be chosen by the user. The resulting performance values are then compared to the specifications and the datasheet of the design is generated, indicating whether all specifications have been met or not.

A generic verification script has been defined for every functionblock (type of circuit), e.g. an OPAMP. As shown in figure 3.17, during verification every circuit is considered as a black box that has a specific functionality. Except for the external input and output pins (this is the functionblock's interface), no signals are monitored inside the circuit. The verification

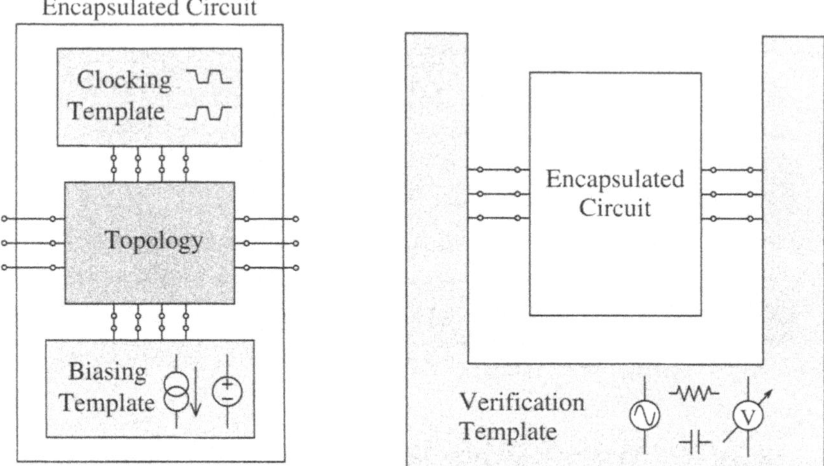

Figure 3.17: The circuit under test, the encapsulated circuit with biasing and clocking templates (topology specific) and the verification template (functionblock and verification task specific) are applied to generate a test harness.

script verifies the requested performance behavior of the functionblock, independent of the actual circuit implementation of that block. Details about the actual implementation and its special properties are therefore encapsulated in a verification harness that is predefined for every schematic. This includes for instance the correct biasing, which varies from topology (schematic) to topology (schematic), the clocking in case of clocked circuits, etc.

It will now be explained how the verification is performed. The verification process is fully automated, and requires no intervention from the user.

3.5.1 Nominal Performance Verification

From the sized schematic a netlist in a format suitable for the selected simulator is created. The schematic is then encapsulated by applying the following schematic-specific templates from the cell library:

1. a biasing template that defines the correct biasing voltages and currents to the circuit schematic. If the circuit is self-biasing from the power supply, no biasing file needs to be created.

2. (in case the circuit is clocked) a clocking template that derives the correct clock signals.

Depending on the functionblock (circuit type) the corresponding verification script is then retrieved from the cell library. Every verification script consists of a sequence of simulation steps. Every simulation step extracts one or more performance values and is composed of the following tasks:

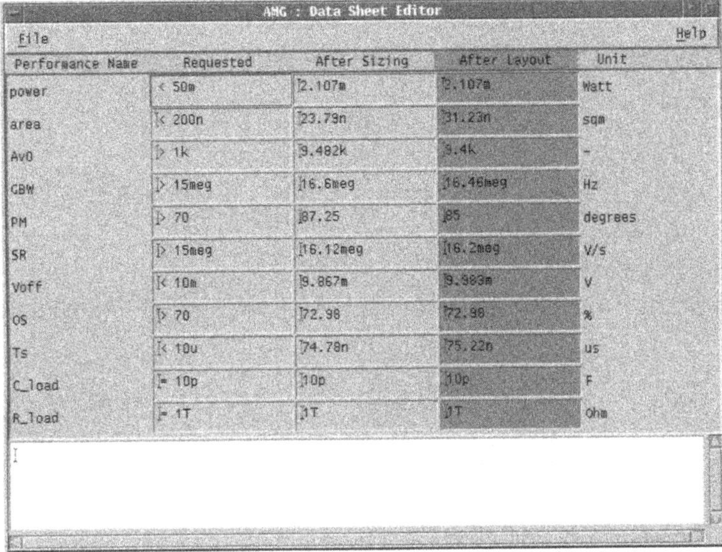

Figure 3.18: The datasheet editor.

1. Define a test configuration depending on the performance characteristic to be simulated (as depicted in figure 3.17). For instance: define the operating conditions (power supply, load impedance, ...), define the feedback configuration (e.g. unity feedback at DC but open loop for AC analysis), define the input stimuli, define the output responses to be captured and calculated (for instance phase margin extraction).

2. Write out all this information into a proper simulation input file including all simulator-specific commands and measurement statements. The device model parameters are added from the technology library according to the selected technology process.

3. Execute the simulator job in batch mode.

4. Extract the desired performance values from the simulator output file. Some characteristics can be obtained directly from the simulation results (e.g. through measurement commands available in the simulator); others will be obtained by post-processing the simulation results in which case general output file browsing functions are used.

5. The obtained performance(s) is stored in the datasheet of the designed circuit and compared to the specifications. Any violations are flagged through a red indication; otherwise the indication is green. A snapshot of such a datasheet is shown in figure 3.18.

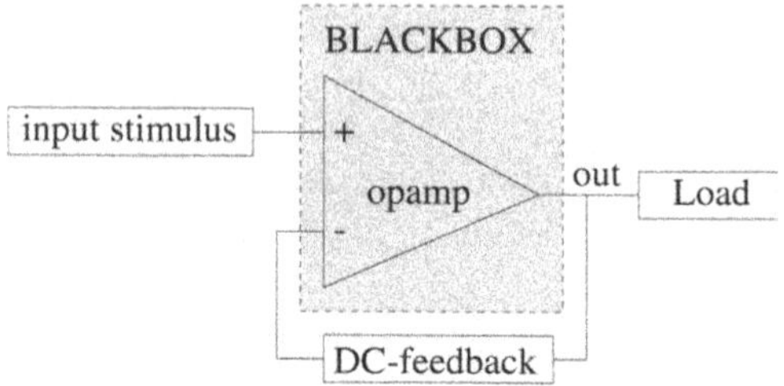

Figure 3.19: The black box OPAMP in its test harness for slew rate analysis.

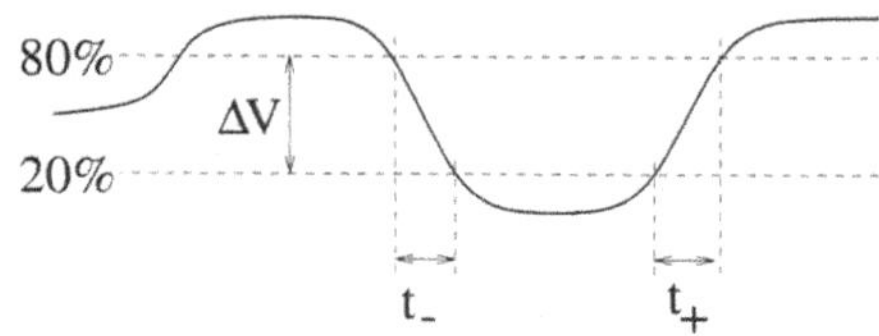

Figure 3.20: Output signal and measurements.

3.5.1.1 Example

An example is now provided to illustrate the general concept of the verification script. The example presented is the extraction of the slew rate of an OPAMP. The script looks as follows.

1. The topology is encapsulated by a biasing and clocking circuit (depicted in figure 3.17). The biasing is realized through current sources and mirror transistors to generate all biasing voltages and currents. The values used have been calculated during sizing and are inserted from the sizing database which is stored in the cell under design.

2. The resulting generic OPAMP is placed in a DC feedback loop, and loaded with the load specified in the specification sheet (as shown in figure 3.19). For a slew rate extraction a square wave is applied. The parameters of the square wave (amplitude, rise time, period) are derived from the slew rate specification. The transient simulation mode is selected. The simulation time is set to one and a half period of the square wave.

3. The transient simulation job is run in batch mode

4. The slew rate specification is extracted from the signal on the output node. The positive slew rate is defined as the slope of the output signal between 20 and 80% of its full swing. The negative slew rate is the slope between 80 and 20% in the negative transition. The slew rate of an OPAMP is the minimum of the absolute value of negative and

positive slew rate:

$$SR_- = \frac{\Delta V}{t_-} \tag{3.53}$$

$$SR_+ = \frac{\Delta V}{t_+} \tag{3.54}$$

$$SR = \min(|SR_-|, |SR_+|) \tag{3.55}$$

The average slopes are extracted by measuring the time elapsed between subsequent threshold passes. This is shown in figure 3.20.

5. The extracted value is stored in the specification sheet and compared to the specifications.

To avoid an expensive simulation run for every extracted specification, all transient and AC (small-signal) jobs are combined into two simulation jobs.

3.5.2 Verification with Mismatches and Technology Spread

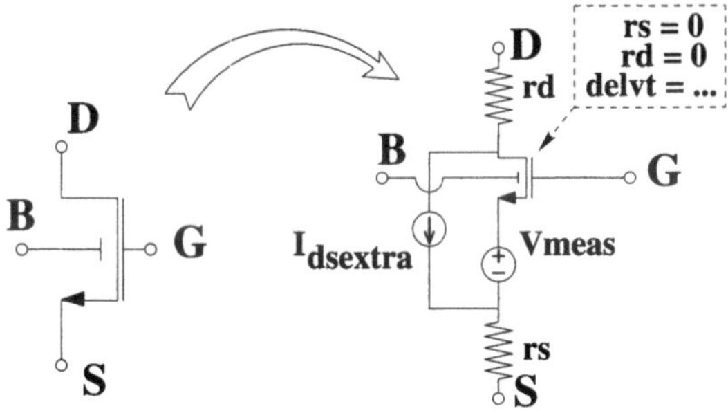

Figure 3.21: For mismatch simulations every MOS transistor is replaced by an equivalent statistical model.

As can be noticed from this approach the nominal performance of the circuit can be verified with only a limited number of simulation jobs. A number of circuit performances are however influenced by device mismatches, which is a statistical phenomenon. Commercial simulators provide Monte-Carlo type of statistical simulation capabilities, but no commercial simulator provides an integrated statistical mismatch model. Therefore, a circuit preprocessor has been developed, called MMPRE [Verha 96, Verha 97] or MIMI, that replaces all MOS transistors in the netlist by an equivalent statistical mismatch model according to the mismatch model of [Laksh 86, Pel 89] as shown in figure 3.21. The mismatch-dependent performance specifications, as for instance the random part of the input offset voltage of an OPAMP, can then be verified by invoking statistical simulations on this modified netlist in the corresponding simulation step in the verification script.

In addition, the statistical technology parameter variations inherent to VLSI production manufacturing also may result in a parametric yield loss. To verify the circuit performance against these technology variations, the technology model parameters are modeled through Principal Component Analysis (PCA) [Joli 86, Chen 93] to extract the correlations between the different parameters. This statistical technology model is then stored in the technology library and can be selected by the user when performing a technology spread verification using for instance Monte-Carlo simulations. Alternatively verification in a limited set of predefined process corners is also supported: slow, fast parameters, minimum or maximum temperature, etc.

3.5.3 Verification over Temperature and Power-supply Operating Ranges

The correct operation of the circuit needs to be verified over the entire operating range for environmental parameters such as temperature, power supply or even radiation (e.g. for space applications). For the temperature, for instance, this is done by repeating the entire verification script while sweeping the temperature from the lowest to the highest value in a user-controlled number of steps. The number of steps is at least three, taking the extreme values and the default value (25° centigrade). Similarly, the supply voltage can be swept. Either these are swept independently, creating a temperature/power supply grid or only the corner points are verified. The average and worst-case performance values are then returned to the user via the datasheet.

3.6 Redesign Wizard

Although a performance-driven design methodology is adopted in the **AMGIE** analog synthesis system, in some cases the tool may not reach a design solution that satisfies all specifications. This may be because the specifications are too tough for the selected circuit schematic, or because simplified models used in earlier design steps incorrectly predicted the actual circuit behavior. Any such specification violations are detected by the tools themselves (for instance the sizing tool flags that it is incapable of meeting the specifications) or by one of the two detailed verification steps. In all these cases the redesign wizard is automatically started. This tool scans the status and the history of the design that failed. It then checks this against a redesign database where different predefined redesign scenarios, which contain procedures to remedy and restart the design process, have been stored. The (possibly multiple) scenarios applicable to the actual design problem are then presented to the user. The user selects an appropriate scenario and is guided step by step to put the design back on track. At present no automatic redesign mechanism has yet been implemented that has the built-in intelligence to automatically choose the best redesign scenario for every possible situation. The redesign scenarios in the database have been added by experienced designers. They are generic, i.e. circuit independent. It is possible for a user to add his own scenarios to a user database.

3.6.1 Example Scenarios

Examples of implemented scenarios are :

- If a design fails during sizing of the cell and if there are alternative topologies, select the next most promising topology. This is the most straightforward redesign scenario.
- If a design fails during sizing of the cell, increase the maximum bounds on allowed power consumption and/or chip area. It is often found that a selected topology can reach the requested performances, but not within the (often arbitrarily) specified power or area bounds.
- If a design failure is detected during verification after sizing and the performance specification causing the failure has been calculated during sizing with an inaccurate approximate formula, restart the sizing with the specification value for this performance tightened with the same amount by which the simulated performance differs from the calculated one.
- If the verification after layout extraction fails, redo the circuit sizing and optimization after updating the estimated layout parasitics with the actually extracted parasitics of the extraction step.

3.7 Summary

In this chapter the inner workings of the **AMGIE** analog synthesis system were discussed in detail. In the previous chapter the **AMGIE** system was presented, including its software architecture and the implemented design methodology: performance-driven, hierarchical (top-down, bottom-up) design. In this chapter the performance specifications and hierarchy were refined. The **AMGIE** synthesis system uses the functionblock concept that was defined in chapter 2. The functional hierarchy that is central in **AMGIE** can be refined by using both structural and geometrical hierarchies when required for a certain topology. It must be noted however that the specifications are only available for the functionblock nodes in this hierarchical decomposition. These specifications are fundamental to the correct operation of the synthesis system. In section 3.1 the specification margins have been defined that are used to drive the different subtools of the **AMGIE** synthesis system. In the subsequent sections the five subtools (Topology Selection, Sizing & Optimization, Layout Generation, Verification, Redesign Wizard) of the **AMGIE** synthesis system were discussed.

In section 3.2 the topology selection tool (TS) has been described. It selects amongst the candidate topologies in the **AMGIE** cell library those candidates that are most suited to achieve the requested specifications. This selection procedure is implemented using three filters that are applied consecutively to the list of all topologies: *boundary checking, interval analysis* and *rule-based ranking*. The first two filters eliminate candidates from the list and do a preliminary sorting. The last filter sorts the remaining candidates into a final list which is returned to the user. The user then has the ability to overrule the selection proposed by the tool or to accept it.

In section 3.3 an overview was given of competitive approaches for sizing synthesis of analog integrated circuits. The approach implemented in the **AMGIE** synthesis system is *improved equation-based circuit optimization.* The approach is supported by the extensive use of off-line/setup tools (ISAAC, SYMBA, DONALD) that speed up the sizing model generation, typically considered a cumbersome task. In the next chapter an experimental comparison will be made between different sizing approaches with inclusion of detailed timing reports. The use of the operating-point driven formulation of these design plans ensures low run-times during synthesis: the time-consuming DC solving of SPICE-like evaluation plans is avoided. By using encapsulated device models full SPICE accuracy is obtained, as far as the small-signal parameters (*gm*, *Cgs*, ...) is concerned. Technology independence is further realized through the use of extensive (technology) modeling: mismatch of devices is modeled with appropriate models, area of active devices (as for instance MOS transistors) is accurately modeled, etc., and the use of technology-independent sizing variables (*logW* and *logL* for MOS transistors). When subblocks are included in the circuit under design, power and area estimators for functionblocks are used to determine their performance specifications. The setup of the cost function has been discussed; depending on the optimization algorithm that is selected by the user, the constraints are added to the scalar cost function (VFSR) or directly handled by the optimization algorithm (SQP). The actual optimization tool (**OPTIMAN**) has a graphical interface informing the user of the optimization run's progress. A practical example shows how a trade-off curve (area-power) can be obtained with the sizing tool.

The layout generation tool (LT) creates a mask-level layout from the sized schematic. In the **AMGIE** analog synthesis system this task is performed by the LAYLA tools [Lam 99]. LAYLA is a *direct performance-driven macro-cell place and route* tool. The layout generation is performed in two steps: device (macro-cell) placement, followed by routing. By using sensitivity information, the degradation of performance specifications directly drives the layout generation process. All important typical analog layout constraints are supported: symmetry, matching, device merging, wire sizing, etc.

The cell under design is verified after sizing and optimization as well as after layout extraction. A fully automated verification tool (VT) has been implemented. It uses *black box* verification. Templates stored with the functionblock apply test harnesses and specify simulation analysis modes; templates stored with the topology apply biasing and clocking signals. Statistical verification for mismatch is provided with MMPRE or MIMI. Technology variations and operating ranges of temperature and power supply are verified using corner analysis. A datasheet is returned and stored in the database for inspection by the user.

If design errors occur, that are either detected by the design tools themselves (for instance topology selection did not find any suitable topology for the requested specifications) or are detected by the verification tool (for instance after extraction the phase margin drops below the requested value), the redesign wizard proposes the novice designer a set of corrective procedures. These corrective actions require the intervention of the user to go back to the design and redo some of the design steps (for instance relaxing the specifications or increasing the layout margin for phase margin) and then the design can be restarted.

Illustrative and representative examples have been added throughout the text to more clearly demonstrate the implemented algorithms and techniques. In the next chapter, chapter 4, experimental results will be presented including fabricated and measured silicon that has been realized using the **AMGIE** system.

Chapter 4

AMGIE Experimental Results

The capabilities of the **AMGIE** system are now illustrated with practical synthesis examples. As already mentioned, the **AMGIE** system can be used both by novice and experienced designers. The examples in this section have been generated by both types of users. The first example is the design of a high-speed OTA that has been sized in three different ways, which allow us to compare the approaches. The second example, the design of an Operational Transconductance Amplifier (OTA), has been generated in a class project on analog circuit design. The third example has been generated by an experienced analog designer, it is the design of an analog signal processing front-end. All examples illustrate that an analog synthesis system like **AMGIE** allows to generate high-performance analog designs in a short total design time, from specification to verified layout. Hence such a system increases both analog design productivity and design optimality, both for novice and experienced analog designers.

4.1 Comparison of Analog Sizing Synthesis: Equation-based vs. Simulation-based

In this example the different sizing synthesis methods are compared for a typical OTA topology. To make the comparison objective, 3 different teams were instructed to optimally size a fixed OTA schematic [Gie 95a, Gie 95c]. Not only the final result, but also the time spent on the different stages of the design was recorded. The three different approaches were:

1. **manual design:** the *experienced* designer could use his or her preferred manual design tools (spreadsheet, simulator, paper and pencil, ...) to design the circuit.

2. **simulation-based optimization:** the *(un)experienced* designer and analog tool user could use (an existing) optimizer in combination with a numerical device simulator (for instance SPICE) to design the circuit.

3. **equation-based optimization:** the *experienced* designer and tool user could use all the tools available for equation-based design (ISAAC, DONALD, **OPTIMAN**, **AMGIE**) to design the circuit.

4.1.1 Design Specifications

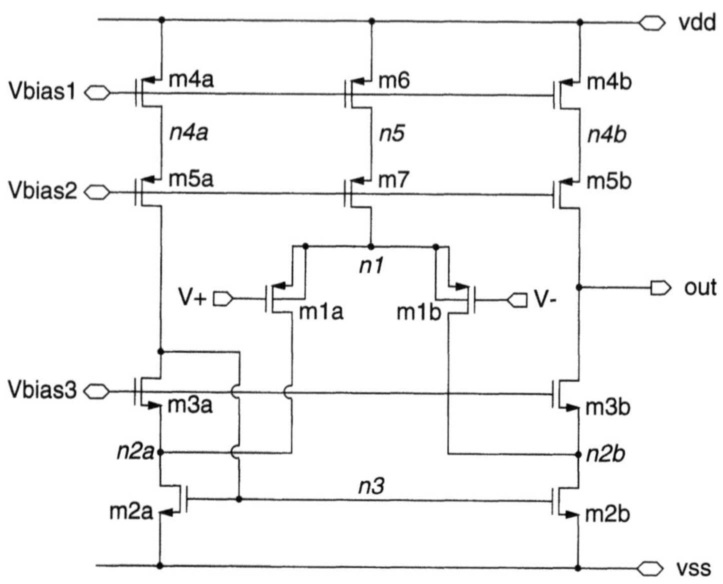

Figure 4.1: Schematic of the high-speed OTA used in the synthesis comparison project.

The synthesis comparison concentrated on the circuit shown in figure 4.1. This is a fairly simple two-stage single-ended OTA. By only using NMOS transistors in the signal path, it is capable of attaining high speeds [Fish 87, Rijns 93, Wu 94].

The performance specifications are summarized in Table 4.1. The design takes place in a 1P2M 0.7μm CMOS technology with a $\pm$2.5V power supply. Note that the objective of the exercise was to optimize the gainbandwidth (*GBW*), within a fixed power budget and additional constraints on stability (phase margin, *PM*), low-frequency gain (A_{v0}), large-signal behavior (slew rate, *SR*, output range, *OR*) and offset (V_{off}) at a given capacitive load (C_{load}). In the last column the obtained performance is summarized: all designs of the three teams approximately reached this (simulated) performance. No actual silicon was made to verify the designs. This was considered unnecessary, since the automated designs can be compared to the manual design of the experienced designer.

The different design approaches are now studied in more detail.

4.1.2 Manual Sizing

The *experienced* designer typically solves the sizing problem as follows. The circuit is analyzed, with a pencil, on paper. Simplified equations are derived linking the performance specifications to currents, device's small-signal parameters and dimensions. The operating regions of all devices (weak or strong inversion, linear or saturation region, ...) are chosen as well as the currents flowing through the branches. Then using a simplified device model [Stey 93] the

Specification	Symbol	Required		Obtained	Unit
Supply current	I_{tot}	<	3	3	mA
Phase margin	PM	>	60	60	°
Low-frequency gain	A_{v0}	>	60	60	dB
Offset voltage	V_{off}	<	5	5.2	mV
Slew rate	SR	>	150	166	V/μs
Output range	OR	>	3	3.2	V_{pp}
Load capacitance	C_{load}	=	10	10	pF
Power supply	$V_{dd},\ V_{ss}$	=	±2.5	±2.5	V
Technology	Θ	=	1P2M 0.7μm CMOS		–
Gainbandwidth	GBW	MAX	–	250	MHz

Table 4.1: Required and obtained performance specifications, the results of the equations-based result are shown.

dimensions (W, L) of the MOS transistors are calculated. Some experienced designers prefer to enter these simplified equations into a spreadsheet to automate the calculation.

This starting point is already a reasonably good design point. The design is then refined using SPICE *simulation in the loop*: the circuit is analyzed (simulated), the specifications are verified, and based on his/her expertise, dimensions of transistors are altered, in order to improve the design. Since a lot of performance specifications are constrained, this is rather difficult for an *unexperienced* designer, since a change of a device dimension affects all performance specifications. Soon a lot of constraints are *active* (i.e. an intermediate solution is found where the values of the specifications are equal to their constrained performance) and it becomes increasingly difficult to find a direction (i.e. a combined change of design parameters) to improve the design.

Nonetheless, all designers participating to the experiment, succeeded in finding the optimal design as defined by the experiment.

4.1.3 Simulation-based Sizing

The previous method fails in the hands of *unexperienced* designers. Especially when a lot of the specifications hit their constrained value, unexperienced designers can not find further improvements and the design process breaks down. Therefore using full automation of the design process is very attractive. The design of simple OTA structures is a waste of time for *experienced* designers anyway.

The most straightforward way of automated design is simply using the same approach the designer uses to refine his design. Use a simulator to evaluate the circuit and explore alternatives. If the designer is replaced by an optimization engine, the full design process is automated.

This has been attempted for this comparison experiment. A characterization harness was created to verify the circuit by numerical simulation and extract all performance specifications. Optimization runs were then started using a global optimization algorithm: Simulated

Annealing. It takes however some optimization runs to get a robust extraction script; this is explained by the fact that with simulated annealing a lot of extreme, strange circuit designs are tried out. For instance, the phase margin seems an easy specification to be measured, but failing circuits sometimes cause strange behavior of the output's phase in the Bode diagram. This causes unstable and unusable designs to be identified as correctly functioning ones, misleading the optimizer. Or a lot of designs are rejected, making it difficult for the optimization algorithm to find a good solution (simulator divergence, ...).

Also this approach succeeded in finding the optimal solution as defined by the experiment.

4.1.4 Equation-based Sizing

The equation-based approach starts with a schematic that is drawn of the circuit. On this schematic symmetrical components are discerned and this symmetry information is added. For instance a differential pair should be symmetric: in figure 4.1 **m1a** and **m1b** should have the same value. This schematic is netlisted to the DONALD [Swi 94, Swi 90, Swi 95] netlist format and the symmetry information is converted into symmetry equations. Next, the independent design parameters are chosen, therefore the approach explained in section 3.3 has been followed. The *logl* (section 3.3.1.2 on page 50) of symmetrical device pairs is such an input parameter of the operating-point driven input set, as are the overdrive voltages (*Vgst*) of device pairs and/or selected node voltages (for instance high-impedance nodes). A few branch currents complete the design parameter set. The properties of this set are: (1) they completely define the circuits sizes and biasing, (2) they allow fast evaluation (no DC operating point has to be calculated), and (3) they are independent, guaranteeing that almost the entire optimization variable space is valid.

The sizing model is at this point limited to a calculation from operating-point (the design parameters) to sizes and biasing. All values of small-signal parameters are available at the end of this calculation. Symbolic equations are now derived using ISAAC [Gie 91b, Gie 89, Gie 91c] to link the performance specifications with the latter. These equations are more accurate (and complex) than the simplified equations of the *experienced* designer. Manually equations are added for output range (*OR*) and slew rate (*SR*).

This model could then be called complete, except for the *design constraints*. The operating region of the devices is checked and penalties are added to the cost function to enforce the correct operating region. Geometric checks are added: sizes are calculated, so the *W* of the devices has to be checked against the technological limit. Also the stability (expressed as *PM*) is further refined: the position of all poles and zeroes is checked; all should be above the gainbandwidth (*GBW*). This counters one of the problems experienced in the previous approach. The phase margin is just a number, it doesn't catch the stability of the circuit completely. If a designer checks a Bode plot, he also looks for strange phase shifts occurring at lower frequencies. An optimizer only does this if it is instructed to do so.

There is one extra design consideration that has not yet been looked at. The proposed OTA circuit contains a local feedback loop [Fish 87, Wu 94], as shown in figure 4.2. This loop is in the signal path, albeit only for half of the signal (there are two parallel signal paths to the output). Any instability in this local loop even at frequencies above the gainbandwidth could cause ringing at the output. To avoid this, the local structure was analyzed and an extra design constraint was added: a phase margin was posed on the local loop. The need for this extra

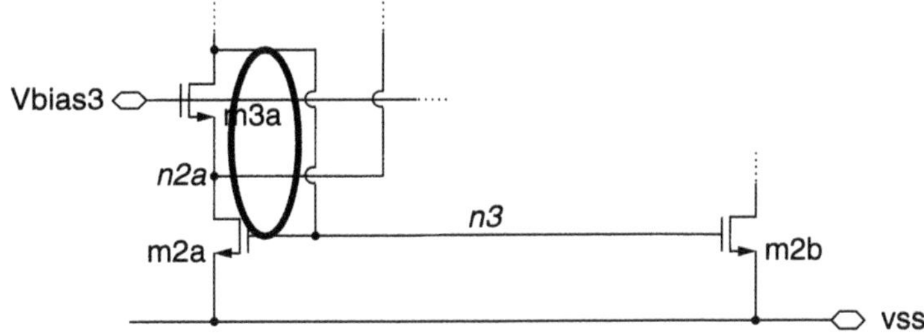

Figure 4.2: Local feedback loop in the high-speed OTA.

constraint is not agreed upon by all experiment participants, since no settling specification was requested. Either way you look at it, defining good design in terms of design constraints or in terms of a specification set that is complete (and would include settling time in this case, that is not disputed), are both hard problems. They require knowledge of circuits and what their behavior is like, to determine exactly what needs to be checked to guarantee correct operation of the circuit inside a system.

At first the equation-based approach did not reach the same GBW value as the other two approaches. Until it became clear that the local stability constraint was not checked by manual designers nor by the simulation-based approach. When this extra constraint was *removed*, the same optimal design as specified by the experiment, was found.

One complete optimization run takes about 5 minutes of CPU time on a SUN SPARC 10 workstation. Figure 4.3 shows the decreasing cost function Φ as a function of the improvement of the design. Three phases can be distinguished in this synthesis run. During the first phase (Penalty on divergence in figure 4.3) the optimizer has not found valid sizing points; in the second phase (Penalty on spec in figure 4.3) the optimizer has found valid sizing points, but the performance specifications have not yet been reached; in the last phase (Objective in figure 4.3) all performance specifications have been reached and the optimizer is maximizing the objective: GBW.

4.1.5 Comparison & Conclusions

The total time to set up all data and complete the equation-based synthesis for the above OTA starting from scratch by an experienced analog designer (library developer) that is familiar with the tools and proposed methodology, was 7 hours. Of these, 5 hours were spent in deriving the analytic equations, also for large-signal characteristics. Ordering the equations and creating the C module with the sequential computational path took 2 hours. A big advantage is that once this modeling effort has been carried out, designs can be optimized for different performance specifications and user-defined objectives in any compatible technology in minutes without changing the model.

The alternative approach using a SPICE-like numerical simulator in an optimization loop is rather easy to set up once extraction of circuit characteristics is automated. The latter setup took around 5 hours. The actual optimization runs with simulated annealing however took

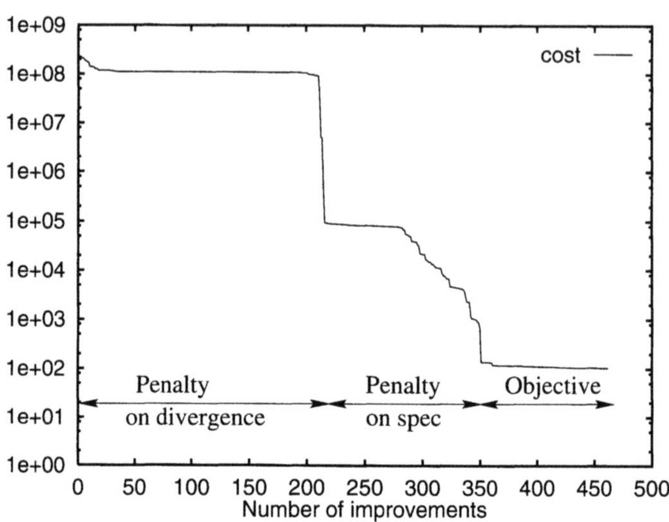

Figure 4.3: Decreasing cost as a function of design improvements.

longer (about 6 hours) because of the call to the simulator at each optimization iteration (which was an implementation issue that in commercial approaches could be overcome). Also, the optimization has to be robust enough to tackle the divergences of some simulation runs.

Finally the same design was also carried out manually by an experienced designer. The expert had derived the knowledge of the circuit by hand, by simulation and using a spreadsheet in approximately 5 hours. In this way, he figured out which device parameters (dimensions) to adjust to fulfill the constraints. The ultimate fine tuning for maximum performance took an additional time of 4 hours.

Time	**Equation-based**	**Simulation-based**	**Manual**
Setup	$7/rf$ hours	$5/rf$ hours	$5/rf$ hours
Optimization	10 minutes	6 hours	4 hours
Total experiment time (no reuse)	< 8 hours	11 hours	9 hours
Total time (reuse factor $rf = 10$)	< 45 minutes	6.5 hours	4.5 hours

Table 4.2: Summary of times spent on the optimal design of the OTA circuit by the three presented approaches, the last row reports the total design time per design with inclusion of the setup time assuming a reuse factor (rf) of 10.

The times reported have been summarized in Table 4.2 [Gie 95c]. All approaches thus approximately took the *same time* to reach the optimal solution. But since the setup times have been included for all methods and the setup time for the equation-based approach is the *largest*, the comparison favors the use of this approach when frequent reuse is expected, i.e.

when many synthesis/optimization runs are expected. The optimization time is considerably lower than with any other of the presented methods. Especially OTAs, OPAMPs and other frequently used circuits are thus ideal candidates for inclusion in the **AMGIE** cell library using the equation-based approach. This result has been achieved by the use of the sizing model generation methodology as presented in section 3.3 that is strongly supported by in-house developed tools.

The sizing model derived during this experiment has been included in the cell library as part of the high-speed topology. It will be used in the next reported experiment.

4.2 Student Exercise: High-speed Operational Transconductance Amplifier

To measure the capabilities of the **AMGIE** synthesis system in supporting inexperienced designers, the following experiment was carried out [VdPlas 01]. A classroom student exercise session (with per definition inexperienced designers) was set up to synthesize an OTA design automatically (steered by the students) for a grid of specifications. In the following subsections the results obtained with this experiment will be reported.

4.2.1 Setup

The **AMGIE** cell library contains a number of topologies implementing the OTA function. With this library a class of EE Master students has generated a number of designs. The class of students were divided in 9 groups, each of which received a different set of specifications. The performance specifications of an OTA that were selected for this exercise session were:

- Low-frequency gain (A_{v0})
- Gainbandwidth product (GBW)
- Phase margin (PM)
- Total offset voltage (V_{off})
- Signal swing (OR, IR)
- Slew rate (SR)
- Settling time ($t_{settling}$)
- Power supply voltages (V_{dd}, V_{ss})
- Load resistance (R_{load})
- Load capacitance (C_{load})
- Power consumption ($power$)
- Area ($area$)

The specifications that were common to all projects are summarized in Table 4.3. The specifications that were different for the 9 groups were the gainbandwidth (GBW), slew rate (SR) and load capacitance (C_{load}). The values are summarized in Table 4.4.

The technology in which the design has to be realized, is a standard 1P2M 0.7μm CMOS technology, the supply voltage was set to $+2.5\text{V}/-2.5\text{V}$.

4.2.2 Session

In this section a summary is given of a typical student exercise session.

Specification	Symbol		Value	Unit
Power consumption	*power*	$<$	50	mW
Area	*area*	$<$	200	nm^2
Low-frequency gain	A_{v0}	$>$	2000	–
Phase margin	*PM*	$>$	70	°
Total offset voltage	V_{off}	$<$	10	mV
Output range	*OR*	$>$	70	%
Input range	*IR*	$>$	10	%
Settling time [0.1%]	$t_{settling}$	$<$	10	μs
Power supply	V_{dd}, V_{ss}	$=$	$\pm$2.5	V
Load resistance	R_{load}	$=$	1.0e12	Ω
Technology	Θ	$=$	1P2M 0.7μm CMOS	–

Table 4.3: Common specifications for all groups.

Groups	$GBW > 5$MHz $SR > 5$V/μs	$GBW > 15$MHz $SR > 15$V/μs	$GBW > 45$MHz $SR > 45$V/μs
$C_{load} = 5$pF	group 1	group 4	group 7
$C_{load} = 10$pF	group 2	group 5	group 8
$C_{load} = 20$pF	group 3	group 6	group 9

Table 4.4: Specification values different for all groups.

Concepts

The students get an exercise document at the start of the session. The first part of this document consists of an introduction to the **AMGIE** and LAYLA tools. The methodology implemented in the tools and concepts are briefly explained. The flow as it has been presented in chapter 2 is also included. The students read these sections first before starting the **AMGIE** environment.

Specification Entry

A typical session then continues with starting up the environment. The first step is filling out the specification values as given in Tables 4.3 and 4.4. Although this seems to be an easy task, often numbers are forgotten or typed wrongly. To avoid this waste of time, basic checks are applied to the values entered. For instance, only positive numbers are acceptable for most of the specification values. If negative numbers are entered an Error is reported to the (novice) user.

Topology Selection

The next step in the design process is the selection of an appropriate topology from the system library. A few topologies are available for the students, among which a simple one-stage OTA, and a few two-stage OTAs. The specification ranges were purposely chosen such that the more complex two-stage OTAs are most appropriate. The students get the advice not to override the candidate selected by the topology selection (TS) tool. The topology which is thus most often chosen is the high-speed OTA topology, which was also discussed in the previous section. If time is left, other topologies can also be explored and some feedback is obtained on the quality of the choice by the topology selection tool. The schematic of the high-speed topology is shown in figure 4.1 on page 74.

Sizing and Optimization

Sizing and optimization (S&O) is the next tool in the design flow. One of the important inputs to the **AMGIE** tool now has to be supplied: the choice of the optimization targets. In this design exercise the aim is to find a high-quality design to implement the requested specifications. High quality can be defined as a design exhibiting an as low as possible power consumption, without sacrificing too much silicon area. As has already been shown in section 3.3.3 on page 57, a combination of *power* and *area* targets can explore the region of interest. By increasing the weight of the *power* target the high quality design point can be found. Remains the problem of estimating the target values of the two specifications.

For experienced designers this does not seem to be a difficult problem. They know how large the area of an OTA could be. This experience has been gained over multiple designs. In fact an area of approximately 50000 square microns is a reasonable guess for the requested specification sets in the used 1P2M 0.7μm CMOS technology. This value has been supplied to the students. The *power* is also easily estimated. An estimator for the lower boundary of the *power* consumption is given by:

$$\begin{aligned} power_{est} &\approx 2I_{gm}(V_{dd} - V_{ss}) \\ &\approx GBWC_{load}(V_{gs} - V_T)(V_{dd} - V_{ss}) \end{aligned} \tag{4.1}$$

In this equation the gainbandwidth and load capacitance is used to estimate the current through the input stage. The only unknown in the equation is the $V_{gs} - V_T$ of the input stage transistor. However a value is readily found: 0.2V. This estimator assumes no current is flowing in the output stage, and thus is certainly a lower bound estimate for the *power*.

The thus obtained *power* and *area* estimates are input to the tool and the sizing and optimization process can be started next. The sizing model, that has been prepared by expert users as has been explained in the previous section, is retrieved from the **AMGIE** cell library. The students thus can not alter the equations used in the sizing model. The first run is primarily used to get feedback on the optimization targets (that have been entered). By adapting the optimization targets and/or weights, the optimization result is influenced. After a few runs (which only take a few minutes per run), a sized design is obtained. In Table 4.5, the sizing and biasing values of the different runs are summarized. As can be seen, the device sizes all have reasonable values, as have the biasing conditions of the devices.

Verification after Sizing

These sizing results are next verified. The verification after sizing and optimization is started. The templates for extracting the performances are retrieved from the library. The simulations

Name	grp1	grp2	grp3	grp4	grp5	grp6	grp7	grp8	grp9	Unit
W_{m1a}	106.7	153.1	290.6	168.5	498.1	645.5	420.2	883.3	1932	μm
L_{m1a}	2.5	1.7	1.7	1.2	2	1.3	1.2	1.2	1.2	μm
$Vgst_{m1a}$	-160	-155	-155	-152	-164	-162	-194	-183	-166	mV
W_{m2a}	29.4	39.6	80.2	53.1	80.3	220.1	136.2	246.8	574.8	μm
L_{m2a}	1.5	1.7	1.5	1.8	0.8	1.6	0.9	0.8	0.8	μm
$Vgst_{m2a}$	203	266	248	297	226	273	259	244	251	mV
W_{m3a}	38.9	49.2	114.3	92.3	190.8	291	162.1	302.1	771.9	μm
L_{m3a}	4.2	3.5	2.7	2.8	2.7	2.5	1.8	2	1.8	μm
$Vgst_{m3a}$	384	441	353	355	342	384	428	445	391	mV
W_{m4a}	174	163.5	227.2	188.9	111.9	355.2	298.9	922	1040	μm
L_{m4a}	3.8	2.5	1.5	2.5	1.5	1.8	1.4	1.5	1.3	μm
$Vgst_{m4a}$	-212	-251	-232	-297	-424	-364	-347	-272	-378	mV
W_{m5a}	29.9	44.1	94.1	74.1	133.7	318.9	304.5	450.8	1115	μm
L_{m5a}	1.7	1.3	1.3	1.3	1.2	1.3	1.2	1.2	1.2	μm
$Vgst_{m5a}$	-342	-349	-347	-342	-339	-330	-313	-349	-344	mV
W_{m6}	186	171.8	225	193.6	119.9	371.7	325.7	1021	864.1	μm
L_{m6}	3.8	2.5	1.5	2.5	1.5	1.8	1.4	1.5	1.3	μm
$Vgst_{m6}$	-212	-251	-232	-297	-424	-364	-347	-272	-378	mV
W_{m7}	33.2	48.6	97.7	79.7	151.3	350.5	350.3	524.8	976	μm
L_{m7}	1.7	1.3	1.3	1.3	1.2	1.3	1.2	1.2	1.2	μm
$Vgst_{m7}$	-338	-344	-342	-337	-334	-325	-307	-343	-339	mV

Table 4.5: Sizing and biasing values of the student design runs.

are run in batch mode.

In figure 4.4(a), the Bode diagram of a typical design (group5) is shown. All non-dominant poles are situated beyond the gainbandwidth. The design is stable and does not contain pole-zero pairs. The transient time response to a pulse input signal is shown in figure 4.4(b). Except for the edges (close to V_{ss} and V_{dd}), the slopes are straight. The slew rate is extracted from 10 to 90% of the full swing.

At the end the students inspect the datasheet editor to verify that no violated specifications are found. If they want to cheat and continue the design process with violated specification values, the **AMGIE** design controller also checks the verified values and refuses to continue the design process.

Sensitivity Analysis for Layout Generation

At the same time the sensitivity analysis tool (part of the LAYLA environment) is run. It relies on the same templates for extracting the performance as the verification tool does. For every node the design has to be simulated once to extract for capacitive degradation, and one global nominal simulation has to be performed to derive the sensitivity (using a finite difference approximation). This is time consuming, especially if transient simulations are required to

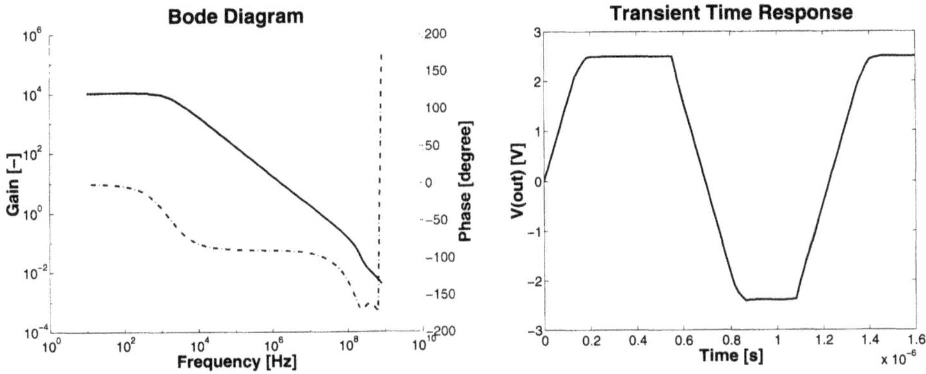

(a) Bode diagram: amplitude and phase response.

(b) Transient time response to a pulse signal.

Figure 4.4: Verification after sizing and optimization of a synthesized OTA (results for group5).

extract a performance specification. To avoid this large time, a representative subset of the specifications is selected: gainbandwidth product (*GBW*) and phase margin (*PM*). These two specifications are strongly influenced by the parasitic capacitance on internal nodes and output node of the circuit and are extracted with a fast AC analysis of a device simulator [1].

In Table 4.6 a typical sensitivity analysis output file is summarized. If we inspect the

	S^P_{n1}	S^P_{n2a}	S^P_{n2b}	S^P_{n3}	S^P_{n4a}	S^P_{n4b}	S^P_{n5}	S^P_{out}	
GBW	0	7e16	1.8e17	4e16	7e16	-6e16	0	-2.85e18	Hz/F
PM	0	-1e10	-1.23e12	-8.6e11	-2e10	-1.5e11	-1e10	7.1e11	°/F

Table 4.6: Sensitivity data.

sensitivity data a few remarks can be made. First of all the sensitivity of *GBW* with respect to the output node (*out*) is the largest. This is obvious, since this OTA is load compensated. The *GBW* is largely determined by the *gm* of the input stage and the capacitance on node *out*. Furthermore, many nodes have opposite sensitivities for *GBW* and *PM*. This also is easily explainable. A lowering of *GBW* with constant non-dominant poles and zeroes improves *PM*, or an increase in *GBW* with constant non-dominant poles and zeroes reduces the *PM*. Notable exception is node *n4b*, which seems to lower both *GBW* but at the same time the non-dominant poles and/or zeroes are lowered even more. What also must be noted is the fact that the sensitivity of the nodes to capacitive loading is asymmetric. Node *n2a* and node *n2b*

[1] The CPU time on a SUN Ultra-1/170 workstation for this extraction process is less than 1 minute. A transient analysis could thus be included to extract slew rate (*SR*), it would however not bring additional insight to the students. It would rather result in much longer sensitivity extraction simulation times.

for instance have different sensitivities both for *GBW* and *PM*, in some cases this difference is more than an order of magnitude.

The power dissipated by the devices, as well as the current flowing through their terminals is also extracted from simulation. These values are input to the LAYLA tool to determine the systematic offset voltage caused by temperature gradients during placement and do appropriate wire sizing during routing to avoid electro-migration effects [Lam 98, Lam 99]. In contrast to the sensitivity data, the circuit behaves symmetrically with respect to power dissipation and current [2].

Therefore the layout directives on the schematic instruct the LAYLA tools to create a symmetric layout. This ensures an optimal offset value. The sensitivity analysis data will guide the layout process towards an acceptable symmetrical layout, although an asymmetric layout could potentially be more advantageous to compensate capacitive degradation due to the differences in sensitivity of symmetric node pairs.

The next step in the design flow is subcell design. Since the high-speed OTA cell is a non-hierarchical (or flat) topology, this step is skipped: there are no subcells to design.

Layout Generation

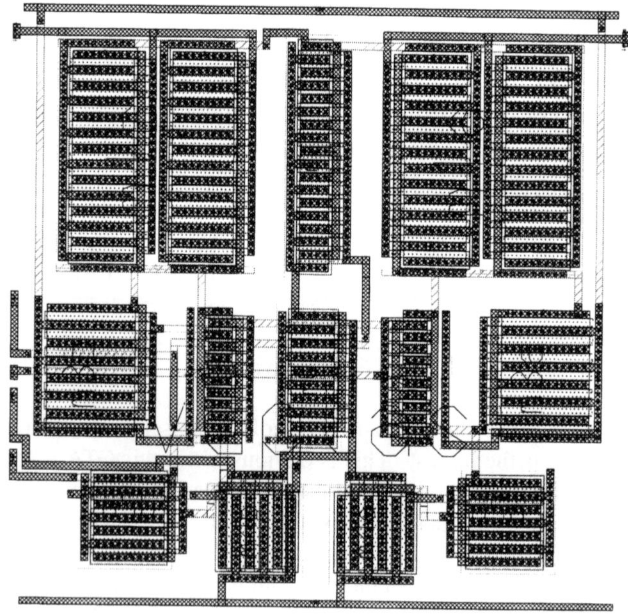

Figure 4.5: Performance-driven generated layout (group5 result).

[2]This is power consumption of all devices in rest state. Depending on the use of the circuit this state might be representative or not. To avoid this an average or application-specific power consumption extraction can be defined, in the library or in the cell under design.

Next the layout is generated by the LAYLA tool. In figure 4.5 a typical layout result (group5) is shown. This layout has been generated using the directives on the schematic, the sensitivity data and device power dissipation and current flowing through the device terminals. The most important user input to the process is the specification of the aspect ratio of the cell. The layout generation process is a two-step procedure. First a performance-driven placement is generated. This fixed placement is then routed using the performance-driven router. Both tools are part of the LAYLA environment. The students were encouraged to experiment with the aspect ratio to find an acceptable layout; there was no fixed layout dimension specified. This would certainly be the case when the OTA is part of a larger system in which a floorplanning step would have determined the optimal extent of the OTA subcell. An overview of the layout results for all groups will be presented in the next section.

Extraction

After the layout has been generated the extraction tool (ET) is started. The extraction tool runs the usual verification checks on the layout: Design Rule Check (DRC), Electrical Rule Check (ERC) and Layout Versus Schematic (LVS) check. Many commercial packages are available to accomplish this. The Mentor Graphics tools [Mentor-Graphics 98] have been used in this exercise session. If all checks are successful, the tool extracts a netlist from the layout, with inclusion of layout parasitics: both capacitive and resistive. Also in this case a commercial package (Mentor's DRCExtract) is used. This extracted netlist is then stored in the runtime database.

Verification after Layout

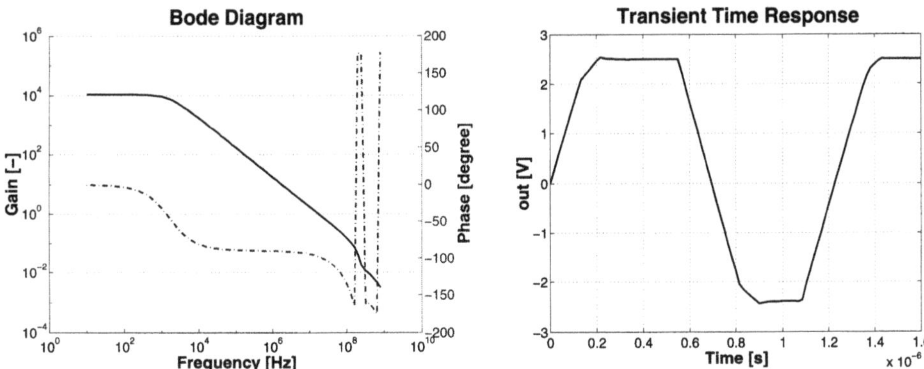

(a) Bode diagram: amplitude and phase response.

(b) Transient time response to a pulse input signal.

Figure 4.6: Verification after extraction of a synthesized OTA (results for group5).

The last step in the design flow is a final verification with numerical simulation. Using the extracted netlist, once again the performance is verified. Now it becomes obvious why a black box approach is required to verify the circuit. The internal nets of the extracted netlist include parasitic resistors and capacitors and are thus entirely different. The verification script can not rely on knowledge of the circuit internals. Typically the simulation time of the circuit is three times larger at this stage than for the verification after sizing and optimization. This is caused by the larger number of devices and nets in the netlist. In figure 4.6(a), the Bode diagram of a typical design (group5) is shown. In comparison to the Bode plot of figure 4.4(a), the poles and zeroes have shifted down. The circuit remains stable however (check the phase margin). The transient time response to a pulse input signal is shown in figure 4.6(b). The circuit now suffers from more overshoot and undershoot around the power supply lines. The signal slopes remain clean however.

4.2.3 Analysis of Results

In Table 4.7 the achieved power consumption is shown for the 9 designs, while Fig. 4.7 shows the layout results. What immediately can be observed from these results is that the layout area doesn't scale in relation to load and speed in the same way as the power does. The power consumption is almost linearly related to the product of speed and load. The area is most evidently not. This is explained by the fact that for the lower load and speed specification values, the input-referred offset voltage specification (< 10mV) puts a lower limit on the area of the active devices. This can clearly be seen from the offset voltage results summarized in Table 4.8. The upper left designs are constrained by the offset voltage specification.

The deviation in the power results for the last column is explained by the stability requirement (phase margin better than 70°). For the first two columns the design is sufficiently stable without spending extra power for pushing non-dominant poles to higher frequencies. The designs with the high speed requirements need to spend extra power for obtaining a stable circuit. This can also clearly be seen from Table 4.9 summarizing the obtained phase margins, the designs in the last column are determined by stability constraints.

Power cons. mW	$GBW > 5$MHz $SR > 5V/\mu s$	$GBW > 15$MHz $SR > 15V/\mu s$	$GBW > 45$MHz $SR > 45V/\mu s$
$C_{load} = 5$pF	0.407	1.25	4.84
$C_{load} = 10$pF	0.808	2.48	8.83
$C_{load} = 20$pF	1.600	5.00	19.6

Table 4.7: Obtained power consumption values.

The simulated performance of a typical result is verified against the specifications in the third column of Table 4.10, and all specifications are satisfied. This classroom project showed that even less experienced designers can generate good designs in a short time with the **AMGIE** system. The only limitation is that enough cells have to be available in the library to have sufficient coverage of typical performance ranges encountered in practical applications.

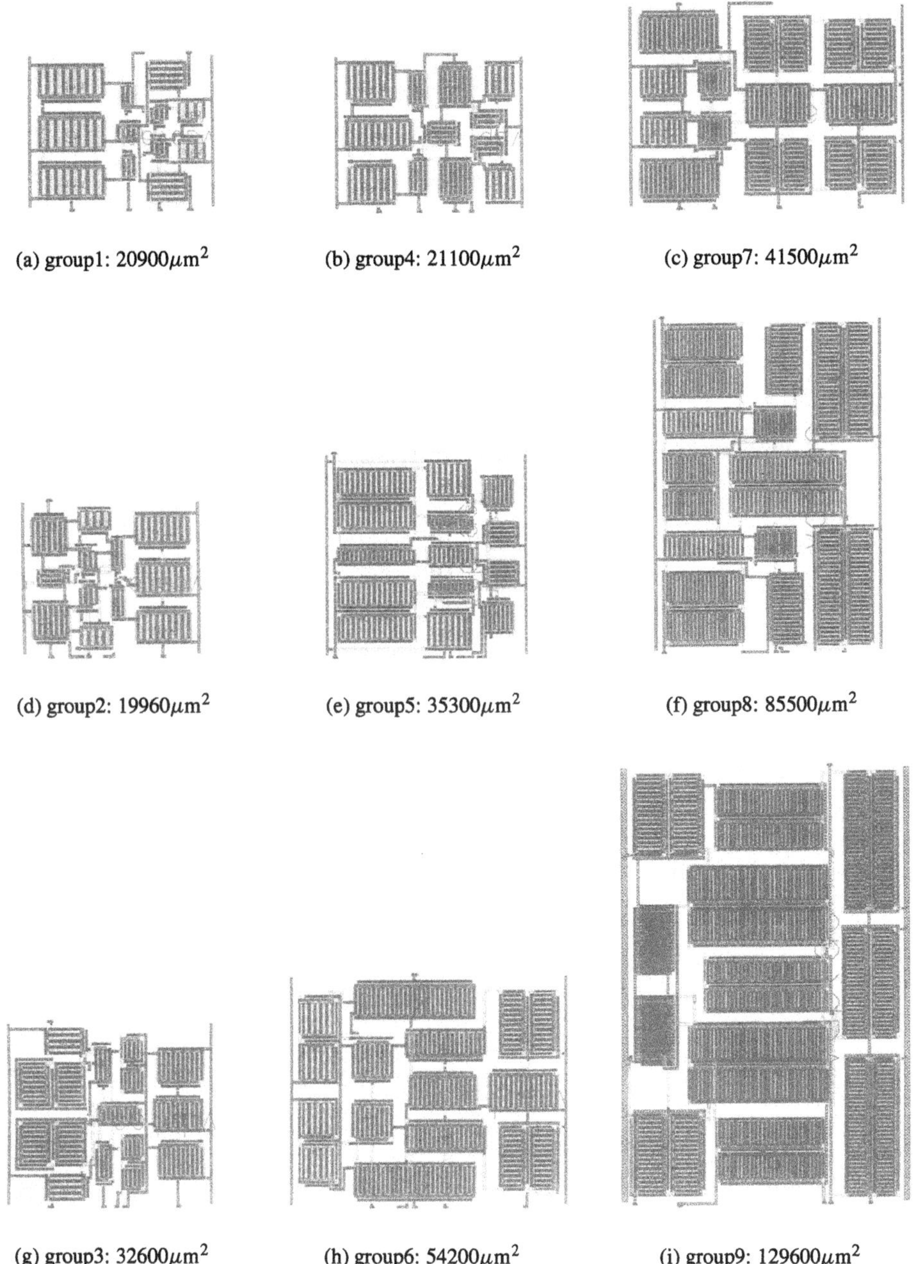

(a) group1: 20900μm^2 (b) group4: 21100μm^2 (c) group7: 41500μm^2

(d) group2: 19960μm^2 (e) group5: 35300μm^2 (f) group8: 85500μm^2

(g) group3: 32600μm^2 (h) group6: 54200μm^2 (i) group9: 129600μm^2

Figure 4.7: Layout results of the exercise session. Note that the smaller layouts have been scaled up slightly to increase visibility. The trend of the area change is however maintained.

Offset voltage mV	$GBW > 5$MHz $SR > 5\text{V}/\mu\text{s}$	$GBW > 15$MHz $SR > 15\text{V}/\mu\text{s}$	$GBW > 45$MHz $SR > 45\text{V}/\mu\text{s}$
$C_{load} = 5$pF	9.98	9.53	8.48
$C_{load} = 10$pF	9.84	7.83	5.63
$C_{load} = 20$pF	9.91	5.76	4.41

Table 4.8: Obtained offset voltage values.

Phase margin °	$GBW > 5$MHz $SR > 5\text{V}/\mu\text{s}$	$GBW > 15$MHz $SR > 15\text{V}/\mu\text{s}$	$GBW > 45$MHz $SR > 45\text{V}/\mu\text{s}$
$C_{load} = 5$pF	82	76	70
$C_{load} = 10$pF	83	77	71
$C_{load} = 20$pF	84	78	70

Table 4.9: Obtained phase margin values.

Specification	**Requested**		**Predicted**	**Simulation**	**Unit**
Low-frequency gain	>	2000	9000	12400	–
Phase margin	>	70	77	79	°
Total offset voltage	<	10	7.83	8	mV
Output range	>	70	70	73	% of supply range
Input range	>	10	80	85	% of supply range
Settling time [0.1%]	<	10	0.075	0.072	μs
Load resistance	=	1	1	1	GΩ
Power supply	=	±2.5	±2.5	±2.5	V
Technology	=	1P2M 0.7μm CMOS			–
Power consumption	<	20	2.5	2.5	mW
Area	<	0.1	0.024	0.035	mm^2

Table 4.10: Specifications common to all OTA designs, comparison with obtained performances after extraction and simulation (design from group 5).

4.2.4 Conclusions

The exercise was performed on standard HP 712/100 workstations. As is evident from the shown data, all groups succeeded in the task. The fastest design team realized the complete design in less than one hour, the slowest team used 2 hours and 15 minutes of the allocated 2 and a half hours to finish the design successfully. An experienced analog designer who is familiar with the **AMGIE** synthesis system, can accomplish the same task in approximately 40 minutes (from specification to layout). This time is an average time, since it must be noted that the design time depends partly on the complexity (size) of the design. The larger (layout) area slows down the bottom up part of the design flow: layout generation, extraction and verification.

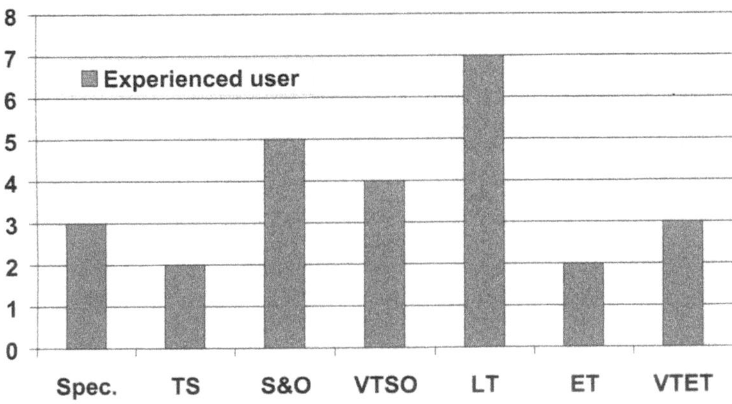

Figure 4.8: Breakdown of the OTA design time, in the case of an experienced tool user and designer. The reported time units are minutes.

A breakdown of the time spent on the design by an experienced tool user is shown in figure 4.8. It shows that the largest time is spent in the synthesis tools: topology selection (TS), sizing and optimization (S&O) and layout generation (LT). The verification steps in the process, verification tool (VT), twice, and extraction tool (ET), require a smaller part of the total design time. The timing information shown has been derived for a typical design (group 5) on a SUN Ultra-1/170 workstation. This machine is slightly faster (50%) than the machines the students had at their disposition.

In the next section, the design by an experienced designer of an analog signal processing chain will be reported. The design of this circuit stresses the **AMGIE** system with respect to the complexity it can handle.

4.3 Charge-Sensitive Amplifier – Pulse-Shaping Amplifier

Charge-sensitive amplifier – pulse-shaping amplifier (CSA-PSA) signal processing chains are an essential building block of particle detector front-ends (PDFEs). These PDFEs are used both in space applications (satellites) and in high-energy particle experiments to detect the energy of incident particles:

1. Every space mission, however short or well shielded, takes place under irradiation. For this reason, radiation is one of the most studied topics in space exploration. At the same time, the volume, weight and power requirements in space are very stringent.

2. In particle experiments, large arrays of detectors are required to measure not only the energy and timing of the particles but also their trajectories. This puts demanding requirements on both the area and power consumption of the individual PDFE chains.

In both applications the environment in which the detector electronics have to function contains high levels of radiation. This is an additional constraint for the design and implementation of solid-state PDFEs. At the same time the PDFE should have a high sensitivity (to detect small energy levels) and a good linearity. The lower boundary of detection is determined by the noise level in the analog front-end. This noise level is typically expressed as the number of equivalent electron charges, for instance a noise level of $1000e^{-}_{rms}$. On the other hand the speed requirements are relaxed. Typical bandwidths for analog front-ends are only a few hundred kHz or a few MHz. These are certainly in reach for CMOS integrated circuits. This bandwidth is limited by the amount of data that can be stored and/or processed upstream. With the advent of commercially available CMOS technologies, that can withstand doses of irradiation encountered in typical applications [Snoey 01], a fully integrated PDFE can be realized at low cost. This offers all the advantages of an integrated solution: lower power consumption, less area and weight, the overall result of which is a cheaper mission or a higher number of experiments that can be shipped on one space mission.

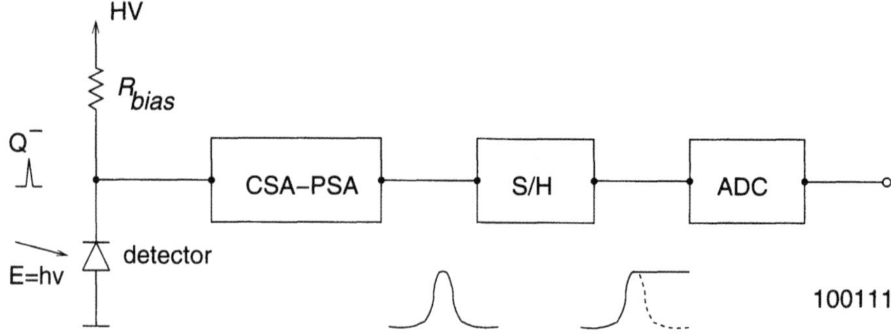

Figure 4.9: Block diagram of a typical particle detector front-end (PDFE).

In figure 4.9, the block diagram of a typical PDFE is shown [Chang 90]. A sensor converts the energy of an incident particle into a charge. The (integrated) size of the charge pulse is a measure of the energy the particle contained and lost in the collision, its timing an accurate representation of the position of the particle in space. In [Chang 90], it has been proven that the processing of this charge pulse is best done with a CSA-PSA. This functionblock converts the hard to measure charge pulse into a semi-Gaussian shaped pulse. The height of the semi-Gaussian pulse is easier to measure, and is an accurate representation of the energy level. By converting the pulse in a semi-Gaussian pulse the noise is optimally suppressed [Chang 90]. The top of the pulse is then sampled and held by a peak-detect sample-and-hold circuit (S/H) for conversion into a digital value with an A/D-converter. Depending on the architecture of the PDFE this A/D-converter is shared amongst multiple analog preprocessing channels or dedicated to one channel [Don 97, Don 98]. The digital output is then optionally processed by a digital signal processor and stored or transmitted.

In the remainder of this section the following topics will be discussed. First the specification set of CSA-PSA circuits will be presented. Next the circuit architecture will be described, and the creation of an equation-based sizing model. Topology selection and sizing synthesis of the CSA-PSA circuit in the **AMGIE** system will then be described. The layout generation will be discussed next. After describing the verification of the circuit, the measurement results of a fabricated prototype detector [Vdbus 98c] will be presented. The obtained results are compared to a previous, manual design in the same technology process. In the last section a breakdown of time spent on the design of this circuit will be discussed and conclusions will be drawn.

4.3.1 CSA-PSA Specifications

Name	Symbol		Value	Unit
Detector capacitance	C_d	=	80	pF
Noise	ENC_{tot}	<	1000	e^-_{rms}
Peaking time	τ_p	<	1.5	μs
Counting rate	*counting_rate*	>	200	kSamples/s
Gain	*sensitivity*	=	20	mV/fC
Max. output range	*OR*	=	2	V
Linearity	*linearity*	<	1	%
Power supply	V_{dd}, V_{ss}	=	$\pm$2.5	V
Technology	Θ	=	1P2M 0.7μm CMOS	–
Area	*Area*	MIN	2	mm^2
Power Consumption	*Power*	MIN	40	mW

Table 4.11: Specification set of the CSA-PSA functionblock.

In Table 4.11 a summary is given of the CSA-PSA specifications. The detector's capacitance value is an important input parameter since it strongly influences the noise performance. In fact, in [Chang 90] it has been proven that a *matched* input stage, that is a CSA having an equal input capacitance, is optimal for noise performance. The noise specification is expressed

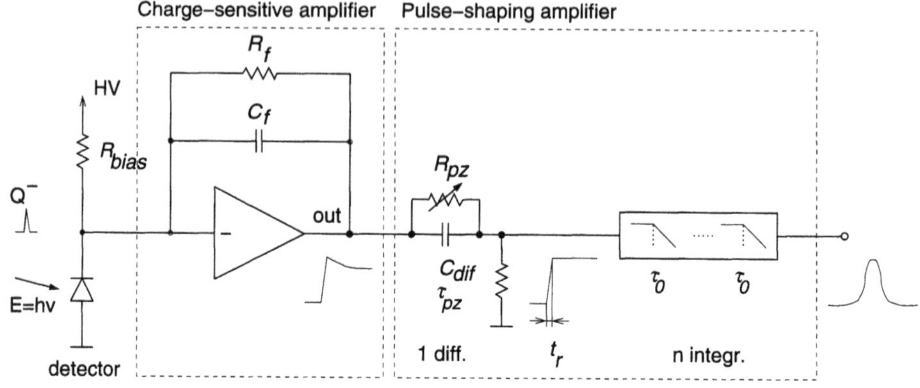

Figure 4.10: Architecture of the CSA-PSA circuit.

as an equivalent charge of electrons. Specifying a charge of $1000e^-_{rms}$ is equivalent with a σ of this energy on the measured energy of the particles (or an accurate error measure). The peaking time is the time between the particle hitting the detector (and immediately creating a charge pulse) and the *peak* of the semi-Gaussian shaped pulse at the output. The counting rate is the maximal amount of particles that, evenly spaced in time, can be handled by the preprocessing chain per second. The gain (or *sensitivity*) is the proportionality factor between the detected charge and the output voltage. The maximal output range puts a limit on the largest detectable particle energy given the gain. It is also an important parameter to interface to the rest of the PDFE. The linearity error must be small enough to accurately determine the particle's energy level. The power supply is limited to a ± 2.5V standard value, for the 1P2M 0.7μm CMOS technology used in the experiment. *Area* and *Power* are to be minimized. The values given in Table 4.11 are reference values extracted from a manually designed CSA-PSA in the same technology. The purpose of the experiment is not only to automate the design of the frequently used CSA-PSA functionblock but also to guarantee the quality of the design, and if possible to improve upon the manual design.

4.3.2 CSA-PSA Architecture

In figure 4.10 the architecture of the CSA-PSA is depicted. The CSA-PSA is composed out of a sequence of a charge-sensitive amplifier (CSA) and a pulse-shaping amplifier (PSA). The CSA converts the charge pulse (a spike) to an (integrated) step voltage at its output, this voltage is stored on C_f. The step signal is differentiated once in the PSA, and subsequently integrated n times, with time constant τ_0. The number of times the differentiated step signal is integrated is a topological parameter that can vary between 1 and 4. This range is found to be sufficient to enclose the optimal value [Chang 90]. The block diagram also contains a feedback resistance across the CSA (R_f) and a pole-zero cancellation block in the PSA. These have been added to solve the integrator's saturation problem. Without R_f, the accumulated

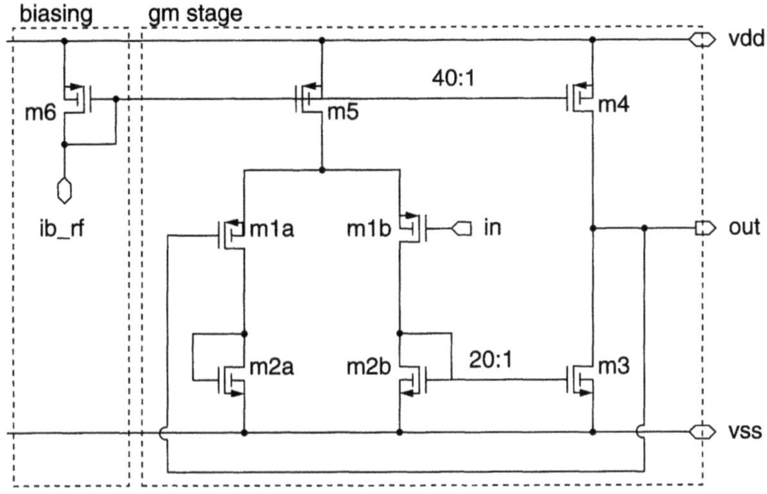

Figure 4.11: Schematic of the 20MΩ active resistor.

charge on C_f would increase steadily, until the amplifier saturates. By adding a high-ohmic resistance, R_f, the charge is reduced steadily. The value of this resistance has been put at 20MΩ. This introduces an extra pole in the transfer function of the CSA. This would lead to errors, unless it is compensated by a zero. This is the function of the pole-zero compensation in the PSA, formed by R_{pz}. The time constant τ_{pz} is equal to the pole created by the feedback resistance R_f and integration capacitor C_f. Since it is hard to match these time constants by matching solely, the pole-zero compensating resistorR_{pz} is made tunable.

The design of the CSA-PSA circuit thus consists of the following blocks: a CSA, a PSA (one differentiator circuit and n integrators), an R_f active resistor (for use in the CSA) and a R_{pz} tunable resistor (for use in the PSA).

In the next paragraphs the derivation of the sizing models for these subcircuits will be discussed. Once the sizing models of the subcircuits are available, equations modeling a selection of performance specifications of the CSA-PSA circuit will be discussed. For a complete description of the sizing model, the reader is referred to [Vdbus 95] or, for the sizing model itself, the cell library of the **AMGIE** system [VdPlas 96b].

The first block that is investigated is the CSA.

4.3.2.1 The Charge-Sensitive Amplifier (CSA)

The CSA is implemented using a folded-cascode structure [Ran 97] with a cascoded active load as depicted in figure 4.12. In addition the feedback resistance, R_f, is also fully integrated. The resistance value of 20MΩ was efficiently implemented using a gm-stage [Stey 91]. In order to achieve the high resistance value a current division of 40 was used (shown in figure 4.11). This subcircuit was manually sized.

In the following paragraph, we will first analyze the open-loop behavior of the CSA, which

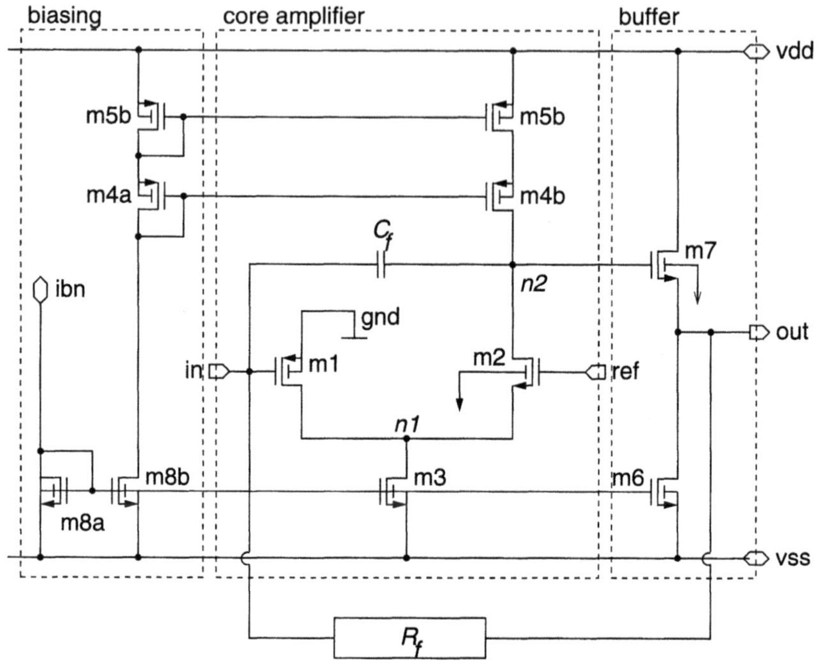

Figure 4.12: Schematic of the folded-cascode charge-sensitive amplifier (CSA).

leads to expressions for the gainbandwidth (*GBW*) and phase margin (*PM*) and allows to derive stability constraints. Afterwards the closed-loop behavior of the CSA is analyzed, which allows us to examine in what frequency range the CSA will function as an integrator. Expressions for the speed (i.e. rise time τ_r) are derived as well.

Because of the nested loop in the circuit (inner loop through the feedback capacitance C_f, outer loop through the feedback resistance R_f), it is not straightforward to derive expressions for the *GBW* and *PM* in open-loop. For this analysis the feedback loop is cut at the gate of the input transistor *m1* of the CSA, shown in figure 4.12.

The core amplifier itself (figure 4.12) has a dominant pole f_d on node *n2* given by:

$$f_d = \frac{1}{2\pi(R_{casc1} \parallel R_{casc2})C_{n2}} \tag{4.2}$$

with

$$R_{casc1} = ro_{m5b} + ro_{m4b}(1 + gm_{m4b}ro_{m5b}) \tag{4.3}$$

$$R_{casc2} = ro_{m1} \parallel ro_{m3} + ro_{m2}(1 + gm_{m2}(ro_{m1} \parallel ro_{m3})) \tag{4.4}$$

$$C_{n2} = C_f + cgd_{m4b} + cdb_{m4b} + cgd_{m2} + cgd_{m7} \tag{4.5}$$

The non-dominant pole f_{p1} on node *n1* is given by:

$$f_{p1} = \frac{gm_{m2} + gmb_{m2} + go_{m2}}{2\pi C_{n1}} \tag{4.6}$$

with $C_{n1} = cgd_{m1} + cdb_{m1} + cgs_{m2} + csb_{m2} + cgd_{m3} + cdb_{m3}$.

The loading of the feedback circuit results in additional poles in the open-loop transfer. The feedback load impedance is given by:

$$Z_f = \frac{1}{sC_{int}} + \frac{1}{G_f + sC_f} = \frac{G_f + s(C_f + C_{int})}{sC_{int}(G_f + sC_f)} \tag{4.7}$$

where $C_{int} = cgs_{m1} + cgd_{m1} + C_{detector}$ is the total capacitance at the input node. This results in a pole in the open-loop transfer function at frequency f_{1f} and a zero at frequency f_{2f} given by:

$$f_{1f} = \frac{1}{2\pi R_f(C_f + C_{int})} \ll f_{2f} = \frac{1}{2\pi R_f C_f} \tag{4.8}$$

The frequency f_{1f} is much lower than f_{2f} as C_f is in the order of fF while the detector capacitance $C_{detector}$ is usually in the order of pF. The frequencies typically differ three decades.

Using these equations, expressions for the open-loop gain bandwidth GBW_{ol} and the phase margin PM can be derived:

$$GBW_{ol} = \frac{GBW_{CSA}}{A_{feedback}} = GBW_{CSA}\frac{C_f}{C_f + C_{int}} \tag{4.9}$$

$$PM \approx \pi - \arctan(\frac{GBW_{ol}}{f_{1f}}) + \arctan(\frac{GBW_{ol}}{f_{2f}}) - \arctan(\frac{GBW_{ol}}{f_d}) - \arctan(\frac{GBW_{ol}}{f_{p1}}) \tag{4.10}$$

with

$$\begin{aligned} A_{feedback} &= \frac{C_f + C_{int}}{C_f} \\ GBW_{CSA} &= \frac{gm_{eq,CSA}}{2\pi C_{n2}} \\ gm_{eq,CSA} &= gm_{m1}\frac{gm_{m2}}{\frac{1+gm_{m2}ro_{m2}}{ro_{m5b}+ro_{m4b}(1+gm_{m4b}ro_{m5b})}+gm_{m2}} \end{aligned}$$

and C_{n2} has been given in equation (4.5).

The open-loop transfer function is depicted in figure 4.13(a) and (b). The positions of the different poles and zeroes identified in the previous calculation have been added to the amplitude plot. At high frequencies a zero, formed by the gate-drain capacitance at the input transistor, occurs (f_{z1}). For a correct operation the CSA should be stable: this is enforced by a $PM > 70°$ and that pole f_d must be higher in frequency than zero f_{2f}. Both these constraints have been added to the sizing model as design constraints.

The closed-loop transfer of the CSA is depicted in figure 4.14(a) and (b). The resulting transimpedance has two important poles:

$$f_{c1} = \frac{1}{2\pi\tau_1} = f_{2f} = \frac{1}{2\pi R_f C_f} \tag{4.11}$$

$$f_{c2} = \frac{1}{2\pi\tau_2} = GBW_{CSA}\frac{C_f}{C_{int}} \approx \frac{GBW_{CSA}}{A_{feedback}} = GBW_{ol} \tag{4.12}$$

The rise time is determined by time constant τ_2 and is given by: $t_r = 2.2\,\tau_2$; τ_1 determines the decay of the CSA (see figure 4.15).

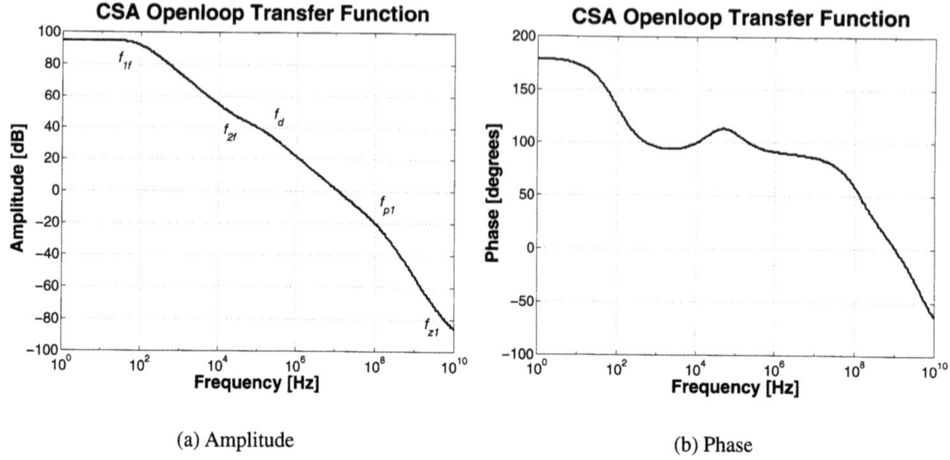

(a) Amplitude

(b) Phase

Figure 4.13: Charge-sensitive amplifier (CSA) open-loop Bode diagrams.

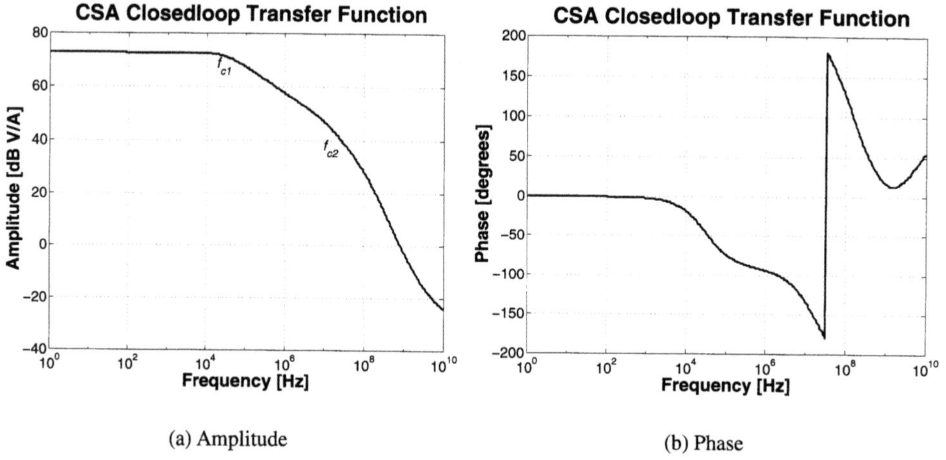

(a) Amplitude

(b) Phase

Figure 4.14: Charge-sensitive amplifier (CSA) closed-loop Bode diagrams.

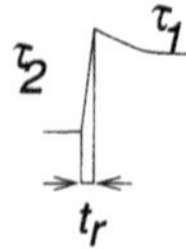

Figure 4.15: Rise time of the charge-sensitive amplifier (CSA).

4.3.2.2 The pulse-shaping amplifier with pole-zero cancellation

The PSA is a bandpass filter consisting of a differentiator and a number of n integrators, as shown in 4.16.

The time constants of the differentiator ($\tau_{differentiator}$) and the integrator sections ($\tau_{integrator}$) are given by (see figure 4.16):

$$\tau_{differentiator} = R_{dif} C_{dif} \tag{4.13}$$

$$\tau_{integrator} = R_{in} C_{int} \tag{4.14}$$

Both time constants are taken equal [Chang 90], or:

$$\tau_0 = R_{in} C_{int} = R_{dif} C_{dif} \tag{4.15}$$

One design parameter of the set R_{in}, C_{int}, R_{dif}, C_{dif} can immediately be determined. The center frequency of the bandpass filter is determined by:

$$f_{cf} = \frac{1}{2\pi R_{int} C_{int}} \tag{4.16}$$

The active amplifier used in the PSA integrator sections is a Miller opamp [LakSan 94a]. The sizing model available in the library has been integrated in the CSA-PSA sizing model. This OPAMP is included in the sizing model of the CSA-PSA to improve the overall optimality of the design. This posed no substantial overhead on the CPU time for the optimization and guarantees a global optimum, that otherwise can not be guaranteed because of the limited accuracy of estimators needed when using an hierarchical approach. The disadvantage of this approach is however that only a Miller opamp can currently be used in the CSA-PSA topology and potentially more advantageous OPAMP topologies are not attempted. Another CSA-PSA topology could however easily be created which uses a generic OPAMP estimator as active element in the PSA integrator sections.

As already indicated, the finite decay time of the CSA ($\tau_1 = R_f C_f$) results in an undershoot at the output of the PSA. This problem is solved by adding a tunable parallel resistor R_{pz} and thus by creating an additional zero in the transfer function of the PSA. This zero compensates for the pole formed by the feedback resistance R_f and the feedback capacitance C_f in the CSA. As R_f varies due to process variations, R_{pz} is to be tuned such that $\tau_{pz} = R_{pz} C_{dif} = R_f C_f$. The tunable resistance R_{pz} is implemented as a gm-stage.

The number of integrators, n, is determined by the optimization in the **OPTIMAN** tool as described later in section 4.3.4.

This concludes the discussion of the derivation of the sizing models of the CSA-PSA sub-blocks. The sizing model of the CSA-PSA circuit is not yet complete. There are a number of performance specifications which need to be derived at the architectural level. In the next two paragraphs the equations for the *sensitivity* and noise of the CSA-PSA will be provided as an example. Please note that for the derivation of these equations the reference work [Chang 90] was used extensively.

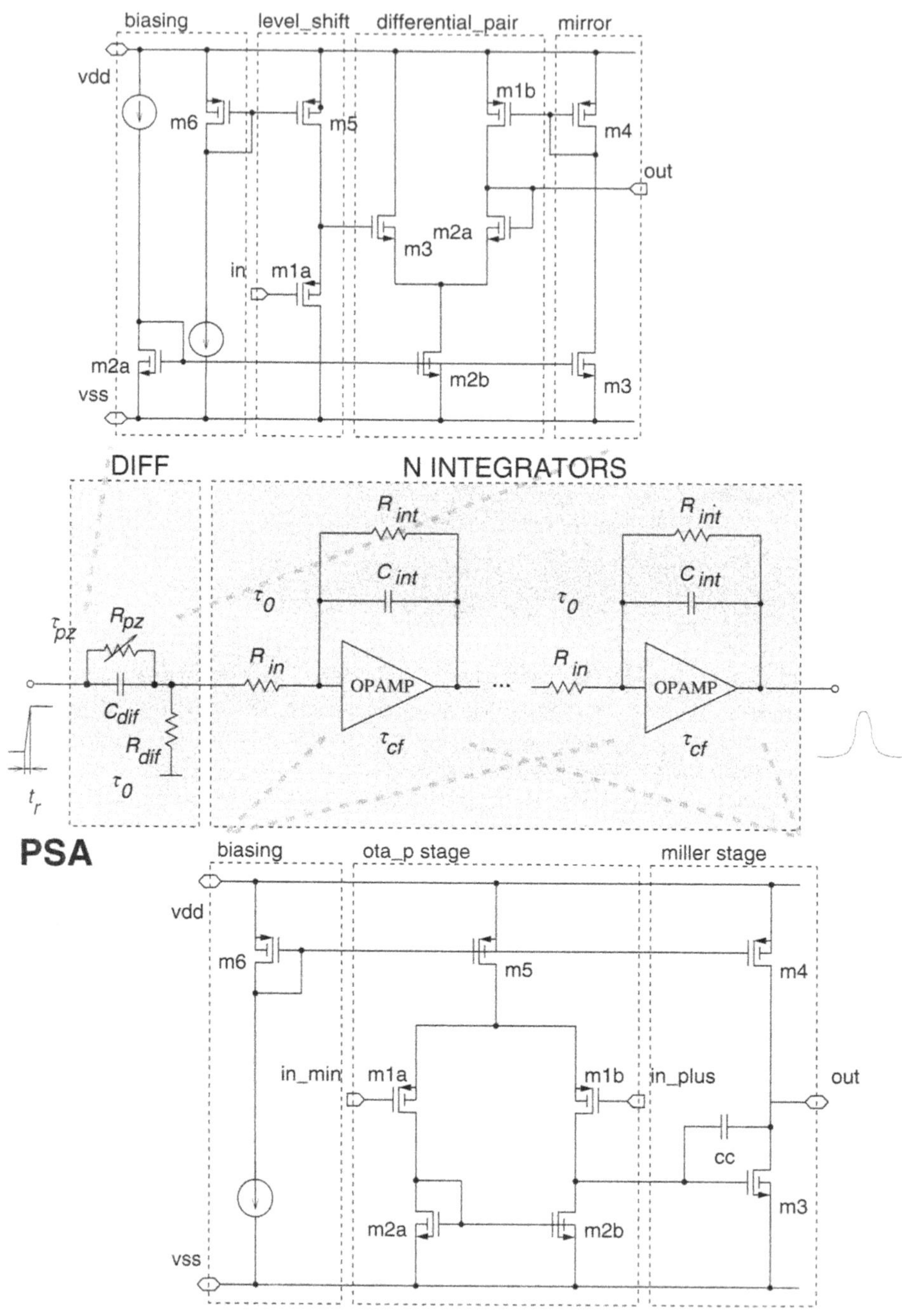

Figure 4.16: Schematic of the pulse-shaping amplifier (PSA) with pole-zero cancellation.

4.3.2.3 CSA-PSA Sensitivity Analysis

In the semiconductor detector world two types of resolution can be distinguished [Chang 90]. One is the **intrinsic detector resolution** associated with the statistical property of the detector itself and the other one is the **electronic resolution** describing the electronic noise in the readout electronics.

The intrinsic detector resolution stems from the fact that not all incident energy (E) is used for generating electron-hole-pairs ($e^- h^+$-pairs). The charge generated by a detector (Q) is given by [Chang 90]:

$$Q = q\,\frac{E}{\varepsilon_C} \tag{4.17}$$

where ε_C is the conversion efficiency, which is for Si at 25° 3.61eV/$e^- h^+$, for Ge at 77K 2.96eV/$e^- h^+$ and q is the charge of one electron.

The charge to voltage conversion of the CSA-PSA circuit is given by [Chang 90]:

$$V_{outp} = \frac{Q}{C_f}\,\frac{A_{v0}^n\, n^n}{n!\, e^n} \tag{4.18}$$

where V_{outp} is the peak output voltage at the output of the CSA-PSA, A_{v0} is the DC gain of one PSA integrator stage, C_f is the feedback capacitor of the CSA and n is the number of integration stages. The sensitivity (or gain) of the CSA-PSA structure (including the detector) is then given by [Chang 90]:

$$sensitivity = \frac{V_{outp}}{E} = \frac{q\, A_{v0}^n\, n^n}{\varepsilon_C\, C_f\, n!\, e^n} \tag{4.19}$$

In this way, the design parameters of the CSA and PSA subblocks (A_{v0}, n, C_f, ...) are translated to the performance of the global CSA-PSA circuit. Together with the noise which is analyzed next, this is one of the most important performance specifications of the CSA-PSA. During sizing the *sensitivity* will be set to 20mV/fC in the presented design.

4.3.2.4 CSA-PSA Noise Analysis

The noise can be reduced to three equivalent noise sources [Chang 90]: (1) the equivalent serial white noise ENC_{SW}, generated by the thermal channel noise of the transistors, (2) the equivalent pink noise ENC_{SF} generated by the transistors, and (3) the parallel white input current noise ENC_{PW}, generated by the leakage current (shot noise) of the detector and the protection diodes of the CSA-PSA and the thermal noise from the biasing circuit of the detector. These equivalent noise sources are given by [Chang 90]:

1. for the parallel white input current noise:

$$ENC_{PW}^2 = K_{PW} C_{PW}(n) \tau_p I_{leak} \tag{4.20}$$

with $K_{PW} = \frac{1}{2\pi q}$ and $C_{PW}(n) = \frac{n!^2 e^{2n}}{n^{2n+1}} \beta(\frac{1}{2}, n + \frac{1}{2})$

and

$\beta()$	:	beta-function
τ_p	:	peaking time (time to reach the peak value of the generated pulse)
n	:	number of PSA integrator sections
I_{leak}	:	detector leakage current

2. for the equivalent serial white noise:

$$ENC^2_{SW} = K_{SW}C_{SW}(n)T_{CSA}\frac{(C_{int}+C_f)^2}{\tau_p gm_{eq,n}} \tag{4.21}$$

with $K_{SW} = \frac{2k}{3\pi q^2}$, $C_{SW}(n) = \frac{n!^2e^{2n}}{n^{2n-1}}\beta(\frac{3}{2}, n-\frac{1}{2})$, $\frac{1}{gm_{eq,n}} = \frac{gm_{m1}+gm_{m3}+gm_{m8}+gm_{m5a}+gm_{m5b}}{gm^2_{m1}}$

and T_{CSA} : temperature of the CSA

3. for the equivalent pink noise:

$$ENC^2_{SF} = K_{SF}C_{SF}(n)(C_{int}+C_f)^2\left(\frac{KF}{WL}\right)_{eq} \tag{4.22}$$

with $K_{SF} = \frac{1}{2q^2C^2_{ox}}$, $C_{SF}(n) = \frac{n!^2e^{2n}}{n^{2n+1}}$ and

$$\left(\frac{KF}{WL}\right)_{eq} = \frac{1}{gm^2_{m1}}\left[\left(\frac{KF}{WL}\right)_{m1} gm^2_{m1} + \left(\frac{KF}{WL}\right)_{m3} gm^2_{m3} + \left(\frac{KF}{WL}\right)_{m8} gm^2_{m8} + \left(\frac{KF}{WL}\right)_{m5a} gm^2_{m5a} + \left(\frac{KF}{WL}\right)_{m5b} gm^2_{m5b}\right]$$

The total noise power, ENC_{tot} is given by [Chang 90]:

$$ENC_{tot} = \sqrt{ENC^2_{SF} + ENC^2_{SW} + ENC^2_{PW}} \tag{4.23}$$

For minimal white noise the capacitance of the input transistor $m1$ (see figure 4.12) should be chosen such that $C_{m1} = \frac{C_{detector}+C_f}{3}$, while for a minimal pink noise contribution, the noise condition $C_{m1} = C_{detector} + C_f$ should be met [Chang 90]. This implies that, as far as pink noise is concerned, either W or L can be chosen freely to meet the optimal noise condition. However, taking into account the requirements for the GBW and the speed of the CSA, a minimal gate length should be chosen for the input transistor. These additional constraints are also taken into account by the **OPTIMAN** tool during optimization.

This concludes the sizing plan derivation. The discussed set of declarative equations is turned into a dedicated design plan, which will then be used in an optimization loop to custom size the circuit while minimizing the power and area consumption. The plan is stored in the cell library of the **AMGIE** system and made available for sizing synthesis. The equations of the sizing model are also the input to the boundary checking and interval analysis models of the topology selection tool and converted to a boundary checking model and interval analysis model as discussed in [Ves 97].

In the next sections the design of the CSA-PSA circuit in the **AMGIE** system will be described. The first step is topology selection.

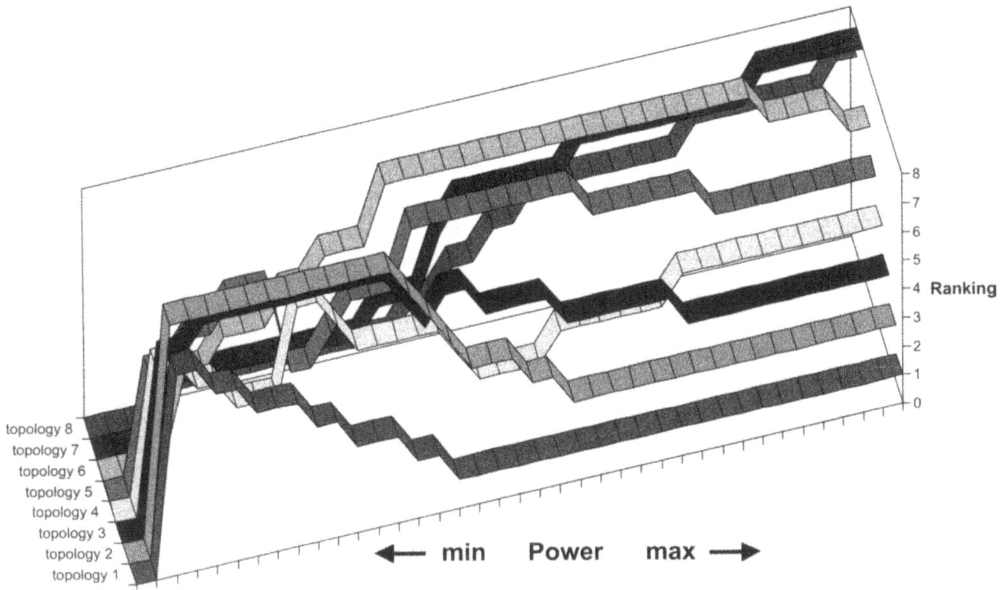

Figure 4.17: Results of topology selection: relative order of the 8 topologies (vertical axis — topology 8 is number 1 in the list) over varying performance specifications as function of the maximum power (horizontal axis).

4.3.3 Topology Selection

The design equations of the CSA-PSA circuit, as derived in the previous paragraphs, have been transformed into topology data: an interval analysis and boundary checking model [Ves 95, Ves 97, VdPlas 01]. Conceptually the model looks as follows:

$$\begin{aligned}
&\text{(noise requirement)} & ENC_{tot} &= f_1(\mathbf{A}) && (4.24)\\
&\text{(speed requirement)} & BandWidth &= f_2(\mathbf{A}) && (4.25)\\
&\text{(power requirement)} & Power &= f_3(\mathbf{A}) && (4.26)\\
&\text{(design equations)} & f_i(\mathbf{A}) &= 0 \quad i = 4, \ldots, m && (4.27)
\end{aligned}$$

here we denote by $\mathbf{A}$ the set of (input) specifications, the topology's design parameters and the technology parameters. The noise requirement, for instance, has been presented in the previous section. Other requirements have not been presented here but are present in the models [Vdbus 95, VdPlas 96b].

These equations have then been used to derive the boundary checking and interval analysis model for 8 different CSA-PSA implementations [Ves 95, Ves 97, VdPlas 01]. The 8 different implementations were obtained as follows: either PMOS or NMOS input transistors for the CSA (i.e. 2 alternatives), each in combination with 4 different orders ($n = 1, \ldots, 4$) for the PSA. Note that in the sizing model the order was a variable (n) and that it has been fixed to an integer value for generating a topology selection model.

The resulting selection order of the topologies depends on the specifications, as shown in figure 4.17. The figure shows in the vertical axis the rank of the 8 topologies from bottom to top as a function of the requirement (performance specifications), on the horizontal axis. The final ranking has been obtained by applying the rule base filter. The rules address topology properties such as complexity, and making a tradeoff between noise and power performance. For the CSA-PSA functionblock approximately 30 rules are included.

It can be observed that the selected topology, the number of rejected topologies and their rank vary significantly with the variation of the input specifications. Furthermore it has been found that each of the 8 used topologies has a region in the performance space in which it is superior to the others [Ves 95, Ves 97, VdPlas 01]. This is explained by the relatively large number of input parameters.

As it turned out, the order of the PSA was easily modifiable into an optimization parameter, so in the library only two different topologies have been included, offering the design quality of the eight topologies modeled in this experiment [Ves 95, Ves 97, VdPlas 01].

4.3.4 Sizing Synthesis: OPTIMAN

The next step in the design flow of the **AMGIE** system is sizing. The corresponding sizing model is retrieved and linked with the **OPTIMAN** tool. After selection of the optimization algorithm (VFSR), the optimization process is started.

For the specifications as listed in Table 4.11, the **OPTIMAN** tool resulted in an input transistor *m1* of the CSA (shown in figure 4.12) with a width of 1623μm and a minimum length of 1.3μm. The predicted power consumption of the core CSA-PSA circuit is only 7mW, which is an improvement by 6 compared to an earlier manual design. The feedback capacitance C_f was optimized to a value of 220fF by the **OPTIMAN** tool, the number of integrators in the PSA (n) was determined by the optimization to be 4. The synthesis resulted in a predicted peaking time (τ_p) of $1.1\mu s$. The complete sizing by the **OPTIMAN** tool takes about 20 minutes on an HP 712/100 workstation. The performance obtained after sizing and verified through simulation is summarized in Table 4.12.

4.3.5 Layout Generation

The CSA-PSA design has been sized and verified. Next the layout has to be generated. The complete schematic of the CSA-PSA is shown in figure 4.18. The LAYLA layout environment [Lam 98, Lam 99] is targeted towards the automated layout generation of OTAs, OPAMPs and general analog circuit. The CSA-PSA circuit does not fall in this category, because of the large number of devices. A *flat* layout solution provided by LAYLA is thus not feasible. However, the building blocks of the CSA-PSA all fall into the targeted application area of LAYLA. Different solutions can be explored to generate the layout with LAYLA. All require hierarchical techniques to build up the final layout, the way in which the process is driven is different amongst the alternatives.

Name	Specified		Synthesis	Unit
Detector capacitance	=	80	80	pF
Noise	<	1000	905	e^-_{rms}
Peaking time	<	1.5	1.1	μs
Counting rate	>	200	294	kSamples/s
Gain	=	20	21	mV/fC
Max. output range	=	2	2	V
Linearity	<	1	0.5	%
Power supply	=	±2.5	±2.5	V
Technology	=	1P2M 0.7μm CMOS		–
Area	MIN	2	–	mm^2
Power consumption	MIN	40	7.2	mW

Table 4.12: Specifications and performance achieved after sizing verification of the synthesized CSA-PSA circuit.

1. a first alternative is to use the LAYLA tools (performance-driven placement and routing) on each building block separately: CSA, R_f, R_{pz} and PSA integrator. The CSA block for example can easily be placed and subsequently routed using the sensitivities of the *CSA* specifications. These were determined during the sizing of the CSA-PSA: for instance the GBW_{ol} or the phase margin, *PM*. This can be done for all subcircuits found in the CSA-PSA. At the CSA-PSA level the subcircuits are placed and routed using the performance degradation on the CSA-PSA specifications.

2. The problem with the previous approach is that the building blocks of the CSA-PSA not necessarily are functionblocks to which specifications can be attributed since no hierarchy was considered during the sizing. In fact only the performance specifications for the entire CSA-PSA circuit can be used to drive the layout process. These have lower bounds on them. To avoid this, the sensitivity of the CSA-PSA specifications to local, subcircuit parasitics can be determined. During the placement and routing of a subcircuit (for instance the CSA), the degradation of the CSA-PSA specifications is then the driving factor. The subcircuit then not necessarily must have specifications associated with it. The drawback of this approach is that the performance specification margin available for a performances, P_j, must be distributed amongst the different subcircuits and the top-level circuit:

$$\Delta \mathrm{P}^{\mathrm{lay}-}_{\mathrm{acc},j} \leq \Delta \mathrm{P}^{lay}_{j} = \Delta \mathrm{P}_{top-level,j} + \sum_{subcircuits} \Delta \mathrm{P}_{subcircuits,j} \leq \Delta \mathrm{P}^{\mathrm{lay}+}_{\mathrm{acc},j} \tag{4.28}$$

Since all subcircuits are separately generated, the available margin for every subcircuit must be limited such that the total degradation, $\Delta \mathrm{P}^{lay}_{j}$, is within the allowed range for every performance specification j. This can be achieved by allocating margins for every specification and subcircuit as is done when allocating allowed net capacitances in the approach of [Chou 90b, Chou 90c]. Since the distribution of margins is not exact, a

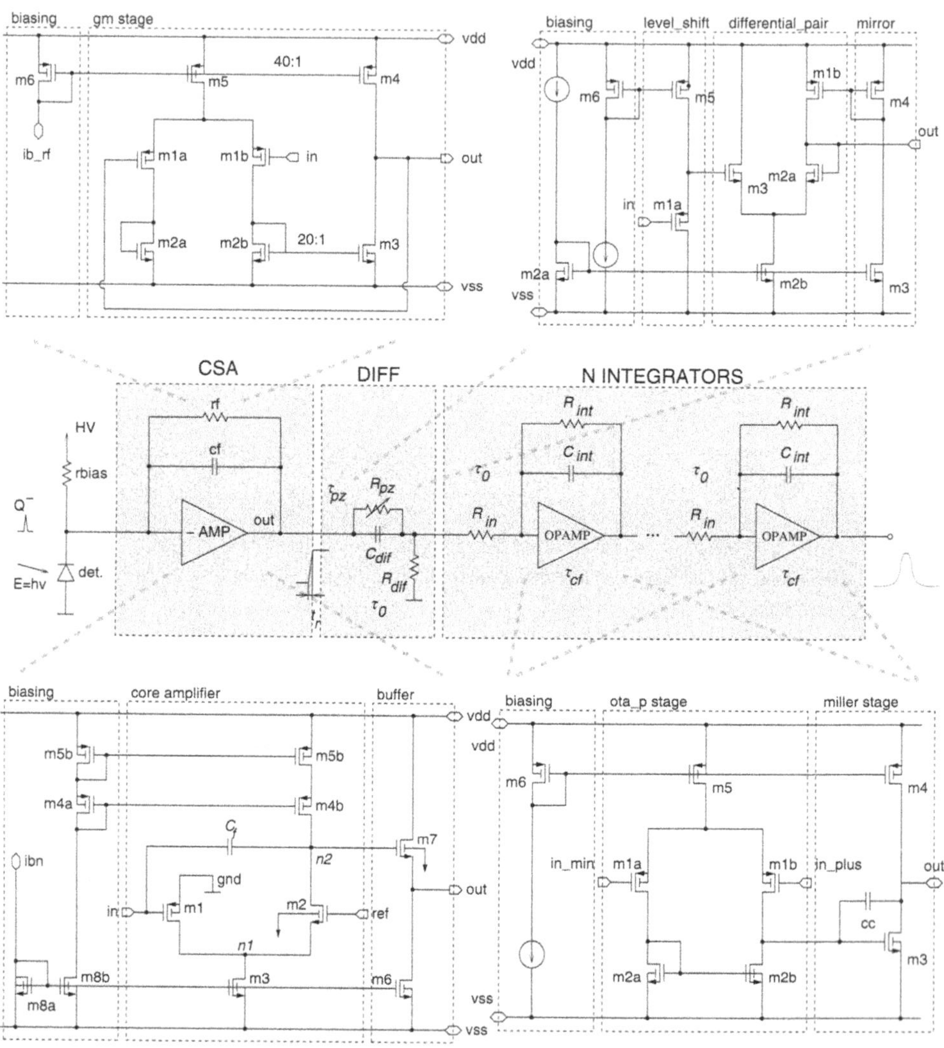

Figure 4.18: Schematic of the charge-sensitive amplifier – pulse-shaping amplifier circuit.

second run with adapted margins might be required to converge to an acceptable layout solution.

3. To solve the problems with the previous approaches, the LAYLA placement tool can be extended to optimize hierarchical circuits. It is possible to simultaneously place all levels of the hierarchy, much as with the sizing and optimization approach used for this design. This approach has however not yet been implemented, but would avoid

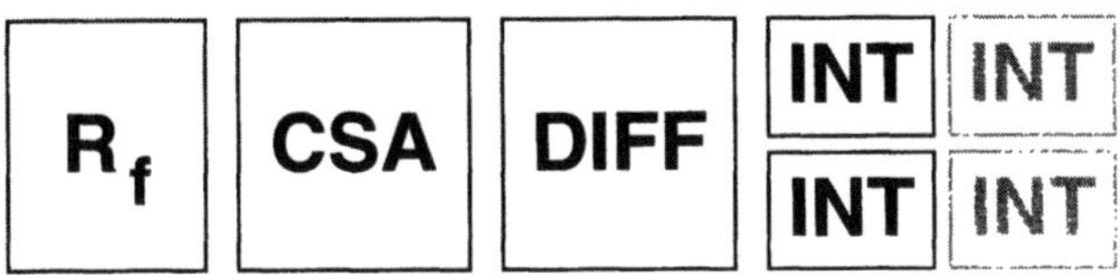

Figure 4.19: Template floorplan for the CSA-PSA topology.

the problems associated with the previous approach: the performance degradations are distributed correctly since all levels are placed simultaneously and subsequently routed.

As already stated, the LAYLA environment currently does not support hierarchical placement and routing in one optimization process (although the implemented methodology does not exclude this approach). Therefore the layout of the CSA-PSA has been generated using approach one. Specifications for the subcircuits have been extracted and their sensitivities calculated [Lam 98, Lam 99].

The CSA-PSA circuit is first decomposed into subcircuits. The CSA and R_f are obvious candidates. They have limited external connectivity and have a specific function (for which specifications can be derived), the PSA differentiator (including R_{pz}) and the integrator (including the Miller opamp) are less obvious blocks. The tunable active resistor or Miller-compensated opamp could have been split off too, but this extra level of hierarchy is not necessary. Hence, four subcircuits need to be placed in the floorplan. Using the area estimates obtained during sizing (sum of individual device areas), a floorplan is created from a template, as shown in figure 4.19. This floorplan has been manually composed. The feedback resistance R_f has been put at the left side. It only interacts with the CSA and thus is not hindering the signal flow to the right. The signal is then processed from left to right. It passes through the differentiator (DIFF) and then an optional number of integrators (INT). On figure 4.19 two integrators are shown, two optional extra integrators have been grayed out.

The layout generation then proceeds as follows:

1. the placements are generated for the four subcircuits.

2. each of the subplacements is routed.

3. the blocks are placed, according to the floorplan. If blocks don't fit, a rerun of placement and routing for a specific block is done with adapted parameters.

4. the top-level layout is routed. Since the router is a general area router and the top-level routing problem is a channel routing problem, manual routing has been preferred[3].

The automated part of the layout generation only took 1 hour of CPU time on a SUN Ultra-1/170 workstation. The complete layout (including top-level routing and DRC, ERC and LVS checks) generation took approximately one day.

[3]J. Vandenbussche and the author did the manual top-level routing.

4.3.6 Verification

After sizing and optimization the CSA-PSA circuit has been verified using numerical simulation. First a nominal verification has been run. The circuit performed well and next a Monte-Carlo simulation has been run to check if the circuit would also function given the unavoidable spread of technology parameters. All samples (40) of the Monte-Carlo run worked, indicating that the parametric yield would be high.

After layout generation the circuit was once again verified: Design rule check (DRC), electrical rule check (ERC) and layout versus schematic (LVS) checks have been run. The circuit passed all these checks successfully. Then the circuit was extracted including parasitics (resistance and capacitance) to be verified with numerical simulation at the device level. Only a nominal verification was run. The circuit functioned once more within spec.

4.3.7 Measurement Results

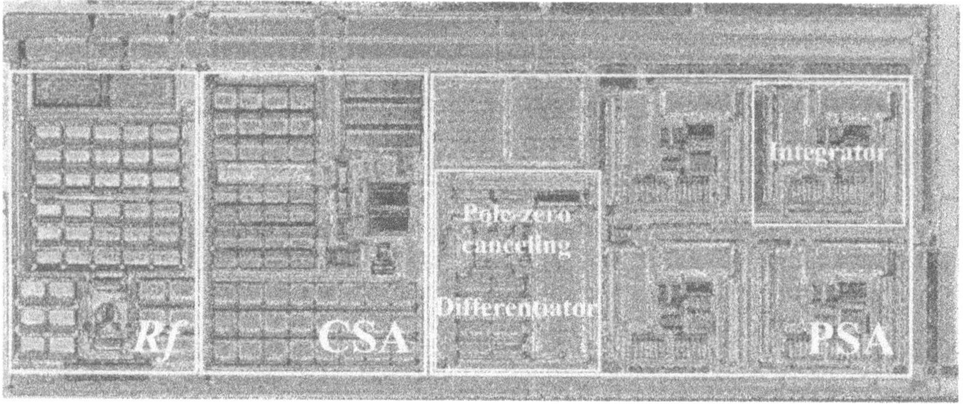

Figure 4.20: Microphotograph of the charge-sensitive amplifier – pulse-shaping amplifier prototype chip.

A microphotograph of the fabricated prototype chip is shown in figure 4.20. The CSA-PSA was processed in a 1P2M 0.7μm CMOS process. The chip was packaged (in a standard ceramic package) and measured. In figure 4.21 the measured time response at the output of the CSA (dashed line) and the CSA-PSA (full line) is shown to an incident particle of 100fC.

The measurement results are summarized in Table 4.13. All specifications have been met or have been exceeded. Furthermore this result was obtained with first silicon. No redesign runs were required. These redesign runs are not unusual when doing analog designs, especially when a new, unknown functionblock is attempted. This success is partly explained by the systematic approach in the design procedure, and partly by the thorough verification that was carried out on the design before fabrication.

The obtained synthesis results are also compared to a previous manual design (in the same technology) in Table 4.13. What is important to note is that the synthesized design outperforms

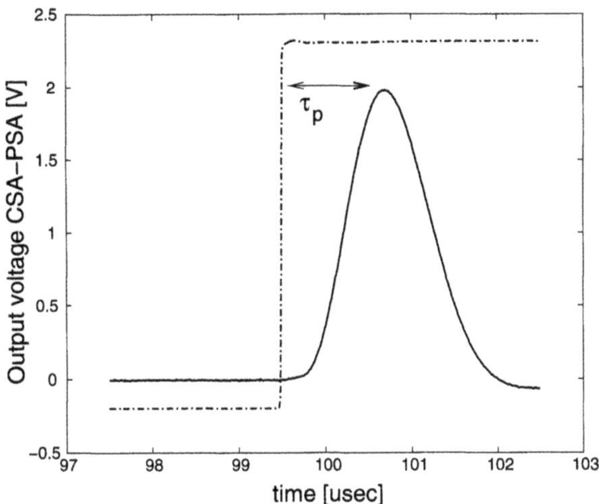

Figure 4.21: Peaking time measurement of the prototype chip: time response to an incident particle with a charge of 100fC.

the manual design in speed, while almost equal noise performance is obtained. Furthermore the synthesized design consumes four times less power in the same technology. It turned out that the manual design was not aggressively optimized with respect to power: standard OPAMP library cells were used instead of custom designed ones. Nevertheless the design time was *not* shorter. The less systematic design process used in the manual design explains why a lot of time was lost in understanding the circuit at the architectural level. No time was left to optimize the complete structure with inclusion of the OPAMPs. The systematic approach used for synthesis requires the designer only to assemble all knowledge in the declarative model. The optimizer then takes over to find the optimal design point.

4.3.8 Conclusions

A fully integrated, low-power CMOS particle detector front-end, optimized for space applications, has been implemented [Vdbus 98c]. Using the **AMGIE** tool the chip has been optimally designed from specification to layout [VdPlas 01]. A breakdown of the setup time is as follows: setting up the sizing model (and the derived topology selection models) took approximately 3 months, setting up the layout generation took 1 day, setting up verification 1 week. Generating a circuit using this topology then takes approximately two days: the optimization run takes 20 minutes, layout generation 1 day, verification takes also 1 day on a SUN Ultra-1/170 workstation.

The chip was processed in a standard 1P2M 0.7μm CMOS process. All performance specifications have been verified through measurements: all values are within spec. With a power consumption of only 10mW (including biasing) and a chip area of 0.6mm^2, the chip compares favorably with a previous manual design and is very well suited for space applications (small volume and weight due to integration and a low power consumption).

Name	Specified		Manual	Synthesis	Unit
Detector capacitance	=	80	80	80	pF
Noise	<	1000	905	952	e^-_{rms}
Peaking time	<	1.5	1.1	1.18	μs
Counting rate	>	200	200	300	kSamples/s
Gain	=	20	20	19	mV/fC
Max. output range	=	2	2	2	V
Linearity	<	1	–	0.5	%
Power supply	=	±2.5	±2.5	±2.5	V
Technology	=	1P2M 0.7μm CMOS			–
Area	MIN	2	0.7	0.6	mm^2
Power consumption	MIN	40	40	10	mW

Table 4.13: Measured performance of the synthesized CSA-PSA prototype chip and a previous manual design.

4.4 Summary

In this chapter, three synthesis examples have been presented that demonstrate the capabilities of the **AMGIE** analog synthesis system. The first example compared three approaches for the sizing synthesis of an OTA circuit: a *manual designer's* approach, a *simulation-based optimization* approach and an *equation-based optimization* approach. The *equation-based* approach implemented in the **AMGIE** system proves to be a valid candidate when the high setup time can be written off over many design runs, since it has the lowest run-time of the three approaches; or, in other words the approach is optimal when a high reuse factor for the circuit is to be expected.

The second example was a true test of how capable the **AMGIE** system is in supporting novice or inexperienced designers. A classroom student exercise session was set up to test the system. The EE Master students divided into 9 groups of 3 persons each, had to design the OTA circuit for a set of performance specification values. The time was limited to 2 and a half hours and despite the inexperience of the designers both in designing circuits and in using the **AMGIE** system, the experiment proved successful: all groups managed to design a functional circuit within the alloted time. Some of the groups even experimented with the system to investigate alternative solutions in the time allocated to the session.

In the third example the design of a charge-sensitive amplifier – pulse-shaping amplifier (CSA-PSA) circuit has been undertaken with the **AMGIE** system. The complexity of this circuit is at the limit of what the **AMGIE** system can handle: approximately 100 devices. Using different hierarchical techniques (as presented in previous chapters) the design of this circuit has been automated. A total setup time of less than 4 months has been achieved, and a synthesis run of this topology takes approximately 2 days. An actual prototype has been fabricated and measured. The resulting device did not only perform within specifications but its power consumption was almost four times lower than a previous manual design with the same performance.

Conclusions

In this first part of the dissertation, the research results on *synthesis of analog integrated circuits* have been discussed. In the first chapter the terminology has been defined that is used in this research area (analog circuit, functionblock, behavioral parameters, behavioral model, functional decomposition, structural decomposition, geometrical decomposition, etc.) culminating in a definition for analog synthesis: **Analog synthesis** *is the process of designing analog circuits from behavioral specification to mask layout, using functional, structural or geometrical decomposition when required, in an automated or semi-automated way.*

Next an overview was given of the research results and current state of the art in analog synthesis. Three generations have been identified. The early work (early and late eighties) primarily relied on using digital algorithms and tailoring them for application to the analog synthesis problem. The use of procedural and artificial intelligence (reasoning) techniques for sizing has been explored in this first generation. The second generation replaced these procedural and artificial intelligence approaches by optimization-based approaches, which proved to be much easier (an order of magnitude) to set up. Performance-driven design methodologies emerged to handle analog constraints more efficiently. The most recent generation of analog synthesis tools continues this trend: optimization-based techniques have de facto been accepted, only the formulation of the problems is still an issue. For sizing synthesis equation-based and simulation-based approaches still compete; for layout synthesis the representation (slicing structure, absolute placement, sequence pairs, etc.) of the intermediate layout solution and the handling of analog constraints (indirect or direct performance-driven) is being explored. A number of representative tools have been discussed, and their advantages and disadvantages have been summarized.

The first chapter then introduced the **AMGIE** analog synthesis system. It is our contribution to the research in the analog synthesis field. It aimed to overcome the major limitations of the earlier tools: it is an *integrated environment*, that covers the *complete design flow* from specification down to layout. It implements a top-down, bottom-up, direct performance-driven design methodology. Complex circuits are decomposed using a functional abstraction. The system uses two libraries: a cell library containing topologies and a technology library containing all relevant technology parameters. The **AMGIE** synthesis system has a modular software structure, defines clear interfaces for design data and design management and can more easily be extended than its predecessors. The objective of the **AMGIE** synthesis system is to automate the design of analog circuits for both novice and experienced designers and in this way increase overall analog design productivity.

In the second chapter the implementation of the **AMGIE** synthesis system has been described in detail. The chapter started with a further refinement of the performance specifications and hierarchy concepts. The *functional hierarchy* that is central in **AMGIE** can be refined by using both structural and geometrical hierarchies when required for a certain topology. It must be noted however that the *specifications* are only available for the functionblock nodes in this hierarchical decomposition. The *specification margins* that are used to drive the different subtools of the **AMGIE** synthesis system have been defined. Then the five subtools (Topology Selection, Sizing & Optimization, Layout Generation, Verification, Redesign Wizard) of the **AMGIE** synthesis system and the algorithms and techniques that were implemented, have been discussed.

The topology selection (TS) tool selects amongst the candidate topologies in the **AMGIE** cell library those candidates that are most suited to achieve the requested specifications. This selection procedure is implemented using three filters that are applied consecutively to the list of all topologies: *boundary checking, interval analysis* and *rule-based ranking*. The first two filters eliminate candidates from the list and do a preliminary sorting. The last filter sorts the remaining candidates into a final list which is returned to the user. The user then has the ability to overrule the selection proposed by the tool or to accept it.

Then the sizing and optimization (S&O) tool was discussed. The approach implemented in the **AMGIE** synthesis system is *improved equation-based circuit optimization*. The approach is supported by the extensive use of off-line/setup tools (ISAAC, SYMBA, DONALD) that speed up the sizing plan generation, typically considered a cumbersome task. The use of the operating-point-driven formulation of these design plans ensures low run-times during synthesis: the time-consuming DC solving of SPICE-like evaluation plans is avoided. By using encapsulated device models full SPICE accuracy is obtained, as far as the small-signal parameters (gm, Cgs, ...) is concerned. Technology independence is further realized through the use of extensive modeling: mismatch of devices is modeled with appropriate models, area of active devices as for instance MOS transistors is accurately modeled, etc., and technology-independent sizing variables ($logW$ and $logL$ for MOS transistors) are used. When subblocks are included in the circuit under design, power and area estimators for functionblocks are used to determine their performance specifications. The setup of the cost function has been discussed; depending on the optimization algorithm that is selected by the user, the constraints are added to the scalar cost function (VFSR) or directly handled by the optimization algorithm (SQP). The actual optimization tool (**OPTIMAN**) has a graphical interface informing the user of the optimization run's progress. A practical example shows how a trade-off curve (area–power) can be obtained with the tool.

The layout generation tool (LT) creates a mask-level layout from the sized schematic. In the **AMGIE** analog synthesis system this task is performed by the LAYLA tools [Lam 99]. LAYLA is a *direct performance-driven macro-cell place and route* tool. The layout generation is performed in two steps: device placement, followed by routing. By using sensitivity information, the degradation of performance specifications directly drives the layout generation process. All typical analog layout constraints are supported: symmetry, matching, device merging, wire sizing, etc.

The cell under design is verified after sizing and optimization as well as after layout extraction. A fully automated verification tool (VT) has been implemented. It uses *black box* verification. Templates stored with the functionblock apply test harnesses and specify simulation analysis modes; templates stored with the topology apply biasing and clocking signals. Statistical verification for mismatch is provided with MMPRE or MIMI. Technology variations and operating ranges of temperature and power supply are verified using corner analysis. A datasheet is returned and stored in the run-time database for inspection by the user.

If design errors occur, that are either detected by the design tools themselves (for instance topology selection did not find any suitable topology for the requested specifications) or are detected by the verification tool (for instance after extraction the phase margin drops below the requested value), the redesign wizard proposes to the novice designer a set of corrective procedures. These corrective actions require the intervention of the user to go back to the design and redo some of the design steps (for instance relaxing the specifications or increasing the margin that the layout tool has for phase margin) and then the design can be restarted.

Illustrative and representative examples have been added throughout the text to more clearly demonstrate the implemented algorithms and techniques. In the third chapter, three synthesis examples have been presented that show the capabilities of the **AMGIE** system.

The first example compared three different approaches for the sizing synthesis of a typical OTA circuit: a *manual designer's* approach, a *simulation-based optimization* approach and an *equation-based optimization* approach. The *equation-based* approach implemented in the **AMGIE** analog synthesis system proves to be a valid candidate when the high setup time can be written off over many design runs, since it has the lowest run-time of the three approaches; or in other words the approach is optimal when a high reuse factor for the circuit is to be expected. One of the most important objections against the *equation-based* approach (its low accuracy and poor design quality), has been overcome by incorporating encapsulated device models (SPICE-accuracy) and deriving high-quality equations for small-signal and large-signal performance specifications in a systematic way with supporting tools.

The second example was a true test of how capable the **AMGIE** system is in supporting novice or inexperienced designers. A classroom student exercise session was set up to test the system. The EE Master students divided into 9 groups of 3 persons each, had to design the OTA circuit for a set of performance specification values. The time was limited to 2 and a half hours (one session) and despite the inexperience of the designers both in designing circuits and in using the **AMGIE** system, the experiment proved successful: all groups managed to design a functional circuit. Some of the groups could even experiment with the system in the time allocated to investigate alternative solutions.

In the third example the design of a charge-sensitive amplifier – pulse-shaping amplifier (CSA-PSA) circuit for space applications has been undertaken with the **AMGIE** system. The complexity of this circuit is at the limit of what the **AMGIE** system can handle: approximately 100 devices. Using different hierarchical techniques the design of this circuit has been automated. A setup time of less than 4 months has been achieved, a design run of this topology then takes approximately 2 days. An actual prototype has been manufactured and measured. The resulting design did not only perform within specifications, but its power consumption was almost four times lower than a previous manual design with the same performance.

The **AMGIE** analog synthesis system is not the work of one person. In total approximately 15 people have contributed to the system. It was the largest software system I have been involved in as a system's integrator and point tool developer. I have been able to acquire a lot of software development skills during this project (structured design, version management, documentation, testing, release management, etc.).

In conclusion, a summary of features of the **AMGIE** system and the most valuable experimental results, is provided here:

- **AMGIE** is an integrated analog synthesis system;
- it automates the design from specifications down to layout;
- it uses a performance-driven top-down, bottom-up, hierarchical design methodology;
- it uses two libraries: a cell library and a technology library;
- it has a modular software structure;
- it supports different types of users: (1) inexperienced or novice designers and (2) expert users or library developers;
- it provides design and data management;
- it offers multiple hierarchical views;
- five subtools automate the different steps in the design process;
- the topology selection tool (TS) selects and ranks candidate topologies using three filters;
- the sizing and optimization tool (S&O) optimizes the selected topology using local and global optimization algorithms towards the given specifications and in the specified technology process;
- it offers an environment for the derivation of the sizing plan;
- layout generation has been automated using the LAYLA tools [Lam 99] that implement a direct performance-driven macro-cell place & route methodology;
- a fully automated verification tool (VT) verifies the circuit after sizing and optimization as well as after layout extraction;
- a redesign wizard helps novice designers to resolve design failures;
- a comparison between (modified) equation-based and simulation-based approaches (for a typical OTA) favors the first when a high reuse factor of the analog circuit topology is expected;
- inexperienced designers can successfully design OTA-type circuits in less than 2 and a half hours using the **AMGIE** system;
- **AMGIE** can handle complex circuits with approximately 100 devices with high design quality while reducing design time considerably;

This concludes part I of this work. In the next part, the research results in the area of *systematic design* of analog circuits will be presented.

Part II

Systematic Design of Analog Circuits

Introduction

In the first part of this work the **AMGIE** analog synthesis system has been described. Experimental results have proven that considerable design time reductions can be obtained by automating the design of analog integrated circuits. The degree of automation is high enough to even allow novice or unexperienced designers to quickly design high-quality analog circuits. However, it must be noted that the successfulness or scope of the **AMGIE** system is limited by its design methodology and point tool algorithms, and by the contents of its library. A high-quality library can cover a large range of the available analog design space. But now and then the current known analog circuit techniques do not suffice. At this point *analog design creativity* (modeling, new schematics, layout techniques, ...) is required to obtain the desired result: a *high-performance* cutting-edge analog design. High performance here not only expresses that a good trade-off in terms of speed–power–accuracy (i.e. extremely high-speed, high-accuracy or all combined) has to be achieved, but also expresses an attribute of the design process itself: the designer has access to the best available design methodology and tools.

The power of the performance-driven top-down, bottom-up design methodology has proven that it delivers high-quality designs. However, the design cannot be automated since a creative contribution of the designer is involved. In addition, for certain circuits, the reuse factor is not high enough to justify the initial model development (analytic equations, sizing plan, etc.) needed for automatic circuit synthesis. In such conditions, tools and methodologies can still be used to support the designer. But an automated integrated synthesis system is not the solution. An experienced designer prefers a set of independent or loosely coupled point tools. These point tools are good at specific tasks in the design process: preferably they give full control over the result to the designer and automate especially the tedious part of the job. A complete set of these tools allows the designer to concentrate on the creative aspect of the design. These point tools have to fit in the design strategy of high-performance analog design. What design methodology can be used ? The top-down, bottom-up, performance-driven design methodology of the **AMGIE** system relies heavily on the use of stored knowledge to automate the design completely and has a fixed design flow. This specific design strategy belongs to the more general category of *systematic design* methodologies. Instead of using **AMGIE**'s *strict design flow* (which is required for automation), the principle of *systematic design* is adopted.

A systematic design methodology requires a rigid design scheme at another level; every design decision/choice needs to be carefully considered: is it appropriate to decide now ? How does the decision influence the behavior and performance of the circuit ? How can this design parameter be linked with one or more performance parameters ? How can these decisions be verified ? etc. Applying a systematic design methodology makes it possible to trace design decisions, to redo the design in another (compatible) technology, debug eventual problems, etc. The definition of systematic design can be formulated as follows: **systematic (analog) design** is the process of designing analog circuits whereby *quantitatively* or *qualitatively* the *design parameters/decisions* (architecture selection/creation, sizing, layout, etc.) are determined/calculated by the *performance specifications* of the requested functionblock in a *traceable*, *explainable* and *verifiable* way.

In the remainder of this dissertation, the research results in the area of *systematic analog design* will be reported. In the following chapter, **Mondriaan** will be presented. **Mondriaan** is an analog layout tool that is complementary to the LAYLA tool [Lam 99]. **Mondriaan** is targeted towards the automatic layout generation of highly regular analog blocks frequently found in analog modules such as A/D-converters, D/A-converters, etc. In the second chapter of this part the systematic design of high-accuracy, current-steering D/A-converters will be discussed. It is a typical application of the systematic design methodology proposed in this text. The resulting design has been fabricated and measured to prove the effectiveness of the design methodology. This work resulted in the first 14-bit intrinsically linear CMOS D/A-converter that does not require tuning or trimming.

Chapter 5

Mondriaan: a Layout Synthesis Methodology for Array-type Analog Blocks

The automation of the physical design task for analog circuits has received a lot of academic research attention. Some of these research results, such as parameterized device generators, are now standard components in commercial EDA frameworks. More complex device generators, that for instance are capable of generating pairs of devices in an inter-digitated form, have been reported in [Rijm 89, Bru 96]. In [Rijm 89, Chou 90a, Cohn 91, Felt 93, Mey 93, Char 94a, Char 94b, Lam 95, Lam 96a, Bru 96, Lam 98, Lam 99] layout environments have been presented that place and route device-level analog circuits following the macro-cell place & route methodology, possibly with a constraint-driven or performance-driven approach [Chou 90a, Cohn 91, Felt 93, Char 94a, Char 94b, Lam 95, Lam 96a, Lam 98, Lam 99]. With these tools layouts of circuit-level blocks such as OPAMPs, OTAs, comparators, etc. can be successfully created. One important class of (analog) layout generation tasks, however, has received less attention. In analog blocks, very often highly regular modules of basic cells are used. Examples of these circuits are flash-type or folding/interpolating A/D-converters [vdPlassche 94], current-steering D/A-converters [vdPlassche 94] or Cellular Neural Networks (CNN) [Chua 93, King 95]. This chapter addresses the layout generation for these regular array-type analog circuits.

Two methods for generating such array-types of (analog) layouts have been used by designers up till now:

1. The layouts are drawn manually. Hierarchy is employed to exploit as much as possible the regularity of the array. For instance, if a number of columns is identical, only one column is drawn and the resulting column cell is instantiated the requested number of times. Connections to neighbors and distribution of power and biasing are in this approach usually realized through abutment of cells. Often, however, some of the cells are special (a reference, a dummy, etc.). These special cases or exceptions to the regular structure destroy the gracefulness of the manual hierarchical cell/instantiation approach. One ends up with more levels of cell/instantiation hierarchy and exceptions than can be over seen. There is little or no reuse possible in this manual layout methodology, except

for copying the result to a new design in its entirety; even a minor change in the basic cells often requires a complete rework, which is a tedious and error-prone job.

2. In [Neff 95, Chang 95b, Neff 96] the synthesis of a specific architecture (row–column architecture) of current-steering D/A-converters has been automated, including the layout generation. The layout is generated from a predefined library template by stretching and tiling a number of basic cell templates [Neff 95, Neff 96]. These templates consist of basic circuit cells on the one hand and pure connectivity cells on the other hand. The stretching of the cells allows tuning of the parameters of the basic cells (wire widths, widths and lengths of MOS transistors, ...) without having to lay them out manually. This approach requires extensive preparation of the basic cell templates such that they can be stretched and that the connections remain correct by abutment for widely varying parameter values. Furthermore the complete architecture needs to be mapped on an irregular cell array (basic circuit cells and pure connectivity cells) which is completely connected through abutment. Although this approach fully automates the layout generation for this particular type of converter, the flexibility and ease of use of the method are severely limited. The creation of the mask-level basic cell templates is not straightforward. Applying this layout approach to other analog circuits is a highly complex task: the library developer needs to come up with a suitable set of mask-level stretchable basic cell templates. No help is provided for this task. The major problem of this approach is thus that the setup of the basic cell template library is extremely difficult. A change of the technology process requires a redesign of the basic cells, which is once again a highly complex and time-consuming job.

In this section a methodology will be presented that offers full flexibility for the layout generation of regular array-types of analog circuit modules. The approach has a small setup time due to the higher abstraction level the layout designer is offered. The goals of the presented layout methodology are: (1) improve designer's productivity, (2) reduce the chance of errors through automation of tedious, repetitive tasks, and (3) provide reusability of layouts. Real-life examples will show a considerable reduction in design time, without sacrificing the design quality. Even more, the methodology allows designers to attempt previously infeasible layout solutions that are capable to push technology limitations. This will be illustrated by the design of a 14-bit current-steering D/A-converter in the next chapter. We believe that these goals have been achieved by combining the following components: a *flexible layout model* and a *layout synthesis methodology*. The presented approach raises the level of abstraction of the analog layout generation process. Instead of pushing polygons at the mask level, the designer inputs the most important and creative part of the mask layout (the position of the cells and how they will be interconnected) at the symbolic level. The back-end part (polygon, mask-level) of the methodology has been fully automated utilizing a tool called **Mondriaan** [1]. Similar techniques have been applied in digital blocks (especially datapaths, ROMs, PLAs, ...) since the early eighties [Joh 79, Cla 80, MeCo 80, Rijnd 88, Rab 96]. This approach has in this work been tailored to generate the layout of high-performance analog blocks.

This chapter is organized as follows. In section 5.1 the scope and the requirements of our new layout methodology will be specified. In section 5.2 the layout model will be discussed,

[1] a Dutch painter of the 20th century famous for his "array-type" paintings [Mont 97]

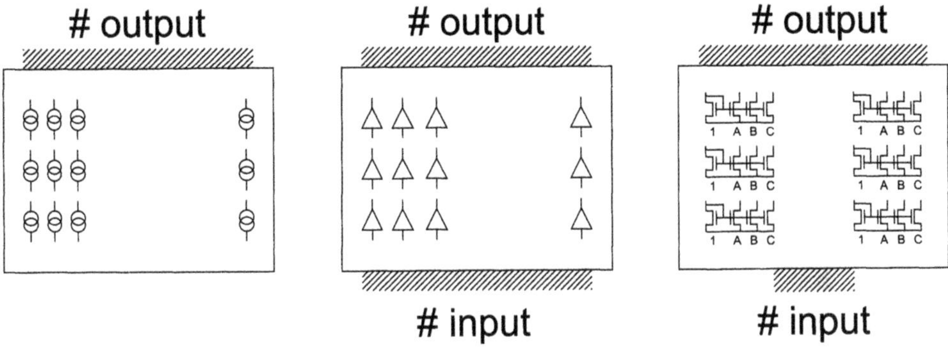

Figure 5.1: Three analog array types: signal generation (current-source array that generates n equal currents), signal processing (n amplification stages, found in flash-type A/D-converters) and signal multiplication and processing (current mirrors, used in interpolation circuits).

i.e. what kind of arrays/connections are modeled in the presented layout methodology. The methodology itself will be explained in detail in section 5.3. It consists of a three-step procedure: (1) floorplanning, (2) symbolic routing, and (3) technology mapping, of which the last two steps are automated in the generic layout tool **Mondriaan** [VdPlas 98]. An illustrative example will in detail discuss the application of the methodology to a (simplified) design example (section 5.4). Experimental results of industrial-strength designs will be presented in section 5.5. Conclusions are formulated in section 5.6.

5.1 Requirements of the New Layout Generation Methodology

The targeted array-like analog layout structures, typically consist of an array of unit cells (potentially with slightly different cell variants). These modules process in a parallel way one or more input signals and steer one or more output signals. Three possibilities are shown in figure 5.1, each represented by a typical example: parallel signal generation (for instance a current-source array that generates n equal currents, found in current-steering D/A-converters), parallel signal processing (for instance amplification of n signals, found in flash-type A/D-converters), and signal multiplication and processing (for instance current mirroring used in interpolation circuits for A/D-converters). This basic layout problem is addressed by the presented methodology.

What requirements should the methodology fulfill ? The degree of automation should be as high as possible, but it should not negatively impact the quality of the result. Not only the run time should be reduced, the setup time should also be as low as possible to improve the ease of use and flexibility. The natural implementation of this circuit type — a regular array of cells — should be the starting point: it makes no sense to implement a circuit that is highly regular on an arbitrarily placed layout structure. The basic cells are

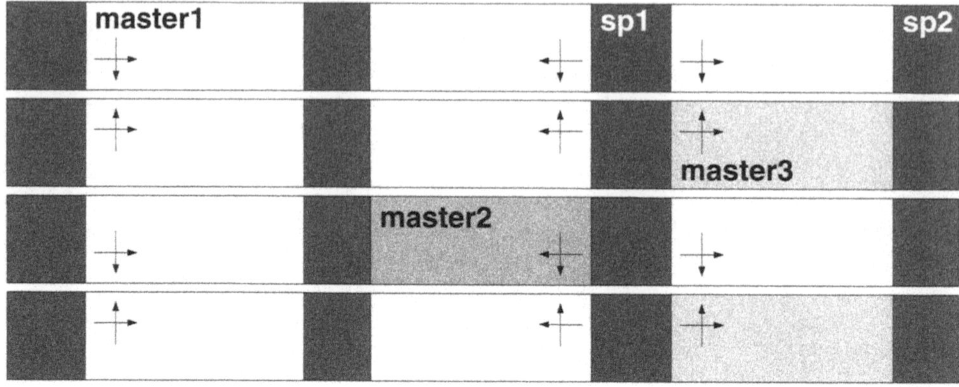

Figure 5.2: Cell array model implemented in the **Mondriaan** tool.

typically small and can either be laid out manually, or by using device-level layout automation [Rijm 89, Cohn 91, Mey 93, Lam 95, Lam 96a, Bru 96, Lam 98, Lam 99], or by using the template stretch approach of [Neff 96, DeRant 00, Vanco 01]. The methodology should support frequently used (analog) layout tricks [MeCo 80, Hast 01]: abutment of array-wide (global) connections, flipping techniques to share signals among neighboring cells, etc. On the other hand, individual connections could be made through abutment; but other ways of making these connections should be provided as well.

All these requirements have led to the layout model which is presented next. The layout model alone does not constitute a working solution. In section 5.3 it will be presented how a regular circuit is mapped efficiently on the layout model using the automatic **Mondriaan** tool.

5.2 Description of the Layout Model

In figure 5.2 the cell array layout model is shown that is used to generate the targeted regular array-type blocks. The basis is a cell array as shown in figure 5.2. A different cell variant (a reference cell, a dummy, ...) can be inserted at any position, as shown in figure 5.2 by the differently shaded individual master cells (**master1, master2, master3**). This overcomes one of the drawbacks of the abovementioned manual hierarchical layout method.

Master cells in the array can be flipped sideways every next column or upside-down every next row or both at the same time (the latter is shown in figure 5.2). These flipping techniques are well-known (analog) layout tricks, used to share lines between neighboring cells [MeCo 80, Hast 01]. In addition, spacer cells can optionally be inserted every next column to improve the array's connectivity. There is one cell for the odd columns (called **sp1**), another for the even columns (called **sp2**), as shown in figure 5.2.

Two types of connections are distinguished: *array-wide* connections and *individual* connections. Array-wide connections are signals that are connected to every cell in the array, such as power, biasing and ground connections. The individual connections connect only to individ-

Figure 5.3: Using spacer cells to extract array-wide connections; the spacer cell is required to realize the asymmetric contacts as shown in the **sp2** cell on the left.

ual cells of the array. Array-wide connections are realized through abutment and feedthroughs in the cells and through spacer cells. The connectivity in the spacer cells used in figure 5.3 cannot be done as part of the master cells (using feedthroughs or abutment), since the contents of the spacer cells are asymmetric (due to the contacts). Individual connections (in and out of the array or internal to the array) are realized through bus and channel routing. As shown in figure 5.4 vertical bus routing channels that cross the cells have been added to the array layout model, and horizontal routing channels have been added in between the cells. Not shown in the figure but also possible are horizontal channels across the cells in designer-specified safe routing regions.

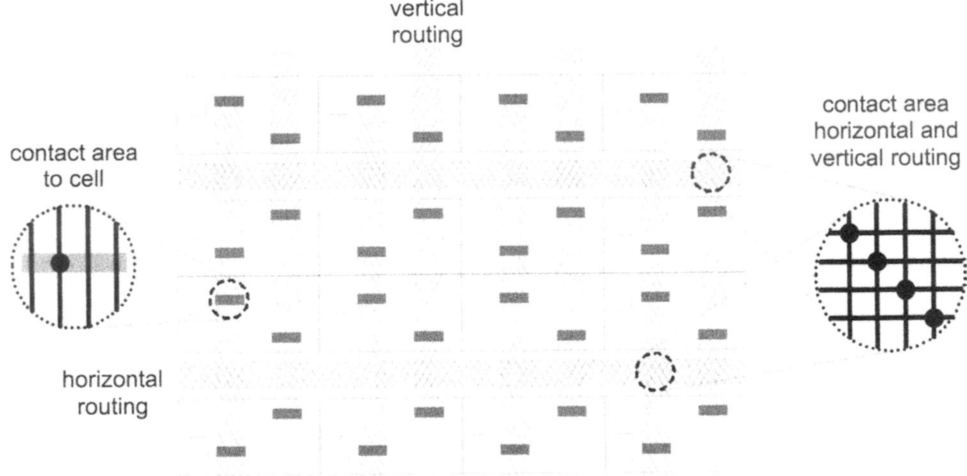

Figure 5.4: Symbolic view of cells and routing channels: *vertical* routing across cells, *horizontal* routing in between cells. Vertical wires connect to the contact areas in the cell, horizontal wires connect to the vertical wires.

Buses in the vertical direction are used to connect wires to the cells; channels in the horizontal direction are used to connect vertical wires with each other. The basic cells contain *contact areas* underneath the vertical bus routing channels. In these areas a connection between the bus and the underlying cell can be made, as shown in figure 5.5, which depicts a

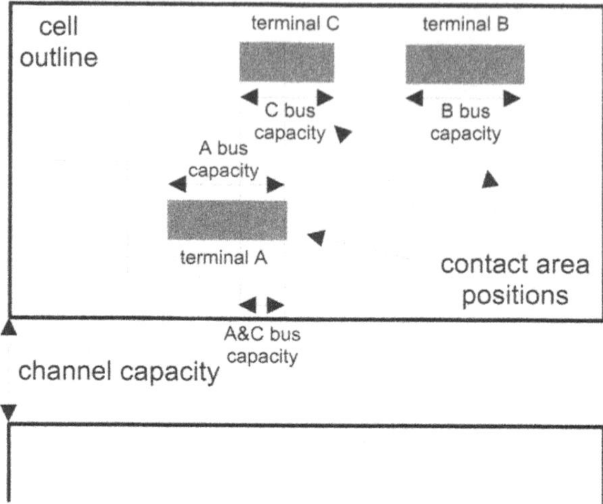

Figure 5.5: Cell outline: cell extent, contact areas and routing channel.

symbolic model of the cell: the *cell outline*. A cell can have multiple user-defined contact areas, which are areas where a connection can be made to a cell. All contact areas in the cells have a *bus capacity*: the number of tracks on a symbolic layer that can pass and connect to the contact area. Sometimes contact areas partly or completely overlap, as is illustrated for contact area **A** and **C** in figure 5.5. In such cases, a bus capacity of the overlap area is defined, this overlap can be used to make connections between different contact areas of different cells. The total *bus capacity* of one column of the cell array is thus defined as:

$$\begin{aligned} column\_capacity = & \sum_{contact\_areas} bus\_capacity_{contact\_areas} \\ & - \sum_{overlapping\_areas} (overlapping\_areas - 1) \times bus\_capacity_{overlapping\_areas} \end{aligned} \tag{5.1}$$

This determines the number of vertical tracks that are available for routing in every column of the array.

The *horizontal channel capacity* is either limited by the space in between the cell rows, or is limited by the channel area allowed by the cell designer across the cell. This capacity determines the number of tracks available for routing horizontally in every row of the array.

The array-generation functionality offered by the above layout model is much more flexible (low setup times, easy to modify or adapt, ...) and is situated at a higher abstraction level than the mask-level stretch and tile approach [Neff 95, Neff 96] described earlier. It covers the requirements of a large variety of analog circuits as will be shown by the examples. This layout model has been combined with a three-step layout generation methodology that utilizes an automated tool called **Mondriaan** [VdPlas 98] for two of the three steps. This methodology is described in the next section.

5.3 Description of the Layout Generation Methodology

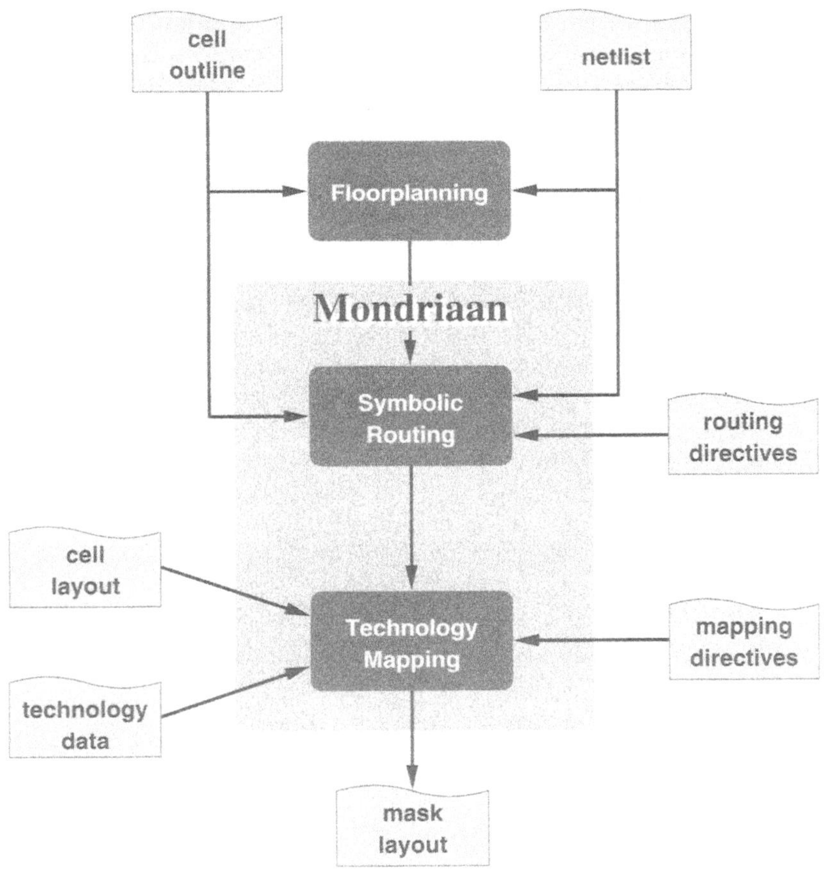

Figure 5.6: Layout generation flow.

Given the presented layout model, the layout generation methodology transforms a module's schematic into a mask layout. The flow chart of the presented methodology is shown in figure 5.6 and consists of three phases: *floorplanning*, *symbolic routing* and *technology mapping*. Although these terms are also used in the digital standard cell place and route methodology, they do not completely express the same concepts here. The targeted modules are analog and the level of control/predictability on the final mask-level layout result must be much higher than what is typically found in standard cell place and route tools. In the presented approach the floorplanning phase represents the generation of a floorplan that comprises all necessary data required to correctly generate a fully placed and routed cell array automatically. What exactly is expressed in the floorplan and how it can be determined will be explained in section 5.3.1. The symbolic routing phase then solves the routing problem given the floorplan, the basic cell outline, the netlist (connectivity information) and the routing directives. In this phase it is determined symbolically in which tracks wires will be created and where connections will be made through contacts. This will be explained in section 5.3.2. The actual mask layout generation in a specified technology process is done in the technology mapping phase described in section 5.3.3. It must be noted that the first phase of the flow, floorplanning, is a *problem-specific* phase that has to be executed by the designer. The second and third phase, however, are *generic* and have been automated in a tool called **Mondriaan** [VdPlas 98]. Please note that the fact that the floorplanning phase has not been included in the generic tool does not preclude automation of the complete process. Full automation of the process can still be achieved, as will be shown in the illustrative example and experimental results sections: it only requires (small) problem-specific programs to be developed; no *generic* solution is possible at this stage unlike for the other two stages.

5.3.1 Floorplanning

During floorplanning cell and pin assignment is performed. In **Mondriaan** a floorplan consists of the following information:

1. cell assignment
   - array dimensions
   - position of every cell in the array
   - flip every next row and/or column of the array; insert spacer cells
2. pin assignment
   - side of the array
   - pin sequence
   - pin grid

The designer determines the position of all cells in the array depending on the specific circuit that has to be laid out and its requirements. He also specifies if the flipping techniques and/or spacer cells are to be used. This is essentially an analog requirement: the placement of the cells is extremely important. It is often optimized (as will be shown in the examples and in the next chapter for a 14-bit D/A-converter) for a specific application and this knowledge must therefore come from the designer. The second part of the floorplan is the pin assignment. This pin assignment information consists of different fields. First of all, the side of the array has to be specified: North, South, East or West. Secondly, the sequence of the pins has to be provided. Together with the pin grid this completely determines the position of the pins. The pin grid is defined as follows: use i tracks of bus **A**, $i \leq bus\_capacity_A$. If i is smaller than the bus capacity, then also the tracks have to be selected, for example: $bus\_capacity_A = 4$, $i = 2$, $tracks = \{1, 3\}$.

At this symbolic level, the designer can easily automate this task using general programming languages (like e.g. C, C++, etc.) or common scripting languages (like e.g. Matlab,

Perl, Python, etc.). However since the floorplanning phase is problem specific, a program will have to be developed by the designer for every specific type of circuit. This will be explained in more detail when some concrete floorplans are generated in the illustrative example and experimental results sections.

5.3.2 Symbolic Routing

The input to the symbolic routing phase is (see figure 5.6):

1. cell outline (including bus capacities of all contact areas)
2. floorplan of the array (cell and pin assignment, cell flipping directives, ...)
3. netlist of the array (connections between contact areas & pins)
4. routing directives

The cell outline and floorplan have already been defined above, in the layout model section and the floorplanning section. The netlist specifies the connections between the cell's contact areas and the pins. The routing directives control the generation of the routing solution. To connect all the contact areas and pins, various solutions are possible. By adding routing directives one solution can be preferred amongst a myriad of different solutions. Two particularly important routing directives are supported:

- use wires that span the complete extent of the column or row (instead of the shortest possible). This directive is used to enforce that all nets have the same capacitive loading and thus have better matching. It also ensures that all nets have a separate track in a bus.
- constrain a net's horizontal wire in a specific row. This allows a designer to determine the sequence of the horizontal wires. This sequence otherwise is completely random in many cases. This can for instance force the routing of one special net in a specific horizontal track. An example of this could be a biasing net in the center of the array.

The routing then proceeds as follows. First, all buses for every column are processed. All connections that can be made between cells and to pins are made in a column. The number of required tracks is minimized by routing wires in the same track of a bus when they don't overlap vertically (and if not prohibited by the routing directives). The resulting required number of tracks is then checked against the bus capacity of all buses. If the bus capacity is not sufficient an error is returned. After processing all columns of the array, all that remains is to generate the horizontal connections. For all vertical wires that need to be connected with each other, tracks are allocated in the horizontal routing channels obeying the routing directives. Once again wires of different nets are routed in the same track (if allowed) to reduce the required number of tracks. Finally, the required number of tracks is checked against the available channel capacity and an error is returned if the capacity is not sufficient. If no horizontal connections are required this step is skipped.

The automatic routing algorithm can be summarized in pseudo code as follows:

```
1) FORALL array columns
      (a) determine #nets:
            based on connections to pins and contact areas of cells
      (b) select track in one or more bus(es) for every net
            reserve complete track if requested by the designer
      (c) if no overlap vertically and in same bus
            route wires of different nets in one track
      (d) if bus capacities are not sufficient
            report error:  bus capacity too low
2) FORALL vertical wires
      (a) determine #nets that need to be connected horizontally
      (b) if #nets > 0
             i. select tracks for every net
                   unless a track has been selected by the user
            ii. if no overlap in horizontal direction
                   merge wires of different nets in one track
           iii. if capacity of channels is not sufficient
                   report error:  channel capacity too low
```

This routing algorithm is fairly simple when compared to channel routing algorithms used in digital applications [Sher 95], but it is targeted to our array layout model (as presented in section 5.2) and it allows to keep full control and predictability on the final result. Analog applications don't benefit from *optimal, digital* routing results obtained with standard channel routers: the optimal analog layout is not minimal worst-case delay or other digital performance measures. More important, analog routing requirements are *equal* capacitance, *equal* resistance, *equal* metal coverage, ... Furthermore the absence of an optimization loop results in fast run times of the routing phase, which encourages interactive use of the tool.

The symbolic routing phase now has determined where wires and contacts will be created in terms of buses and contact areas, but the actual mask layout in a specified technology process has yet to be generated. This is done in the technology mapping step.

5.3.3 Technology Mapping

Using actual technology data and the physical cell layout, the automatic technology mapping step tiles the mask-level cells based on the floorplan. It realizes all array-wide routing (such as power supply, biasing and ground connections) by abutment. The optionally requested spacer cells are physically inserted between the columns to connect to the basic cells horizontally and route vertically out of or into the array. The symbolic layers are then mapped on physical routing layers in the selected technology process, the physical vertical and horizontal wires are inserted and contacts are added to generate the connectivity. Since symbolic layers have been used in the symbolic routing phase, multiple metal layers can be used to create a wire. This reduces the resistance of the connection in technologies that have a high number of metal layers available. The final result is a mask layout, which is DRC-error free, and the final placement of the pins (not only the mask-level layout coordinates and the mask-level pitch but also their sequence). This sequence is important: it can be input to the floorplanning phase of a module connected to the one just generated as part of a larger circuit. This will be illustrated in the illustrative examples (section 5.4). The routing and technology mapping phase have been separated in **Mondriaan** to allow easy porting of analog modules between different technologies. If cell outlines are compatible in different technologies, only the technology mapping step has to be rerun to generate a new layout.

In this way the layout of cell arrays used in A/D-converters, D/A-converters and other parallel, regular analog structures can be generated in a technology independent way. The connections between the different modules of a larger circuit are easily realized by the use of bus generators (as shown in figure 5.7). The distribution of clock signals, power and biasing is best realized by the use of tree generators (as shown in figure 5.8) [Bern 98]. A set of these generators is part of the **Mondriaan** layout tool and is discussed next.

5.3.4 Bus and Tree Generators

In figure 5.7 the six types of bus generators are shown. Bus generators are *n*–to–*n* type connections. Obvious implementation types are corner (figure 5.7(a)), splitter (figure 5.7(b)), level and pitch change buses (figure 5.7(c), (d), (e)), with 45° routing if allowed in the specific technology (figure 5.7(f)). All of these are available in the form of flexible device generators. One type of bus, **S** (Serpentine) type (figure 5.7(c)), has a special property. Although a pitch change and corner are combined, the length of all wires in the bus is equal. This results in an equal delay on all lines, and an equal voltage drop and capacitance. This type of bus is used (1) to carry signals between modules when resistance and capacitance is extremely important, or (2) to distribute clocks (by merging all lines on one side of the bus [Bern 98]) or (3) other delay-sensitive signals.

Three types of 1–to–*n* type tree generators are available as shown in figure 5.8. The unary variant (figure 5.8(a)) is used most often for distributing biasing and power. Its voltage drop along the tree is given by:

$$V_k = \sum_{j=1}^{k} \left(R_{trunk,j} \sum_{i=j}^{n} I_i \right) + R_{tap,k} I_k \tag{5.2}$$

where k is the position on the tree starting from the root, $R_{trunk,j}$ is the resistance of the trunk between $j-1$ and j, I_i is the current drawn from tap i and $R_{tap,k}$ is the resistance of tap k. By using a tapered variant (as is shown in figure 5.8(a)) and assuming that I_i is equal for all i, the voltage drop is approximately linear; a uniform width tree would have a voltage drop curve that is approximately quadratic. Of course trees not carrying any DC current (voltage biasing for instance) do not suffer from this parasitic effect. The binary tree (figure 5.8(b)) and **H** tree (figure 5.8(c)) of [Bern 98] have the advantage of offering 1-D or 2-D equal resistance and delay distribution of signals, albeit at a higher resistance and capacitance for the same covered distance.

All bus and tree generators generate mask-level layout structures when given values for their structural parameters: wire lengths, wire widths, wire pitches, corner directions, ... In addition they return valuable information as for instance total capacitance, resistance or expected voltage drops at their taps given the current that is carried (see equation (5.2) for an example). This allows an early check of the voltage drops in the lines and avoids costly redesigns that would occur if the problem would only be detected during final extraction and verification.

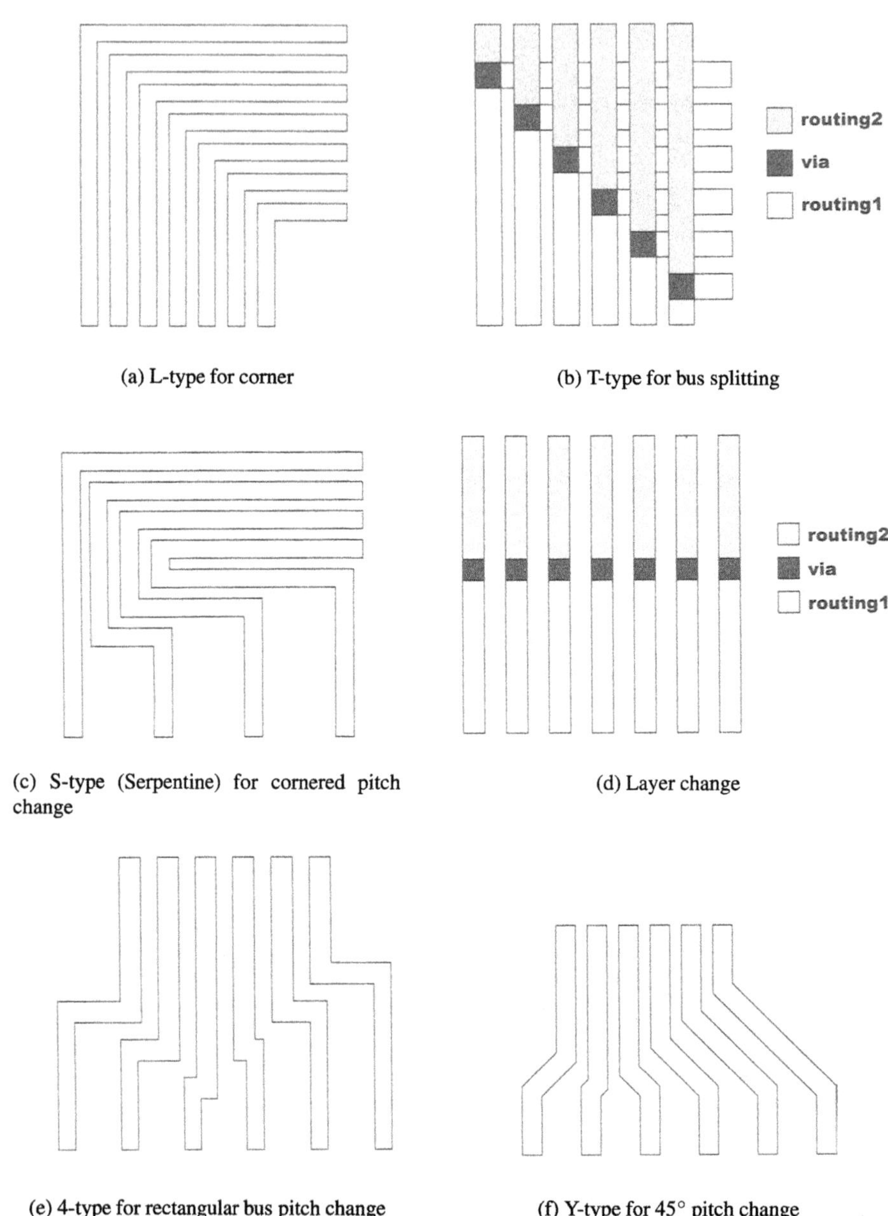

(a) L-type for corner

(b) T-type for bus splitting

(c) S-type (Serpentine) for cornered pitch change

(d) Layer change

(e) 4-type for rectangular bus pitch change

(f) Y-type for 45° pitch change

Figure 5.7: Bus device generators.

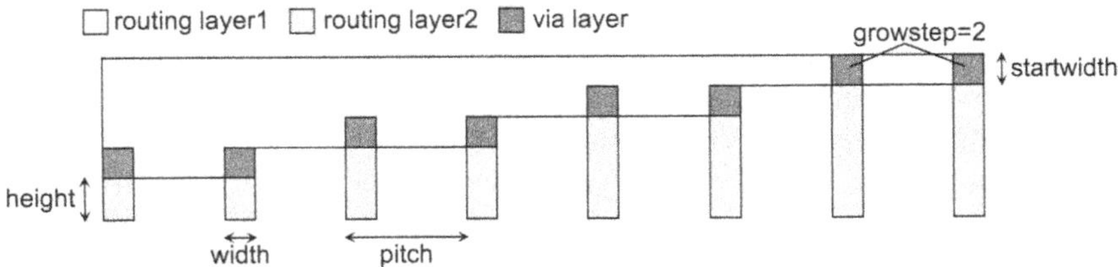

(a) Unary tree, tapered to have a linear voltage drop along the length

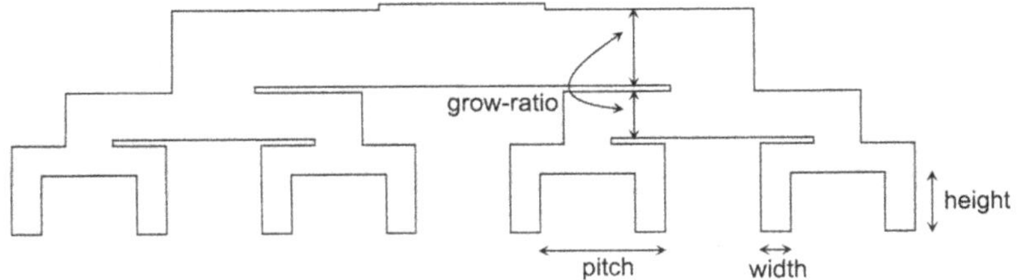

(b) Binary tree (equal delay/resistance for distribution in one dimension)

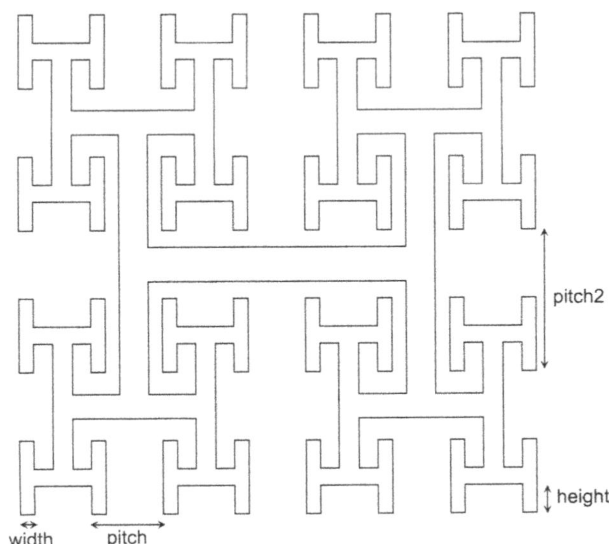

(c) **H** tree [Bern 98] (equal delay/resistance for distribution in two dimensions)

Figure 5.8: Tree device generators.

5.4 Illustrative Example

The example given here is not a real-life example and serves solely as an illustration of the introduced layout model and synthesis methodology. The analog core of a 4-bit current-steering D/A-converter [vdPlassche 94, Vdbus 99a, Vdbus 99b] was chosen to demonstrate how the methodology is used to create the layout of a D/A-converter, in a 1P2M 0.5μm CMOS process. This analog core consists of two modules [vdPlassche 94, Vdbus 99a, Vdbus 99b]: the *current source* array and the *switch/latch* array. Both arrays will be generated separately, they will then be assembled and connected using the bus and tree generators. The complete layout generation process will be covered; emphasis has been put on how the designer exploits the methodology to lay out the analog core by reasoning at a higher symbolic level than the physical polygon level. The actual physical layout generation methodology will then be performed by **Mondriaan** as has been explained above. First the generation of the 4-bit current source array is discussed; next the switch/latch array will be generated and at the end the two modules will be assembled. It is important to understand that due to the use of the presented layout methodology the designer lays out at the symbolic level; no polygon-level editing is required. Cell and pin assignment, and pitches are the entities the designer manipulates. This is where the methodology creates the much wanted flexibility: a designer can go back, find a new cell assignment, a new floorplan, etc. and the tool generates the actual layout from that input. As the back-end process (routing and technology mapping to the polygon level) has been automated, it is extremely fast to allow multiple iterations if needed until the designer is satisfied with the result.

5.4.1 Current Source Array

In this low-complexity example, the current source array module consists of 15 equally sized current sources and one reference current source, as shown in figure 5.9(a) and (b).

Cell Assignment The current sources are each split in four units, which are connected in parallel, and are realized using a common-centroid placement; common-centroid placement is a well-known analog layout technique that is often used to compensate systematic gradients [Vit 85, Bast 96a, Hast 01]. Also the switching sequence [VdPlas 99b, Cong 00] is an important factor and must be under full control of the designer. In our example a *spiral* switching sequence has been chosen by the designer. In addition, a layer of dummy cells surrounds the cell array to avoid the unequal surroundings effect [Vit 85, Pava 94, Hast 01]. The cell assignment (floorplan data) can be automated using the following pseudo code, this pseudo code is usable for the general case of an n-bit current source array where n is even:

1. make an array of $2^{n/2}$ by $2^{n/2}$
2. place the reference cell in the top-left position
3. let $i = 0$
4. until $i < 2n - 1$ do
    (a) move to the south, east, north or west, (in this order) to find an unused entry in the array
    (b) place current source i, increment i

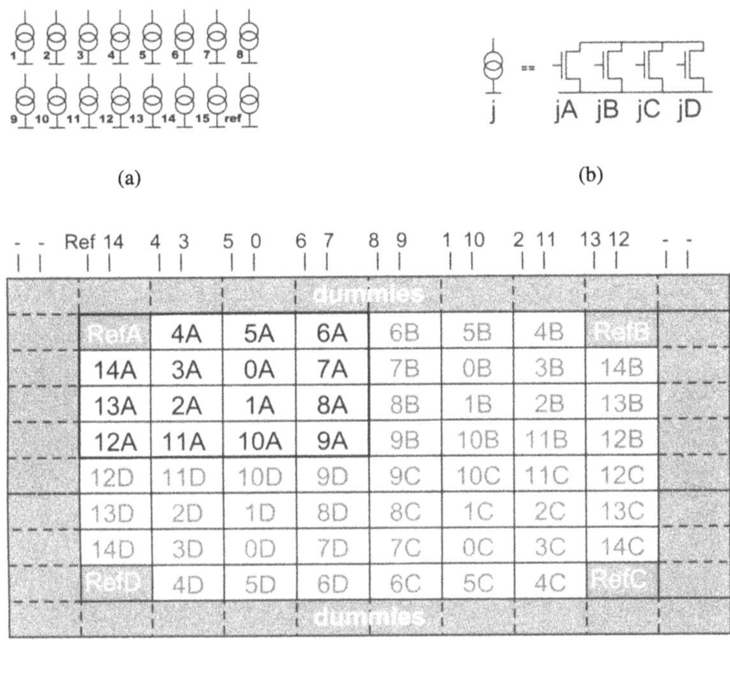

Figure 5.9: Schematic of current source array: 16 equal current sources (a), each current source is split in four units (b), and the floorplan (c).

```
5. mirror the cell array both horizontally and vertically and
   add A,B,C and D suffixes in the process
6. add rows and columns of dummies on every side of the array
```

The resulting cell assignment for the 4-bit current source array, a 10 by 10 cell array including the extra dummies, is shown in figure 5.9(c). No rows or columns are flipped, all cells have only been translated. This is required to obtain the best possible matching of MOS transistors [Vit 85, Pava 94, Hast 01].

Pin Assignment The second part of the floorplanning step is the pin assignment. The current source array has 16 outputs, 15 equal currents and a reference current output. The 15 current outputs connect to the second module, the switch/latch array, which will be placed on top of the current source array in the final layout. Therefore the current-source array's pins are to be placed at the north side of the array. Furthermore it should be easy to connect to the switch/latch array. If we assume that the width of the current source array and switch/latch array are approximately equal, the connections between the modules are most easily realized when they are spaced regularly and span the north side of the array completely. Since from

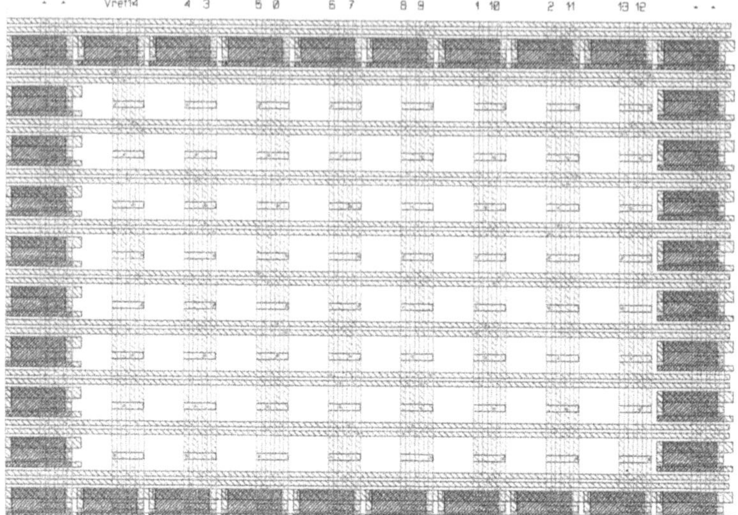

Figure 5.10: Automatically generated 4-bit unary current-source array. For reasons of clarity the actual current-source cells have not been displayed except for the dummy cells surrounding the array. The pins are shown at the top of the figure.

the basic cell outline it is known that the cell contact area has a bus capacity of 4, the total number of vertical tracks available is:

$$\sharp\, vert\_wires_{cursrc\_array} = bus\_capacity_{cursrc\_unit,\ pin\_contact\_area} \times \sharp\, columns_{cursrc\_array} \qquad (5.3)$$

For this example this results in 4 times 10, i.e. 40 tracks. Only 16 connections are required, so 16 out of 40 must be selected. This can easily be done: take half of the wires in every column and do not use the first two and last two wires (these are on columns of dummy devices anyway). Given this specification, the only missing piece of the floorplan is the sequence of the pins. This sequence can easily be derived using the cell assignment. If the first unconnected cells in the columns are used to determine the column's pins, the following sequence is found (it is also shown on top of the array in figure 5.9(c)): {–, –, Ref, 14, 4, 3, 5, 0, 6, 7, 8, 9, 1, 10, 2, 11, 13, 12, –, –}. This can also easily be automated for an n-bit array with the following pseudo code:

```
1. initialize an empty pin list
2. for every column in the cell array do
3. let i = 1

    (a) until i == 3 do
    (b) for every current source do

         i. if the pin is already in pin list, continue
        ii. else add pin to pin list and increase i
```

Layout Generation The actual physical generation of the current-source array then proceeds with the automated routing using **Mondriaan**. The routing directive to use full-length wires has been specified to ensure equal routing (except contacts) for all current sources. After the automated technology mapping step, the mask layout shown in figure 5.10 is obtained; the cell's content has not been displayed in the figure to more clearly show the routing. As can be seen on the figure, the routing is extremely regular except for the contacts making connections to the contact areas and connecting the vertical wires with the horizontal wires. This is one of the constraints for accurate matching of the sources: the array should be identical for every source, including the metal coverage. The pin placement is shown at the top of the figure: the pin sequence was already specified by the designer, the mask-level pin pitch of the current-source array is given by:

$$pitch_{cursrc\_array} = \frac{width_{cursrc\_array}}{\sharp\, wires_{cursrc\_array}} \tag{5.4}$$

which in our example results in a mask pitch of 4.2μm (a connection every 4.2μm). In the vertical direction the second metal routing level was used, since metal level one was used internally in the horizontal direction to distribute the power and biasing of the cell by abutment. The parallel devices of each current source have been connected in the horizontal direction by wires in between the cells since metal level one had already been used internally. If a third metal layer would have been allowed or available in the technology, the height of the array could have been reduced substantially by routing the horizontal wires across the cells. Using the presented methodology and tools a change like this could be done in a matter of minutes, where as the manual method or stretch and tile approach would require extensive reworking. Note that the wires run on to the edges of the cell array. This has been done to achieve equal metal coverage across the entire array for matching purposes [Tuin 97, VdPlas 99a].

5.4.2 Switch/Latch Array

Let us next consider the switch/latch array of the 4-bit analog core.

Floorplanning The current-source array has already been generated down to the mask layout level. So the exact size of the array and position of the pins is available. The switch/latch array consists of 15 equal switch/latch driver cells. It is preferred that, in order to ease connecting the two resulting modules, the *pitch* of input and output buses is unchanged. If it is assumed that we require a **spacer2** cell (every odd column) to extract array-wide signals, the number of rows in the switch/latch array (every switch/latch cell is connected to one current source) is determined by the mask-level pin pitch of the switch/latch array (which is taken equal to the pin pitch of the current-source array) and the width of the basic cells according to the following equation:

$$\sharp\, rows_{switch/latch\_array} = \frac{width_{switch/latch\_cell} + \frac{1}{2} width_{spacer2}}{pitch_{switch/latch\_array}} \tag{5.5}$$

$$= \frac{width_{switch/latch\_cell} + \frac{1}{2} width_{spacer2}}{pitch_{cursrc\_array}} \tag{5.6}$$

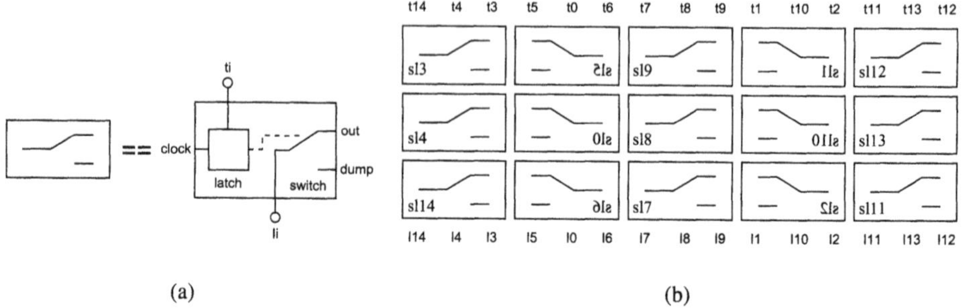

Figure 5.11: The switch/latch cell contains a digital latch driving a switch (a). The routing-driven assignment result: the pins at the bottom of the figure have been input, the assignment of the switch/latch cells and output pins (at the top) have been derived by propagating the connectivity (b).

In this equation the number of rows of the switch/latch array ($\sharp\, rows_{switch/latch\_array}$) has to be an integer value. For the given width of the basic cell, three rows is optimal for our example. The **spacer2** cell width has been adapted to fill up the space and collect the array-wide signals *out* and *dump* out of the array vertically. Since in total there are 15 cells (one for every current source), an array of 5 by 3 as shown in figure 5.11 is used. Note that the switch/latch cells have been mirrored sideways every next column as indicated symbolically in figure 5.11. This allows for the output currents of neighboring cells to be collected in the **spacer2** cell (which itself is not symmetric), and carry it vertically out of the array without crossing digital signals.

Cell Assignment Of course, the switch/latch cell assignment is now not determined completely independently by the designer. The pin sequence of the current source array has already been determined. If we want to connect the pin to the correct cell, the cell needs to be assigned in a column above the pin. To find a consistent cell assignment, the columns are scanned from bottom to top for odd columns and top to bottom for even columns to assign cells: the cell connected to the encountered pin takes the first free slot. The floorplan shown in figure 5.11(b) shows the resulting cell assignment for the switch/latch array.

Pin Assignment There are two pin sets to this array: the current source outputs (pins *out*, *dump* and I_i) and the digital control lines (pins t_i). Since the current-source array is placed below the switch/latch array and the digital decoder will be placed above the switch/latch array in a complete D/A-converter, the current-source connections are placed at the south side of the switch/latch array; the digital control lines at the north side of the array. Two separate contact areas are available in the cells, one for the current source output, one for the digital control line. The out/dump pins are array-wide connections and use abutment through spacer cells. Only two signals need to be assigned in the floorplan: the digital steering signal t_i and the connection to the corresponding current source cell I_i. Each are assigned a separate track, resulting in two tracks for each cell (there are no spare tracks in this case). Thus both pin sequences select all available tracks in their respective buses. The pin sequence for the digital control lines results from the cell assignment and is the same as the pin assignments of the current sources. Both sequences are also shown on the floorplan in figure 5.11(b). Both these steps (cell and pin assignment) can once again easily be automated for the n-bit case.

Layout Generation After floorplanning, routing and technology mapping is done automatically using the **Mondriaan** tool [VdPlas 98]. In figure 5.12 the resulting layout is shown. In this array wires end where they are connected. Accurate matching is not required for digital control signals. This limits the load and delay on the digital signal wires. The gnd, vdd and clock signals have been routed horizontally across the array through abutment.

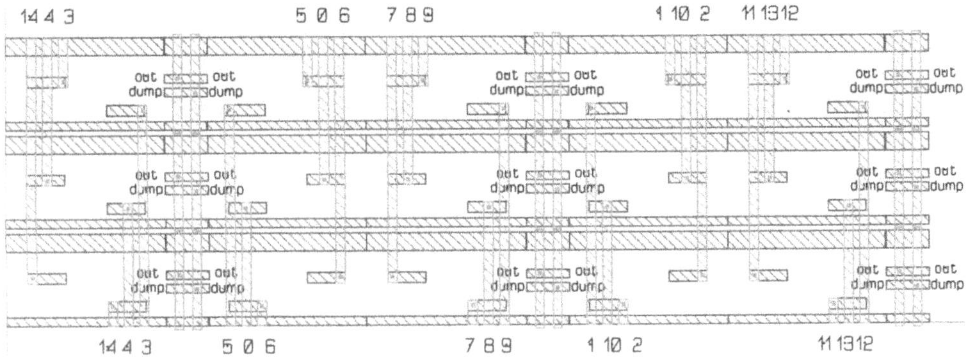

Figure 5.12: Layout of the 4-bit switch/latch array. For reasons of clarity the switch/latch cells' contents have not been displayed. The pins are shown at the bottom and at the top of the figure. At every odd column of the latch cell columns, spacers have been inserted to collect the output currents.

5.4.3 Assembly

All that remains now to finish the layout of the analog core of the D/A-converter, is vertically connecting all power and biasing lines using the tree generators, and generating appropriate buses for connecting the two modules together. In figure 5.13 the final result is shown: the power, ground, clock and out/dump connections have been realized using unary trees, the modules have been connected using buses. Of course, for this illustrative 4-bit example no tool is really needed. But this is no longer true for data converters of higher resolution as encountered in industrial practice. In that case, the manual generation of the layout is a time-consuming and error-prone task.

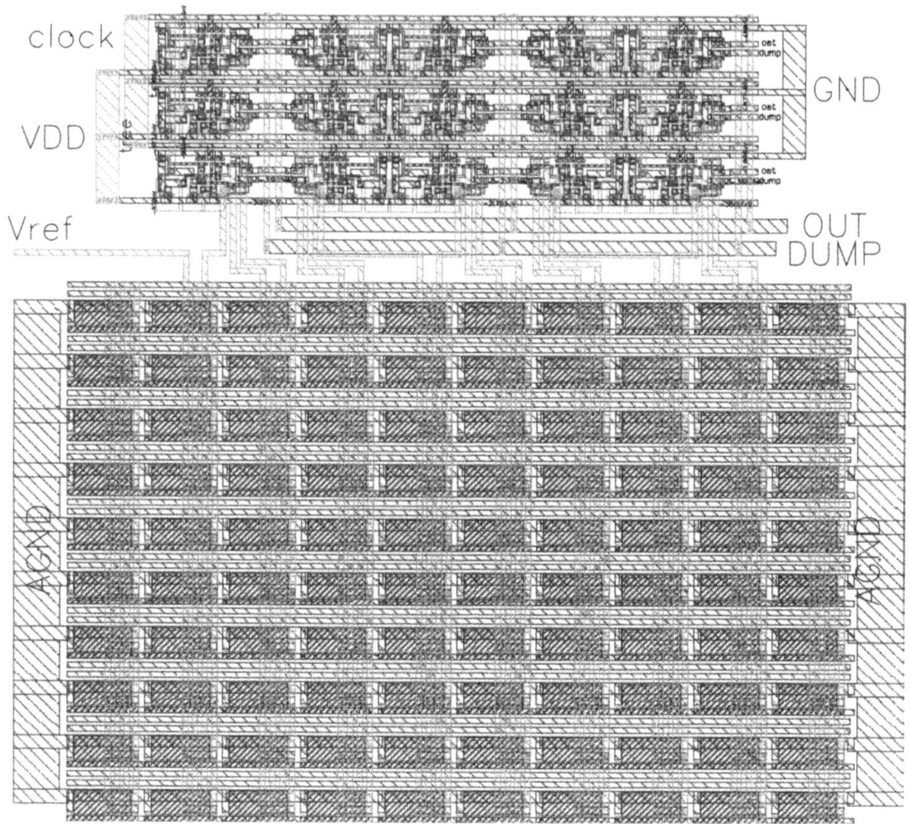

Figure 5.13: Complete layout of the 4-bit analog core. The current source array and switch/latch array have been placed and the array-wide and individual signals have been connected using trees and buses.

5.4.4 Conclusions

In this section the presented layout methodology has been applied to the layout generation of a 4-bit analog D/A-converter core. It has been shown how the designer operates to build flexible module generators for the two modules using the layout methodology and the **Mondriaan** tool. The designer does not manipulate any mask-level polygon structures directly. The abstraction level has been raised: cell assignment, pin assignment, pin pitches, abutment for array-wide routing, core-level floorplanning, module assembly, ... are the problems the designer can concentrate on. These are also the most important problems: it is at this level that the layout can be optimized; the lower level (mask-level array layouts) has been automated in **Mondriaan**.

5.5 Experimental Results

Let us now present some real design examples. The proposed methodology and the **Mondriaan** tool have been applied to the physical design of high-speed folding/interpolating A/D-converters and high-resolution current-steering D/A-converters.

5.5.1 Folding/Interpolating A/D-converter Modules

Folding/interpolating A/D-converters combine high speed and accuracy with moderate power requirements [vdPlassche 94]. The important modules of this converter type are: the input stage generating the folding signals, the intermediate block generating the interpolated signals, the comparator string discriminating the interpolated signals, and a (ROM-based) encoder [Uytt 00]. Since the comparator array can easily be generated by tiling and since dedicated tools exist for generating a digital encoder, only the folding and the interpolation modules are left [ThoLoo 97]. It will now be shown how these modules are generated with the presented approach.

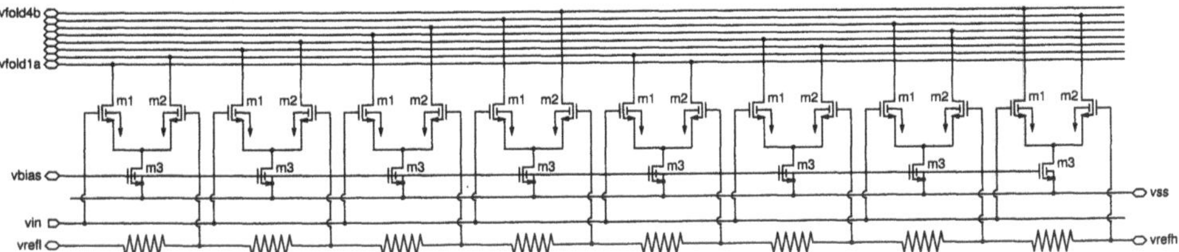

Figure 5.14: Generating folding signals by cross-coupling the input stages in a high-speed A/D-converter.

In figure 5.14 the schematic of an input stage of a folding/interpolating A/D-converter is shown. It consists of a set of differential pairs, of which one of the inputs is connected to the input of the A/D-converter and the other input is connected to a resistor string generating a set of reference voltages. The outputs are cross-coupled to a bus of folding signals. In this case four differential folding signals are generated, each having two folds. Depending on the architectural requirements of the A/D-converter, the number of folding signals (F) and the number of folds (N) are determined during architectural sizing. The layout of an array of FN input stages then has to be generated. The position of the instances is completely determined and, as can be seen, extremely simple. The pin sequence is also very simple: use all tracks in the bus, put the folding signals one after the other.

A generated layout is shown in figure 5.15(a), in which the number of folding signals F equals 4, while the number of folds N equals 9. A zoom in of this input stage is also shown in figure 5.15(b), which corresponds exactly to the schematic of figure 5.14: four folding signals each having two folds. Please note that both the layouts have been rotated 90° with respect to **Mondriaan**'s layout model: the vertical folding signal bus runs horizontally. The rotation was done to make the layout correspond to the schematic of figure 5.14. The generation of this input stage module was completely automated including the layout generation of the basic

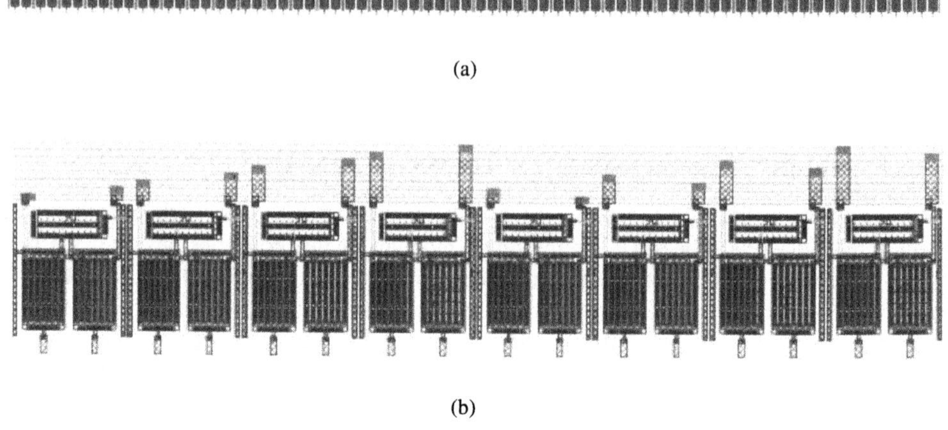

(a)

(b)

Figure 5.15: Full layout (a), and zoom in on one fold of a folding input stage (b).

cell. The basic cell, which consists of a differential pair and current source, was generated by using the analog place and route tool LAYLA [Lam 99] in approximately 5 minutes of CPU time (on a standard SUN Ultra-1/170 workstation) including the time needed to start up the commercial Mentor Graphics environment [Mentor-Graphics 98]. The basic cells were then tiled using the presented methodology and **Mondriaan** in approximately 10 seconds of CPU time on the same machine. The technology process used was a standard 1P2M 0.5μm CMOS technology. The pseudo code for automating the floorplan generation of the folding input stage for F folding signals and N folds is:

1. make a cell array of 1 column of $F*N$ rows
2. let $i=1$
3. until $i==N$
   (a) let $j=1$
   (b) until $j=F$
      i. place inputStage i_j at position $i*F+j$
      ii. increment j
   (c) increment i
4. create empty pin list
5. let $k=1$
6. until $k==F$
   (a) add pin vfoldk_a to pin list
   (b) add pin vfoldk_b to pin list
   (c) increment k

The folding signals are then input to the interpolation block. Interpolation is achieved by using weighted current mirrors that combine signals from neighboring folding signals. This

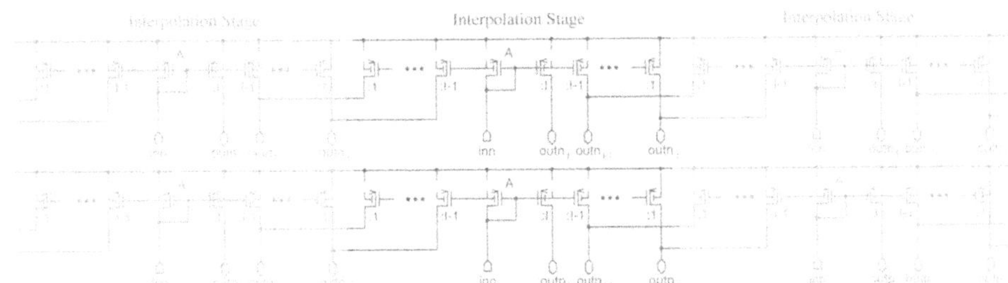

Figure 5.16: Generating interpolated signals by using weighted current mirrors in a high-speed interpolating A/D-converter.

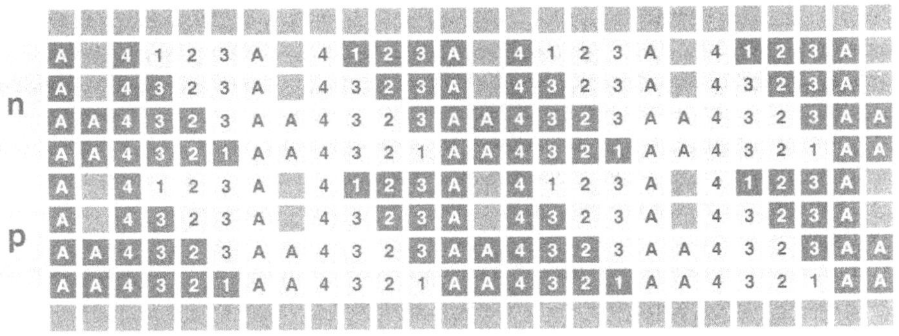

Figure 5.17: Floorplan of interpolating current mirrors. The numbers indicate the interpolation signal being generated, the greyed out cells are dummies (surrounding the array and filling up empty slots).

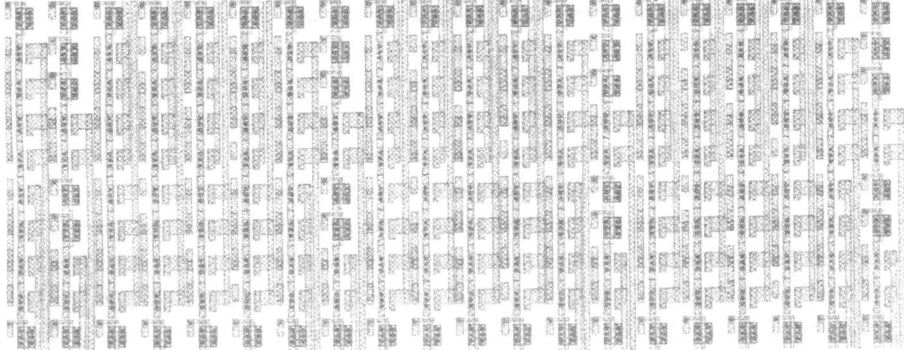

Figure 5.18: Layout of interpolating current mirrors. This layout corresponds to the floorplan shown in figure 5.17.

is shown in figure 5.16. When I interpolated signals are to be generated, current mirrors with ratios from 1 to $I-1$ are added to current mirrors of the neighboring folding signal of $I-1$ to 1. One mirror of ratio I is used to transfer the folding signal itself as output signal. The current-mirror diode has a different scaling factor (A) to tune the frequency behavior of the overall structure. Because of matching requirements the current mirrors are implemented using equally sized transistors which are placed in parallel to obtain the requested ratio. In figure 5.17 the floorplan of the proposed interpolation circuit is shown. Every column of cells combines an interpolated signal, except for the columns containing the current-mirror diodes (A). The greyed out cells are dummies, filling up empty spots and surrounding the complete array to ensure equal surroundings. The vertical routing is then used to input the folding signals, to output the interpolated signals and to connect the gates of the current mirrors. The gates of the current mirrors are connected horizontally with the second metal layer. The input parameters for the generation of the interpolation block are the number of interpolated signals, I, and the number of folding signals, F. These determine the number of interpolation stages that will be generated. Once again the floorplanning step could easily be automated to build a module generator for a generic interpolation circuit that, in combination with **Mondriaan**, automatically generates the layout of this converter module. In figure 5.18 the synthesized layout of the interpolation module is shown, the technology used was a standard 1P2M 0.5μm CMOS technology. The actual transistors have not been displayed in the cells to more clearly see the routing. The total CPU time on a SUN Ultra-1/170 workstation to generate this layout is less than 10 seconds.

Both these modules all together can thus be generated in less than 10 minutes of CPU time; doing manual layout this would at least take several hours. The resulting layouts can then be inspected early on in the design cycle and late engineering changes (e.g. due to a change in the process parameters) can easily be handled. If important architectural changes are required (for instance a change of the number of input stages), regenerating these layouts also takes little time in the presented approach. To complete the overall layout, the bus and tree generators in **Mondriaan** can then be used to speed up the assembly of all the converter's modules.

5.5.2 Current-Steering D/A-converter Modules

Figure 5.19 shows the block diagram and floorplan of a 14-bit current-steering segmented D/A-converter (see for a detailed description chapter 6). The current-source array (lower part of figure 5.19) contains all the current sources (both the unary and the binary-weighted current sources). The binary-weighted sources have been realized by putting some of the current source transistors in series, as shown in figure 5.20.

The floorplan of the current source array is shown in figure 5.21. The unary current sources are implemented by placing 16 MOS transistors in parallel (Quad Quadrant), in this way averaging technology gradients [Vdbus 99a, VdPlas 99b]. The binaries are inserted in two columns, at approximately 1/4 and 3/4 of the current-source array. Although the array consists of identical transistors, the routing of the binary sources is entirely different (MOS transistors are put in series). Including the dummy current sources surrounding the array (4 rows and 3 columns), over 5000 cells have been placed and routed. This certainly precludes the use of manual layout in this case. The pin assignment resulting from the current-source array generation, drives the placement of the switches (center part of figure 5.19) as explained

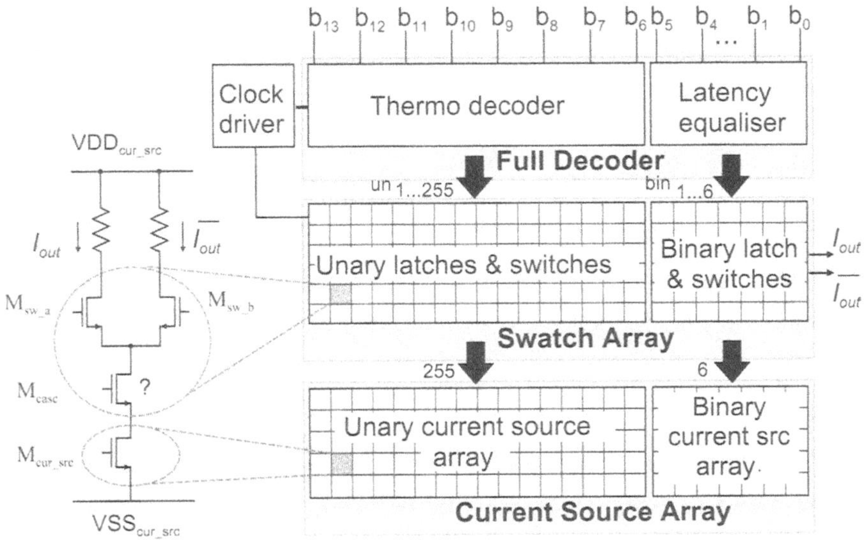

Figure 5.19: Block diagram and floorplan of the proposed D/A-converter architecture.

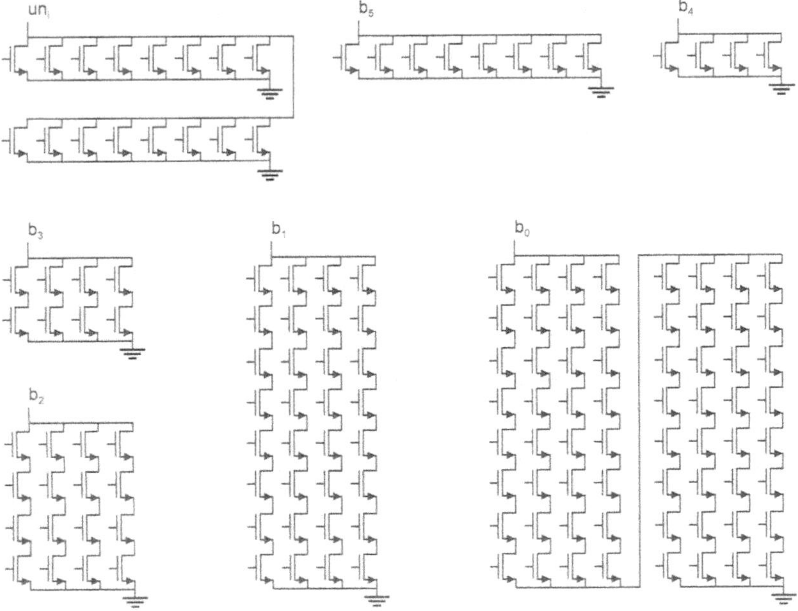

Figure 5.20: Schematic of the current-source array of the 14-bit current-steering D/A-converter.

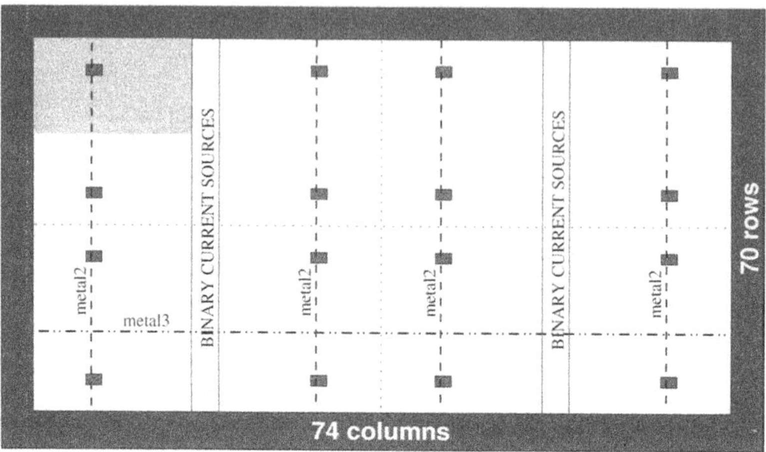

Figure 5.21: Floorplan of the current source array of the 14-bit current-steering D/A-converter.

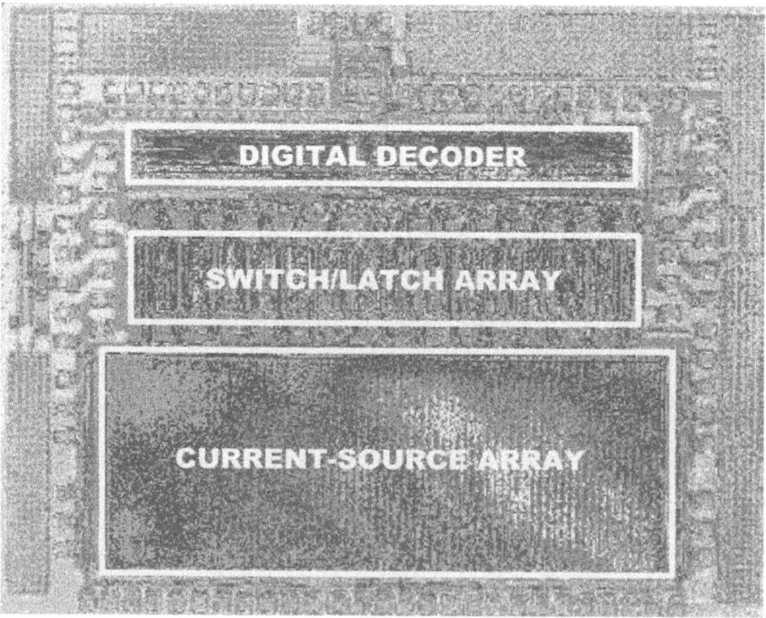

Figure 5.22: Automatically generated layout of the 14-bit current-steering D/A-converter.

in the illustrative example section. The binary switches have different widths and are placed vertically above the binary current sources (this is a result of the cell assignment). The digital control line sequence output resulting from the switch/latch array placement is then input to the standard cell place and route tools used to generate the digital standard cell decoder (top of figure 5.19).

All the modules have been connected using the bus generators. The wiring pitch from the digital decoder down to the current sources is constant. This also ensures that all modules approximately have the same width, resulting in an elegant chip-level layout. All power, clock, ground and biasing distribution has been realized using the tapered and binary tree generators. Except for the layout creation of the basic cells and for the chip assembly (placing bondpads and connecting them), no editing at polygon level was required in this layout. The total CPU time required to generate the current-source array was 1 minute on a standard SUN Ultra-1/170 workstation. The CPU time for generating the switch/latch array on the same machine was less than 20 seconds. The chip photograph of the generated chip is shown in figure 5.22. The technology used was a standard 1P3M 0.5μm CMOS technology.

In total three high-accuracy D/A-converters were synthesized with the **Mondriaan** tool. The design of these converters will further be described in the next chapter, chapter 6. Design time of an earlier manual design of a similar current-steering D/A-converter [VdBosch 98] and of the new approach are listed and compared in Table 5.1. Note that the use of the presented methodology and the supporting tool **Mondriaan** allows to reduce the layout generation time from 19 to approximately 8 working days (of 8 hours). Of this, one day was used for the analog modules, four days for the digital place & route (which was out-sourced) and three days for the final assembly. The resulting chip was not only designed much faster, it was at the time of publication also the first intrinsically linear 14-bit D/A-converter in CMOS technology to be published, indicating that the use of CAD tools does not necessarily imply low performance.

Task	**Manual design**	**Automated design**
floorplan	2 days	1 hour
current-source	3 days	1 hour
switch/latch array	5 days	7 hours
thermocoder	5 days	4 days
assembly	4 days	3 days
Total person effort	**19 days**	**8 days & 1 hour**

Table 5.1: Time spent on layout for a manual design and a design using the proposed methodology, showing the realized productivity gain.

5.6 Conclusions

A layout synthesis methodology has been presented which targets the layout generation of regular array-type analog blocks. The approach takes in consideration *typical analog requirements*, supports frequently used *analog design* and *layout techniques*, and is *very flexible* (low setup and run times). A three-step procedure (*floorplanning*, *symbolic routing* and *technology mapping*) raises the abstraction level compared to other existing approaches by automating the last two phases in a tool called **Mondriaan**. Full control and predictability of the result is guaranteed. Not only does the methodology result in a considerable design productivity boost, it also enlarges analog layout capabilities which can be exploited by the designer to surmount the technological boundaries for layout-driven designs. The layout synthesis problem of these regular blocks is solved in a *fast* and *technology independent way*, promoting *layout reuse*. A set of bus and tree generators completes the presented tool set. Industrial-strength examples have demonstrated the applicability and usefulness of the implemented approach. In the next chapter this layout methodology is applied to the design of high-accuracy current-steering D/A-converters.

Chapter 6

Systematic Design of Current-Steering D/A-converters

Current-steering D/A-converters are frequently used analog functionblocks. A typical application is found in video processing systems where they are used to convert a digital video signal to an analog RGB signal. Another typical application is in telecommunication systems where they are used to generate data signals (for instance xDSL). The specification ranges that are found in these applications vary: low to medium accuracy (8 bit or higher) for video applications, high accuracy (10 bit or higher) for telecommunication applications; update rates of a few tens of MHz to a few hundreds of MHz; total signal to noise and distortion ratio (SNDR) requirements of 50 to 80dB, or spurious free dynamic range (SFDR) requirements of 60 to 80dB; glitch energy of a few pV.s; etc.

The SoC (Systems-on-a-chip) paradigm requires that these blocks can be integrated in a standard (digital) CMOS technology. And in fact, the implementation of these converters typically does *not* require analog extensions to the CMOS process (high-quality resistors, capacitors, ...). In this sense the design of these current-steering D/A-converters is of importance for real-life SoCs and a representative example for the application of mixed-signal design methodologies and tools developed for the SoC era that are the subject of this work.

In this chapter the systematic design of current-steering D/A-converters that have a high accuracy (up and above 12 bit) and a moderate to high update rate (approximately 200MSamples/s), is investigated. The research presented here resulted in the publication of the first 14-bit current-steering D/A-converter in CMOS technology known to the authors, that achieved full static linearity without tuning or trimming [Vdbus 99a, VdPlas 99b].

In the presented research the design itself was not the only objective. Of course an important objective of the work was to design, manufacture and measure prototype D/A-converters, to prove that this type of converter can be realized with the targeted performance specifications. But next to this design problem that had to be solved, the most important objective of the research work was to refine and verify the design methodology that is proposed in this work: *systematic design*. This systematic design methodology will be explained and applied in the remainder of this chapter [VdPlas 00, Vdbus 01]. Important to note is that the systematic design methodology has resulted in high-quality designs [VdBosch 98, Vdbus 99a, VdPlas 99b] and in the creation of point tools (one of which was already discussed in chapter 5), automating part of the design process. The design methodology has also allowed a design productivity increase. This productivity gain has been measured across the different prototypes that have been designed (by the same design team). This productivity gain did not compromise design quality. The latter is one of the most often heard objections expressed by designers when automation of analog design is proposed. One of the most important conclusions of this research is that given the necessary conditions, *analog design automation* does not sacrifice *design quality*.

The scope of this chapter not only extends to the design of the blocks and the methodology that has been utilized. In addition the derivation of the specifications of the block in its SoC environment (or any other enclosing environment) will be discussed. The approach taken makes use of behavioral modeling techniques. A generic analog behavioral model has been built using an analog hardware description languages (such as VHDL-AMS, Verilog-AMS, SpectreHDL, EldoFAS, Saber's MAST, ...). This generic model can then be used for system simulation by selecting appropriate values for the parameters of the D/A-converter behavioral model. In this sense this chapter forms an exception in this book. All other discussed methodologies for synthesis start from the *given* specifications, in this chapter a means on how to derive these specifications has been included. At the back-end of the design process the same extension has been added. A behavioral model is extracted, modeling the implementation as closely as possible for inclusion in system-level verification simulations. It will be explained how the generic behavioral model has been adapted and the parameters can be extracted.

Current-steering D/A-converters have most successfully been implemented using a segmented architecture combined with row–column decoders [Miki 86]. In this chapter a novel segmented architecture will be presented [VdBosch 98, Vdbus 99a, VdPlas 99b]. The design flexibility of this novel architecture is much higher than the row–column decoder based traditional architecture; the proposed segmented architecture uses a modular design: the design consists of three modules that can be designed independently. The switching sequence, one of the most important implementation parameters of a current-steering D/A-converter is also completely flexible. These properties of the novel segmented architecture facilitate the application of the *systematic design* methodology.

The outline of this chapter is as follows. First the design flow of analog functionblocks is reviewed, and it is applied to the design of a mixed-signal converter circuit. Next the operating principle of current-steering converters and the specification table with typical performance values are presented. In the next section the novel segmented converter architecture is proposed. The actual design trace is then described: each design step (sizing, layout, verification) is discussed in detail. Next the prototypes are presented and the measurement results are discussed. In the last section conclusions are drawn summarizing the research results.

6.1 Functionblock Design Flow

In the design of analog functional blocks as part of a large system on silicon, a number of phases are identified. These are depicted in figure 6.1. The first phase in the design is the *specification phase*. During this phase the analog functionblock is analyzed in relation to its environment, the surrounding system, to determine the system-level architecture and the block's required performance specifications. With the advent of standardized analog hardware description languages (VHDL-AMS [VHDL-AMS 99], Verilog-A/MS [Verilog-AMS 98]), the

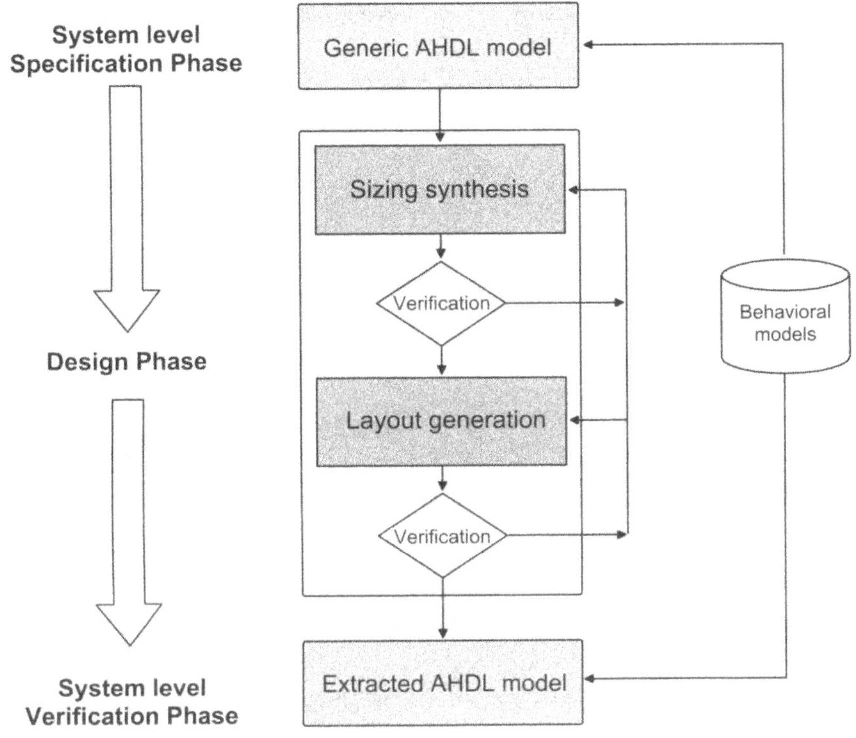

Figure 6.1: Converter functionblock design flow.

obvious implementation for this phase is a generic analog behavioral model [ElTa 89, Getr 90, Anta 95, Sale 96, Fitz 98]. This model is parameterized with respect to the performance specifications of the functionblock.

The next phase in the design procedure is the design (synthesis) of the functionblock, shown in the center of figure 6.1, this phase consists of sizing synthesis and layout generation. The design methodology used is the top-down, bottom-up performance-driven design methodology [Chang 95b, Gie 95b]. This design methodology has been accepted as the de facto standard for systematically designing analog building blocks [Lin 98, Sam 99]. In [Neff 95] the design of current-steering D/A-converters has been automated following this methodology for one specific architecture. This architecture is however only usable for 8- or 10-bit D/A-converters. In this chapter higher accuracy D/A-converters are designed by using an improved converter architecture. The novel architecture will be presented in section 6.2.2.

When the converter design is finished and verified, the complete system in which the functionblock is utilized, must be verified, as shown in figure 6.1, by system-level simulations. Once again the technique of behavioral modeling is applied. This time the actual behavioral parameters are extracted from the finished design, and used to verify the functioning of the block within the system.

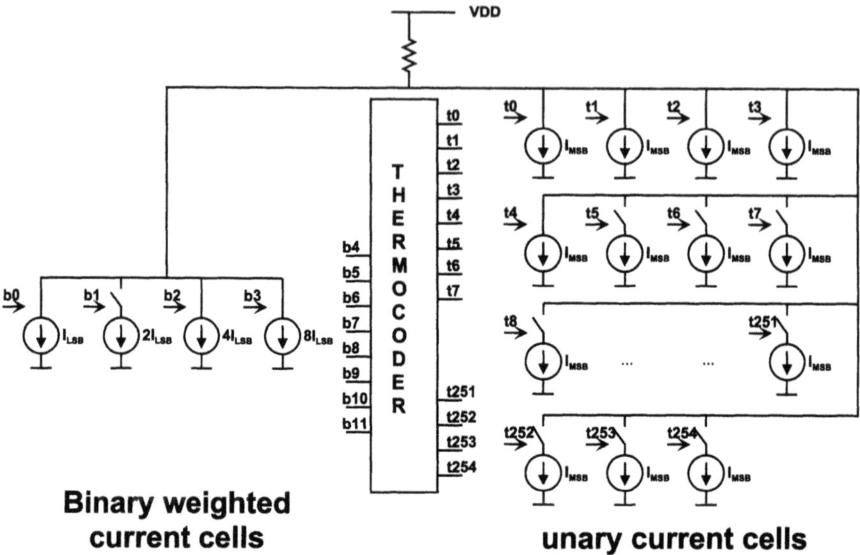

Figure 6.2: Operating principle of a segmented current-steering D/A-converter.

In the next sections the following topics will be discussed: the generic behavioral modeling, the sizing synthesis, layout generation and behavioral model extraction steps in the design flow for high accuracy D/A-converters. First the specifications of current-steering D/A-converters, the novel D/A-converter architecture and its complete set of design parameters are described.

6.2 Current-Steering D/A-converter Architecture

6.2.1 Operating Principle and Specifications

For high-speed, high-accuracy D/A-converters, a segmented current-steering topology is usually chosen as it is intrinsically faster and more linear than competing architectures [vdPlassche 94, Raz 95] such as resistor-string D/A-converters [Pel 90].

The conceptual block diagram of this type of D/A-converter is shown in figure 6.2: the l least significant bits are implemented using binary-weighted current sources while the m most significant bits steer a unary array of equally sized current sources. The binary switches are directly steered by their respective bit-lines. The unary switches are steered by a thermometer decoder. The decoder converts the given binary code to a corresponding number of active lines at the output. Why this segmented architecture (a combination of binary weighted and unary current sources) is accepted as a standard will become clear later on.

The general specification list for a current-steering D/A-converter is given in Table 6.1. The specifications can be divided into four categories: static, dynamic, environmental and op-

	Specification	Symbol		Value	Unit
Static	Number of bits	n	=	14	
	INL	INL	<	0.5	LSB
	DNL	DNL	<	0.5	LSB
	Parametric yield	$Yield$	>	99	%
Dynamic	Glitch energy	E_{glitch}	<	1.0	pV.s
	Settling time [10–90%]	$t_{settling}$	<	10	ns
	SFDR@500kHz	$SFDR$	>	80	dB
	SNR	SNR	>	84	dB
	Sample frequency	f_s	=	100	MS/s
Environment	Output range	V_{out}	=	1	V
	Load	R_{load}	=	50	Ω
	Digital levels	V_{dig}		CMOS	
	Power supply	V_{dd}	=	2.7	V
	Technology	Θ	=	1P3M 0.5μm CMOS	–
Optimization	Power consumption	$power$	MIN	200	mW
	Area	$area$	MIN	15	mm^2

Table 6.1: Specification table of current-steering D/A-converters with typical values.

timization specifications. In the case of a D/A-converter the **static** parameters include static accuracy (i.e. number of bits), integral non-linearity (INL), differential non-linearity (DNL) and parametric yield. The **dynamic** parameters include settling time, glitch energy, spurious-free dynamic range (SFDR), signal-to-noise ratio (SNR) and sample frequency. The **environmental** parameters include the power supply, the digital levels, the load and the output range. The power consumption and area need to be **minimized** for a given technology. This specification list serves as input for the design process that will be explained in the sections on the design of the D/A-converter.

6.2.2 Proposed Architecture and its Design Parameters

The conceptual block diagram of figure 6.2 is implemented by the proposed segmented architecture shown in figure 6.3. The current source is implemented either as a single MOS transistor (M_{cur_src}) current source, a cascoded (M_{casc}, M_{cur_src}) current source or (not shown on figure 6.3) any other type of MOS current source. The currents generated by the current sources are switched to one of the two differential output nodes by switch transistors M_{sw_a} and M_{sw_b}. These are steered by a latch, providing the optimal switching signals to the MOS transistors. The full decoder comprises both the thermometer encoder (thermocoder), that generates the steering signals for the unary latches from the digital input word, and a latency equalizer block for the binary control signals. This latency equalizer block ensures correct timing for the steering signals of the binary latches. One of the important architectural choices is how many input bits are implemented using binary-weighted current sources and how many using unary-weighted ones (degree of segmentation): l bits are implemented binary, m bits are

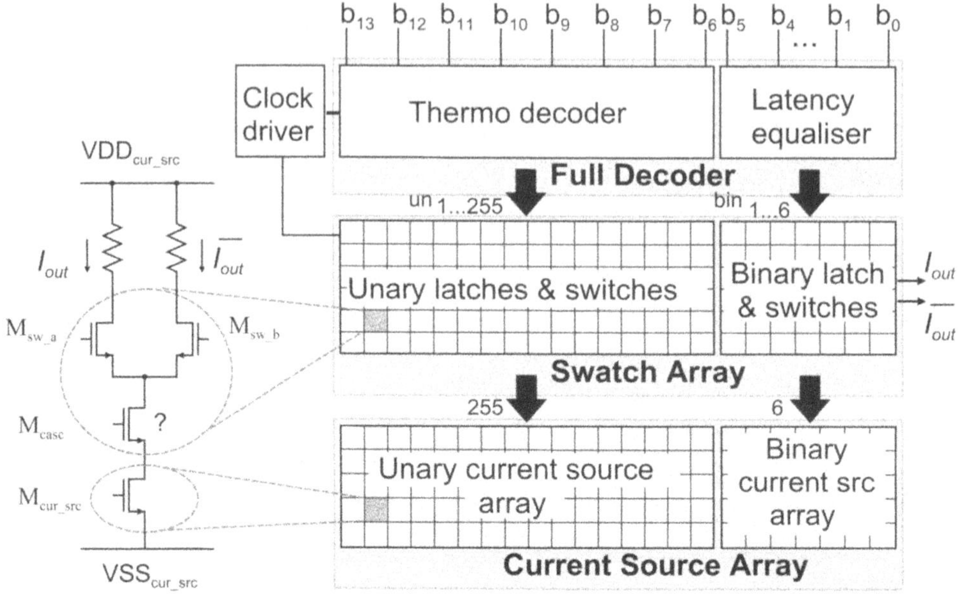

Figure 6.3: Block diagram and floorplan of the proposed D/A-converter architecture.

implemented unary, this gives n bits in total:

$$n = l + m \tag{6.1}$$

The basic floorplan of the proposed architecture is also shown in figure 6.3. The switches and latch are implemented as one unit cell, and placed in an array, referred to as the *swatch* array in the middle. The current source transistors are also placed in an array, the *current source array* at the bottom. The *full decoder* block is at the top. The three large modules (full decoder, swatch array and current source array) are connected by signal buses. A *clock driver* completes the D/A-converter.

An important design parameter of a current-steering D/A-converter is the *switching scheme*. The switching scheme has three components. A unary current source consists of *one* or *more parallel* units spread out over the current source array, as shown in figure 6.4(a), (b) and (c). By splitting the unary current sources the spatial errors are averaged, which is necessary for high-accuracy applications. The number of units used, j, and the *spreading* of these units across the array determines to what extent spatial errors are compensated or reduced. The second parameter of the switching scheme is the *switching sequence*. In [Miki 86] it is shown that the remaining spatial errors are not accumulating when the current sources are switched on in an optimal way. The here proposed architecture differs from previously used architectures in that the switching sequence is fully flexible and can be programmed (when generating the layout) to optimally compensate for systematic errors that would otherwise deteriorate the targeted linearity. It is also different from the competing architectures in

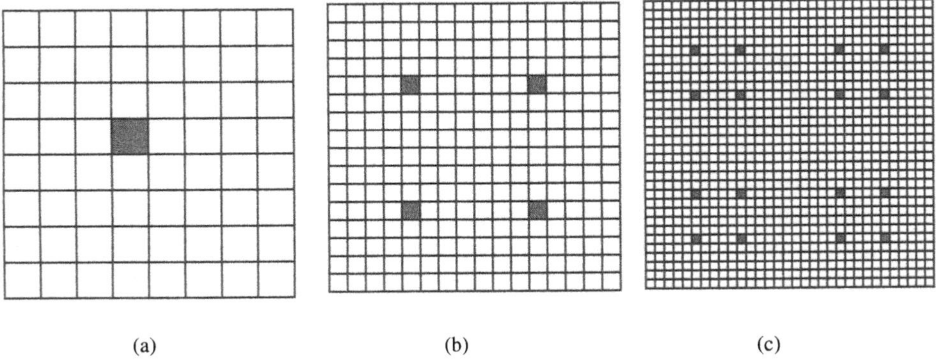

Figure 6.4: Three different switching schemes: (a) unary current source implemented as 1 unit, (b) unary current source implemented as 4 units in parallel, (c) unary current source implemented as 16 units in parallel.

that it decouples the three main functions of the design: the static accuracy of the converter is realized in the current source array, the dynamic switching of the currents is realized in the swatch (switch/latch) array and the decoding is done in the digital decoder. Each module can independently be optimized for its function. This is not the case for row–column-based architectures [Miki 86] where the three functions are mixed, leading to a monolithic design.

	Design parameters of the architecture
Architectural level	l (number of LSBs)
	m (number of MSBs)
Module level	j (number of units for unary current source)
	spreading of units across array
	switching sequence
Circuit level	$W_{\mathrm{M_{cur\_src}}}$, $L_{\mathrm{M_{cur\_src}}}$, $(V_{gs} - V_t)_{\mathrm{M_{cur\_src}}}$
	insert $\mathrm{M_{casc}}$ or not ?
	$W_{\mathrm{M_{casc}}}$, $L_{\mathrm{M_{casc}}}$, $(V_{gs} - V_t)_{\mathrm{M_{casc}}}$
	$W_{\mathrm{M_{sw}}}$, $L_{\mathrm{M_{sw}}}$
	latch transistor sizes
	clock driver

Table 6.2: Design parameters of the presented D/A-converter architecture.

The design parameters of the proposed segmented architecture are summarized in Table 6.2. Determining these parameters based on the performance specifications is the goal of the design process. Next, it will be explained how values for the performance specifications of the D/A-converter can be derived using behavioral modeling for the specification phase.

6.3 Behavioral Modeling for the Specification Phase

By using a complete hardware description language model of a D/A-converter, the designer can explore different solutions on the system level in terms of performance, power and area consumption [Vdbus 98b, Vdbus 99b]. In this way the high-level specifications of the system can be translated into specifications for the D/A-converter, as well as for the other blocks.

The generic behavioral model of the D/A-converter [Vdbus 98b, Vdbus 99b] is divided into a digital thermocoder (which performs the translation from binary to thermometer code) and an analog core which incorporates the latches and switches and the current source arrays. For the analog core SpectreHDL [SpectreHDL 98] was used to implement the model. The digital decoder was implemented in VHDL and simulated with Synopsys [Synopsys 98]. As an example the generic AHDL models for the dynamic behavior (glitch energy and settling time) and static behavior (INL and DNL) are presented next.

6.3.1 Dynamic Behavior

For the dynamic (transient) behavior of the D/A-converter, two specifications are taken into account: settling time $t_{settling}$ and glitch energy E_{glitch}. The settling time is mainly determined by the capacitance on the output node C_{out} and can be modeled as such in the behavioral model.

The glitch is not only dependent on the number of current sources switched when going from $level_i$ to $level_j$, but also on the choice of the number of bits l which steer the binary-weighted current source array.

A generic model of the glitch can be obtained by superposition of an exponentially damped sine and a shifted hyperbolic tangent [Vdbus 98b, Vdbus 99b]:

$$
\begin{aligned}
i_{out} = {} & A_{glitch} \sin\left(\frac{2\pi}{t_{glitch}}(t - t_0)\right) \exp\left(-\text{sign}(t - t_0)\frac{2\pi}{t_{glitch}}(t - t_0)\right) \\
& + \frac{level_j - level_i}{2} \tanh\left(\frac{2\pi}{t_{glitch}}(t - t_0)\right) + \frac{level_j + level_i}{2}
\end{aligned}
\tag{6.2}
$$

in which i_{out} is the output current, A_{glitch} is the amplitude and t_{glitch} the period of the glitch signal and $level_i$ and $level_j$ are the code levels between which the converter switches.

The glitch energy is defined as the integrated difference between the ideal and the measured response. This integral is approximated as the integral of half a period of the damped sine-wave minus the gray shaded triangle as depicted in figure 6.5. Using equation (6.2) this difference or glitch energy can be approximated by:

$$
\frac{E_{glitch}}{2R_{load}} nr_{switched} = \left[A_{glitch} \sin\left(\frac{2\pi}{5}\right) \exp\left(-\frac{2\pi}{5}\right) + \frac{level_j - level_i}{4} \left(\tanh\left(\frac{2\pi}{5}\right) - 1\right)\right] \frac{t_{glitch}}{4}
\tag{6.3}
$$

where $nr_{switched}$ is the number of current sources switched when going from $level_i$ to $level_j$, R_{load} is the resistive load applied to the converter and E_{glitch} is the glitch energy.

The results of this behavioral model of the glitch energy are depicted in figure 6.6. At time t_1 one current source is switched on; at time t_2 a larger number of current sources is switched on, which results in a larger glitch as can clearly be seen on figure 6.6. Notice also that at time

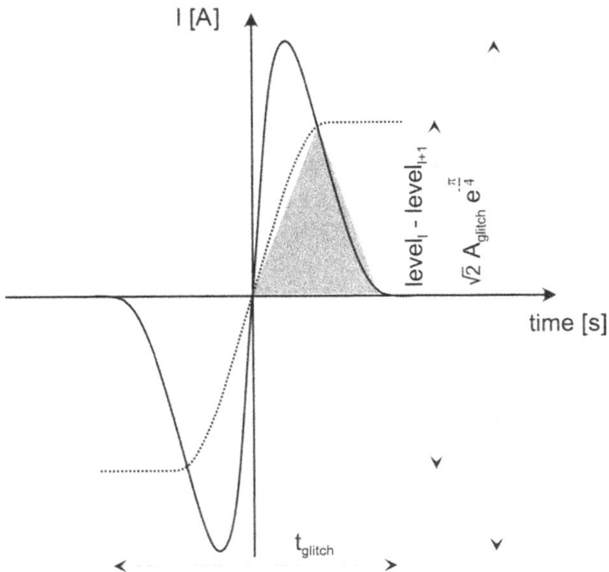

Figure 6.5: Calculation of the amplitude of the damped sine A_{glitch} in terms of the glitch energy E_{glitch}.

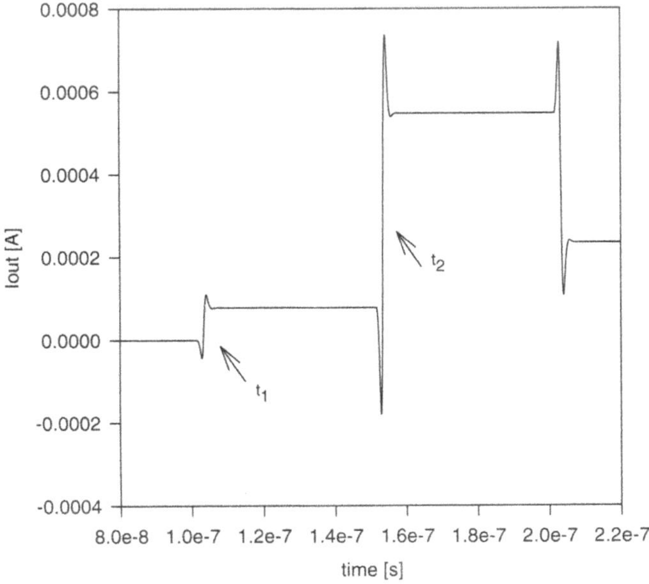

Figure 6.6: Time response of the behavioral model: at t_1 one additional current source is switched on; at t_2 several additional current sources are switched on.

t_1 as well as t_2 the overshoot of the glitch is smaller than the undershoot which is due to the settling behavior that was also incorporated in the model.

6.3.2 Static Behavior

The static behavior is determined by the INL and DNL specifications. These are modeled using a stochastic process, as follows. Let **p** be a vector of $2^n + w - 1$ independent random variables with a variance of 1. Then the statistical nonlinearity of the converter can be modeled as follows:

$$\Delta level_i = p_i + A \sum_{j=i+1}^{j=w+i+1} p_j \tag{6.4}$$

in which A is a real value, and w is an integer value.

The standard deviation of $\Delta level_i$ is then given by:

$$\sigma(\Delta level_i) = \sqrt{1 + (w-1)A^2} \tag{6.5}$$

and the standard deviation of $\Delta level_{i+1} - \Delta level_i$:

$$\sigma(\Delta level_{i+1} - \Delta level_i) = \sqrt{2(1 - A + A^2)} \tag{6.6}$$

Since

$$\text{INL} \propto \sigma(\Delta level_i) \tag{6.7}$$

$$\text{DNL} \propto \sigma(\Delta level_{i+1} - \Delta level_i) \tag{6.8}$$

the values of the unknowns A and w can be derived given values of INL and DNL. When the D/A-converter is simulated using this generic statistical model, it *statistically* exhibits the requested INL and DNL.

In this way the acceptable specifications for the D/A-converter can be derived by performing simulations at the system level. The design now continues with the synthesis part of the design flow, as shown in the center of figure 6.1 on page 147.

6.4 Synthesis Flow of the D/A-converter

Figure 6.7 shows the synthesis flow resulting from applying the hierarchical design methodology [Chang 96, Lam 98, Don 98] to the targeted high-speed, high-accuracy D/A-converter. It is a mixed-signal design and thus contains analog and digital design tasks.

The analog design flow is grouped on the left, the corresponding digital flow is grouped on the right. The analog flow consists of a hierarchical sizing at two levels: the architectural level and the device level. The digital synthesis completes the sizing part of the mixed-signal design. The design steps are verified using standard approaches (numerical verification with a simulator, at the behavioral, device or gate level).

In the bottom-up phase, the floorplanning is done jointly for analog and digital blocks. After this the layouts of the analog modules are generated using the **Mondriaan** tool [VdPlas 98],

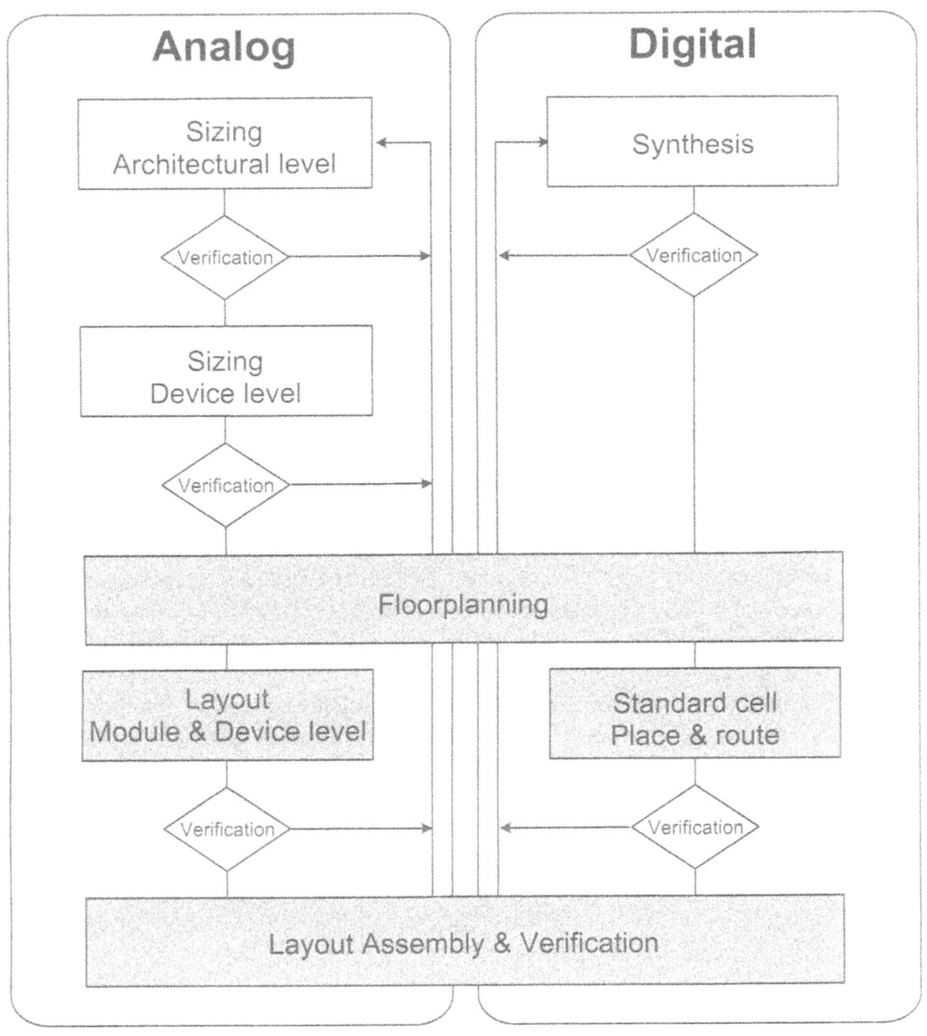

Figure 6.7: D/A-converter synthesis design flow.

which has been discussed in chapter 5 of this work. The decoder layout is created using standard cell place & route tools. Both layouts are separately verified. The blocks are assembled at the module level and again a module-level verification is done with standard tools.

Large parts of this design flow have been automated. To achieve this high degree of automation, both commercial EDA tools (simulators, digital synthesis tools, standard cell place & route tools, etc.) and general mathematical tools (Matlab) as well as in-house developed dedicated tools (**Mondriaan**, MIMI, C-optimizer, etc.) have been used.

6.5 Sizing Synthesis

The specifications that have been derived during the specification phase, are input to sizing synthesis. The design of the converter is performed hierarchically, as indicated in figure 6.7. Firstly some decisions on the architectural level have to be made. Thereafter the sizing of the transistors at the device level has to be done.

6.5.1 Architectural-level Synthesis

The two architectural-level parameters (l, m) are determined during architectural-level sizing synthesis. Two important performance criteria as listed in Table 6.2, are taken into account: *static* and *dynamic* performance.

6.5.1.1 Static Performance

The static behavior of a D/A-converter is specified in terms of INL and DNL. A distinction has to be made between *random* errors and *systematic* errors. The random error is determined solely by mismatch. The systematic errors are caused by process, temperature and electrical gradients. In optimally designed D/A-converters the INL and DNL are determined by random errors (i.e. *mismatch*) only. A small safety margin (20% of INL) is reserved to allow for *systematic* contributions. The DNL performance is by definition not higher than 2 × INL and is thus also automatically minimized. The *systematic* errors are layout determined and thus are minimized during layout generation by optimizing the switching scheme. This optimization is explained in section 6.6. Sufficient for now is that these systematic effects will be compensated for. The bounds on the random error effects are handled now.

The acceptable *random* error can be calculated from Monte-Carlo yield simulations. The tolerable relative standard deviation of current matching $(\sigma(I)/I)$ can thus be calculated [Bast 96b]. Figure 6.8 depicts the yield simulation for a 14-bit D/A-converter. The plot shown in figure 6.8 has been calculated using a Matlab [Matlab 99] program.

In the meantime in [VdBosch 00] an analytic formula has been presented that replaces the time-consuming Monte-Carlo simulations:

$$\frac{\sigma(I)}{I} < \frac{1}{2A\sqrt{2^n}} \tag{6.9}$$

where the tolerable relative standard deviation of current matching $(\sigma(I)/I)$ is linked to the number of bits n and a yield-determined parameter A, which is given by:

$$A = inv\_norm(0.5 + \frac{Yield_{\text{INL}}}{2}) \tag{6.10}$$

here *inv_norm(argument)* is the inverse function of the normal cumulative function integrated from *−argument* to *+argument*. The $Yield_{\text{INL}}$ is the wanted yield for an INL better than 0.5LSB. Consult [VdBosch 00] for a table with pre-calculated values of parameter A.

For a yield of 99.7%, the required relative current matching $(\sigma(I)/I)$ is 0.063% for a 14-bit D/A-converter calculated with the Monte-Carlo simulation and confirmed by the analytical formula, equation (6.9) of [VdBosch 00].

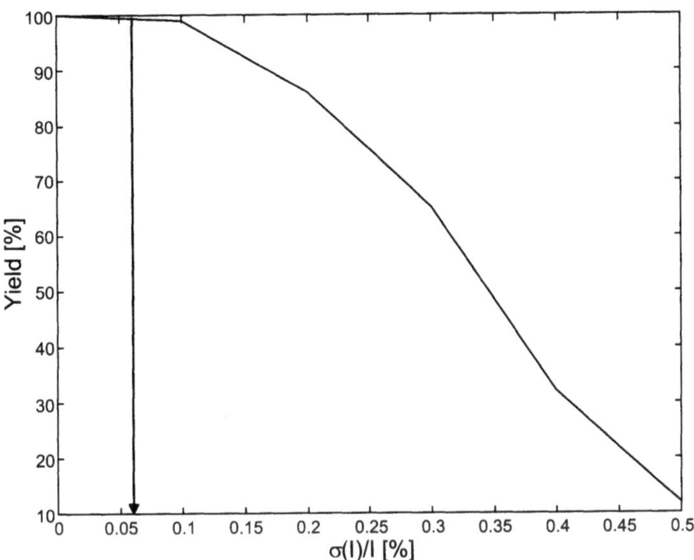

Figure 6.8: Yield as a function of unit current cell variance for a 14-bit D/A-converter (INL better than 0.5 LSB).

From the full swing (V_{out}), the number of bits (n) and load resistance (R_{load}) the current of one LSB (I_{LSB}) is calculated:

$$I_{\mathrm{LSB}} = \frac{V_{out}}{R_{load}\,(2^n - 1)} \approx \frac{V_{out}}{R_{load}\,2^n} \tag{6.11}$$

Then, an estimate for the active area of the current source transistor can be calculated based on the MOS mismatch model [Laksh 86, Pel 89]:

$$W_{\mathrm{LSB}} \times L_{\mathrm{LSB}} = \frac{I^2_{\mathrm{LSB}}}{2\,\sigma^2(I_{\mathrm{LSB}})}\left[A^2_\beta + \frac{A^2_{V_T}}{(V_{gs} - V_T)^2}\right] \tag{6.12}$$

where $\sigma(I_{\mathrm{LSB}})/I_{\mathrm{LSB}}$ is the unit current source standard deviation and A_β , A_{V_T} are technology mismatch constants [Laksh 86, Pel 89]. For minimal area the $V_{gs} - V_T$ is maximized. The lower bound for the area is given by:

$$(W_{\mathrm{LSB}} \times L_{\mathrm{LSB}})_{lowerbound} \approx \frac{I^2_{\mathrm{LSB}}}{2\,\sigma^2(I_{\mathrm{LSB}})} A^2_\beta \tag{6.13}$$

The total current source array area ($area_{cur\_src,est}$) can then be estimated:

$$area_{cur\_src,est} \approx 2^n\, f_{routing}\,(W_{\mathrm{LSB}} \times L_{\mathrm{LSB}})_{lowerbound} \tag{6.14}$$

where $f_{routing}$ is the routing overhead factor ($f_{routing} > 1$). The static performance places a strict constraint (lower bound) on the area of the current source array.

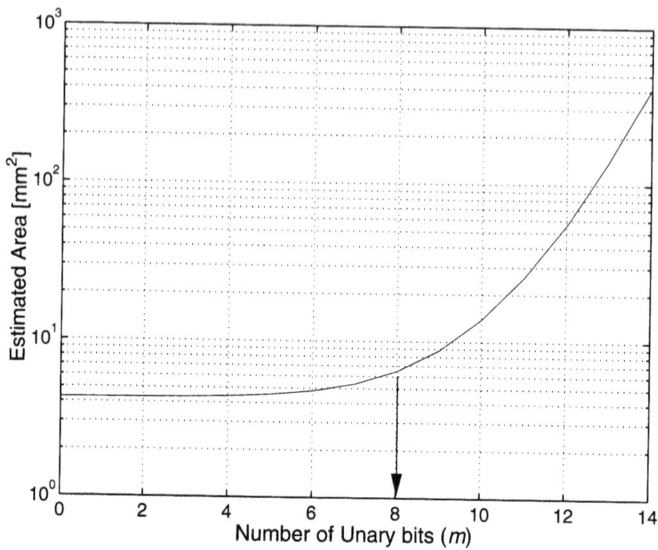

Figure 6.9: Estimated area of the D/A-converter as a function of the number of unary bits (m).

6.5.1.2 Dynamic Performance

The nonlinear *dynamic* behavior of a D/A-converter is usually specified in terms of admissible glitch energy. This specification is mainly determined by (1) the number of bits implemented binary/unary (l, m), and (2) the way the current sources are synchronized when switched on/off. The largest glitch will occur when switching off all binary implemented bits and switching on the first unary current source. This implies that the decision on the number of bits l to be implemented binary and the number of bits m to be implemented unary, determines the worst-case glitch.

The lowest possible glitch energy is obtained when a full unary implementation is chosen [Lin 98]. This would however result in a large area increase. The total core chip area ($area_{core,est}$) is estimated by:

$$area_{core,est} = area_{cur\_src,est} + area_{swatch,est} + area_{decoder,est}(l, m) + area_{routing,est}(l, m) \quad (6.15)$$

The area of the current source array is fixed by equation (6.13) as is the area of the swatch array ($area_{swatch,est}$). However, the area of the thermocoder increases ($\propto 2^m$), as does the size of the routing buses connecting the three modules, if the number of unary bits (m) is increased. Figure 6.9 shows that in submicron technologies (in this particular case 0.5μm) an optimal number of unary-implemented bits is 8, otherwise the total area of converter grows unacceptably due to the increase of the decoder (digital standard cell count) and routing area components. This choice will ultimately limit the *dynamic* performance of the D/A-converter.

The quantization noise of the D/A-converter can readily be calculated since the number of bits is specified. An ideal n-bit D/A-converter has a peak *SNR* (over the Nyquist band) given in dB by:

$$SNR_{ideal} = 6.02 \cdot n + 1.76 \tag{6.16}$$

assuming uniform quantization steps and a full-scale sinusoidal input [vdPlassche 94, Raz 95]. This value is the upper limit of SNR that can be obtained. The thermal noise, caused by the transistors (section 6.5.2.2 on page 160), will be added to the quantization noise and result in the total SNR of the D/A-converter.

6.5.2 Circuit-level Synthesis

The circuit-level synthesis determines the circuit-level design parameters, as shown in Table 6.2. Again the two performance constraints (*static* and *dynamic*) are taken into account.

6.5.2.1 Static Performance

The active area of the unit current source array has been calculated from mismatch constraints (see equation (6.12)). A high biasing voltage ($V_{gs}-V_T$) is preferred for mismatch reasons. The upper limit for the biasing voltage is determined by the output swing (switching transistors M_{sw} need to be in the saturation region) and the power supply. From equation (6.11) and (6.12), W_{cur_src} and L_{cur_src} can be calculated given a choice of $V_{gs} - V_T$:

$$\left.\begin{array}{l} \frac{2\sigma^2(I_{\text{LSB}})}{I^2_{\text{LSB}}} = \frac{A^2_\beta}{W_{\text{LSB}} \times L_{\text{LSB}}} + \frac{4\,A^2_{V_T}}{W_{\text{LSB}} \times L_{\text{LSB}} (V_{gs}-V_T)^2_{\text{LSB}}} \\ (V_{gs} - V_T)_{\text{LSB}} \approx 1\,\text{Volt} \end{array}\right\} \Rightarrow W_{\text{LSB}} \times L_{\text{LSB}} \tag{6.17}$$

$$I_{\text{LSB}} = KP \frac{W_{\text{LSB}}}{L_{\text{LSB}}} \frac{(V_{gs} - V_T)^2}{2} \quad \Rightarrow \quad \frac{W_{\text{LSB}}}{L_{\text{LSB}}} \tag{6.18}$$

A second source of nonlinearity is the finite output impedance of the current source. The output impedance of the D/A-converter is given by [Raz 95]:

$$R_{output} = R_{load} \parallel \frac{R_{cur\_src}}{\text{code}} \qquad \text{code:} \quad 0 \rightarrow 2^n - 1 \tag{6.19}$$

where R_{load} is the load resistance, code is the number of sources switched on to the output and R_{cur_src} is the output impedance of the current source (including switch transistor) given by:

$$R_{\text{cur\_src}} \approx gm_{\text{M}_{\text{sw}}} ro_{\text{M}_{\text{sw}}} ro_{\text{M}_{\text{cur\_src}}} \tag{6.20}$$

This nonlinear impedance causes deterioration of the INL given by [Raz 95]:

$$\text{INL} \approx \frac{R_{load}\,(2^n - 1)^2}{4\,R_{cur\_src}} \tag{6.21}$$

The optional cascode transistor M_{casc} is inserted if the output impedance is too low.

These calculations resulting in the sizing of the current source transistors (M_{cur_src} and M_{casc}) have been implemented in a Matlab [Matlab 99] script. For a 14-bit D/A-converter this gives a W of 1.125μm and an L of 104.5μm in a standard 1P3M 0.5μm CMOS technology.

6.5.2.2 Dynamic Performance

In order not to deteriorate the *dynamic* performance, the following factors are taken into account in the circuit-level synthesis [Wu 95, VdBosch 98]: (1) synchronize the control signals of the switching transistors, (2) reduce voltage fluctuation in the drains of the current sources, (3) carefully switch the current source transistor on/off. The synchronization of the control signals is achieved by adding a latch immediately in front of the switching transistors M_{sw} (shown in figure 6.3 on page 150). The voltage fluctuation at the drain changes the current from the current source because of the finite output impedance of the current source transistor M_{cur_src}. The problem can be solved by using a large channel length for the current source transistor, and tuning the crossing point of the switching control signals such that both switches are never switched off simultaneously [VdBosch 98, Vdbus 99a].

Using a device-level simulator (for instance Hspice [Hspice Manual 99]) in an optimization loop, the latch and the switches are sized, taking the crossing point and speed as constraints in the optimization process. This determines the sizing of the switches and latch.

The influence of circuit noise on the circuit can be approximated as follows [Wikn 99]:

$$\text{SNR} \approx 3n - 6 + 20\log(I_{LSB}) - 10\log(\overline{i_{LSB}^2}) \tag{6.22}$$

where the SNR is expressed in dB and I_{LSB} is the current of one LSB and $\overline{i_{LSB}^2}$ is the total noise power corresponding to one LSB.

The basic circuit is a current source, be it a single transistor or cascode current source [Wikn 99]. If the impedance of the cascode is low enough, the only contribution to the noise is coming from the current source transistor:

$$i_n^2(f) = 4kT\frac{2}{3}g_m \approx 4kT\frac{2}{3}\frac{2I}{V_{gs} - V_T} \tag{6.23}$$

where $i_n^2(f)$ is the noise spectral density caused by a transistor in saturation. The total normalized noise power for a given bandwidth (BW) is then:

$$\overline{i_{LSB}^2} = i_n^2(f) \cdot BW \approx 4kT\frac{2}{3}\frac{2I_{LSB}}{(V_{gs} - V_T)_{LSB}} \cdot BW \tag{6.24}$$

Substituting equation (6.24) in equation (6.22) gives for the SNR [Wikn 99]:

$$\text{SNR} \approx 3n - 6 + 10\log(I_{LSB}) - 10\log\left(\frac{8}{3}kT\frac{2}{(V_{gs} - V_T)_{LSB}}BW\right) \tag{6.25}$$

For a 14-bit D/A-converter with a I_{LSB} current of 1.22μA, bandwidth (BW) of 75MHz and biased as calculated in the previous paragraph this gives a (theoretical) thermal SNR of 94dB. The thermal SNR is in reality thus dominated by quantization noise. This performance constraint does not influence the design, as predicted by [King 96b]. In [King 96b] it is stated that mismatch requirements are stronger than noise requirements in 2.5μm to 0.7μm technologies for A/D-converters and filters. Theoretically (i.e. calculations based on linear single transistor stages), when the mismatch requirements for accuracy are achieved, the thermal noise level is approximately 20dB lower or better and this performance specification (SNR) is automatically fulfilled. This is confirmed in this design for current-steering D/A-converters, although the margin is only approximately 10dB: the thermal SNR is 94dB, the mismatch accuracy for a static linear 14-bit converter (INL $<$ 0.5LSB) is 86dB.

This concludes the circuit-level sizing synthesis of the analog blocks: the current source and swatch cells. The digital decoder is synthesized next.

6.5.3 Full Decoder Synthesis

Since the architectural parameters (l, m) and the latch transistor sizes are now known, the thermocoder can be synthesized.

In our case the number of output lines of the thermo encoder increases with 2^m, where m is the number of bits, resulting in complex logic and large input capacitance, which have to be carefully buffered. This complexity exceeds the behavioral synthesis capabilities of commonly used commercial tools like Synopsys, and a special VHDL implementation using lookup tables was developed. The encoder is realized in two steps: coarse and fine encoding. An example will clarify this.

0	**1**	**2**	**3**	**4**	**5**	**6**	**7**	**8**	**9**	**A**	**B**	**C**	**D**	**E**	**F**
1	1	1	1	1	1	1	1	1	1	1	1	1	1	1	1
0	1	1	1	1	1	1	1	1	1	1	1	1	1	1	1
0	0	1	1	1	1	1	1	1	1	1	1	1	1	1	1
0	0	0	1	1	1	1	1	1	1	1	1	1	1	1	1
0	0	0	0	1	1	1	1	1	1	1	1	1	1	1	1
0	0	0	0	0	1	1	1	1	1	1	1	1	1	1	1
0	0	0	0	0	0	1	1	1	1	1	1	1	1	1	1
0	0	0	0	0	0	0	1	1	1	1	1	1	1	1	1
0	0	0	0	0	0	0	0	1	1	1	1	1	1	1	1
0	0	0	0	0	0	0	0	0	1	1	1	1	1	1	1
0	0	0	0	0	0	0	0	0	0	1	1	1	1	1	1
0	0	0	0	0	0	0	0	0	0	0	1	1	1	1	1
0	0	0	0	0	0	0	0	0	0	0	0	1	1	1	1
0	0	0	0	0	0	0	0	0	0	0	0	0	1	1	1
0	0	0	0	0	0	0	0	0	0	0	0	0	0	1	1
0	0	0	0	0	0	0	0	0	0	0	0	0	0	0	1

Table 6.3: Truth table for the thermometer encoder ($m = 4$)

Table 6.3 gives the thermometer encoder specification in case of four bits ($m = 4$). If we look at the truth table from a high level (*coarse* encoding) three different $2^{m/2} \times 2^{m/2}$ submatrices can be distinguished: the lower diagonal matrices which consist completely of zeros (6 submatrices in Table 6.3); the upper diagonal matrices which consist completely of ones (6 submatrices); and finally the diagonal itself (4 submatrices), the truth table of which

(a)

00	01	10	11
x	1	1	1
0	x	1	1
0	0	x	1
0	0	0	x

(b)

00	01	10	11
1	1	1	1
0	1	1	1
0	0	1	1
0	0	0	1

(c)

00	01	10	11
1	0	0	0
0	1	0	0
0	0	1	0
0	0	0	1

Table 6.4: Truth table for the different coders ($m = 4$): (a) coarse encoder, (b) fine encoder, (c) address decoder.

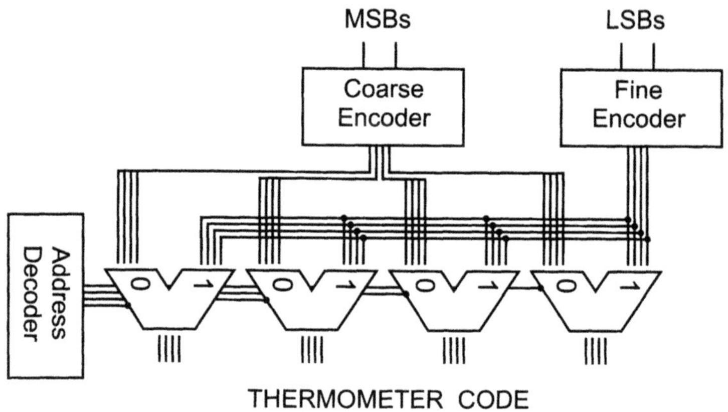

Figure 6.10: Schematic of the table look-up based thermometer encoder.

will be referred to as the *fine* encoding. The truth table for the overall *coarse* encoding is depicted in Table 6.4(a), where a **zero** stands for lower diagonal, **one** stands for upper diagonal, and **x** stands for fine encoding. The truth table for the fine encoding is given in Table 6.4(b).

The implementation of the thermometer encoder using *fine* and *coarse* encoders is schematically shown in figure 6.10: the address decoder decides whether at the coarse level the diagonal submatrices, the upper diagonal submatrices (**ones**), or the lower diagonal submatrices (**zeros**) are used. The address decoder steers the different multiplexers, resulting in the correct thermometer code. The truth table for the address decoder is given in Table 6.4(c).

This two step look-up table implementation of the 8-bit thermometer encoder ($m = 8$) was synthesized with a standard cell library. An additional pipeline was inserted to meet the timing constraints. The remaining l LSBs are delayed by the equalizer block to have the same overall delay. The full decoder is synthesized using Synopsys [Synopsys 98] starting from a VHDL description.

6.5.4 Clock Driver Synthesis

The clock driver generates the clocking signals for the full decoder and swatch array. Both these modules (decoder and swatch array) have been sized already and thus their capacitive clock input load is known. Two inverter chains (scaled exponentially) have been designed to drive the required load including the wiring capacitance. One drives the analog latches, the other drives the digital decoder. Both are synchronized with each other to ensure proper data transmission between the two blocks.

6.6 Layout Generation

Current-steering D/A-converters are a typical example of layout-driven analog design. The sized schematic alone does not constitute an operational converter. An important part of the performance is determined by the handling of layout-induced parasitics and error components (i.e. systematic errors).

All classical countermeasures for avoiding coupling from the digital blocks to the analog blocks [Su 93, Ghar 96, Ing 00] (guard rings, shielding, separate supplies, ...) and standard matching guidelines (equal orientation, dummies, ...) have been applied and will not be further discussed. We will concentrate here on the extra required layout measures.

6.6.1 Floorplanning

The floorplan proposed in figure 6.3 is now refined. The relative position of the blocks is already fixed, what still has to be to determined are the aspect ratios of the different modules and most importantly the pitch of the buses connecting the modules. From equation (6.15) the estimated area of the converter is available, as are the area estimates of the three modules. When this area estimate is combined with the wanted global aspect ratio (*aspect_ratio*) the *width* and *height* of the D/A-converter core can be calculated:

$$width_{core,est} = \sqrt{area_{core,est} aspect\_ratio_{core}} \tag{6.26}$$

$$height_{core,est} = \sqrt{\frac{area_{core,est}}{aspect\_ratio_{core}}} \tag{6.27}$$

Typically the wanted $aspect\_ratio_{core}$ is 1, or a square chip layout is requested. From the thus obtained $width_{core,est}$ the wire pitch of the buses connecting the modules in the D/A-converter core can then be determined:

$$pitch \approx \frac{width_{core,est}}{\#wires} \tag{6.28}$$

where the $\#wires$ is given by the degree of segmentation or the number of bits l that are implemented binary and the number of bits m that are implemented unary:

$$\#wires = l + 2^m - 1 \tag{6.29}$$

This results in a *pitch* of approximately 10μm in the case of the 14-bit D/A-converter in a standard 1P3M 0.5μm CMOS technology. This value is not yet *final*, it is a reference value that will be utilized to obtain a high-quality layout. The layout of the current source array is generated first, since it is the most critical and largest module, and it will determine the final value of the *pitch*. Once this final pitch value is determined, the layout generation of the different modules is *decoupled* and can take place in parallel.

6.6.2 Current Source Array Layout Generation

The sizes of the LSB current source (W_{LSB} and L_{LSB}) have been determined. From this the sizes of all other weighted current sources and the unary current source are easily derived. To have optimal matching properties, the current source must be built up from identical basic units.

How these units are connected and where they are placed, the cell assignment, are the last design parameters of the design, see Table 6.2. The error sources that cannot be eliminated by design (sizing) and therefore must be compensated by the switching scheme, are:

- voltage drops in biasing wires, power supply wires, ...
- edge effects
- metal coverage
- temperature gradients
- distance effect
- technology process gradients

In this list a number of categories can be considered. First there are systematic effects of which the size is known precisely (such as voltage drops). Secondly there are systematic effects of which the exact size is not known (edge effects, metal coverage, temperature gradients). Thirdly there are random effects (distance effect, process gradients [Maly 86, Chang 00]) of which the size is not exactly known, but their profile shape does give extra information.

The current error caused by the voltage drop in the ground lines [Miki 86, Naka 91] can be approximated by a quadratic curve:

$$(\frac{\Delta I}{I})_{voltage\_drop} = \sqrt{gmR_{gnd}}\,\frac{\cosh(\sqrt{gmR_{gnd}}\,x)}{\sinh(\sqrt{gmR_{gnd}})} \approx a_0 + a_2 x^2 + \ldots \tag{6.30}$$

where x is the coordinate (or position) of the current source, gm is the transconductance of the current source, R_{gnd} is the resistance of the ground line, and it is assumed that the current source array has a horizontal supply line, connected on both sides.

In [Bast 98a] the effect of the switching sequence on the contribution of the ground line voltage drop to the INL specification has been investigated. For the sequential switching sequence of [Miki 86] the following $\mathrm{INL}_{seq,gnd}$ is obtained:

$$\mathrm{INL}_{seq,gnd} \approx \frac{gmR_{gnd}}{9\sqrt{3}} \tag{6.31}$$

In order to have an INL error of less than 0.5LSB, the ground line resistance must then be smaller than 3.8Ω for a 12-bit D/A-converter. This value is *not* met when using minimal width metal wires with a length of 1 to 4mm (this length is imposed because of MOS matching constraints on the minimal dimensions of the transistors). In this calculation it has been assumed that the metal sheet resistance is approximately 50mΩ/□, a typical value for submicron processes.

The symmetrical switching sequence of [Naka 91] reduces the problem of ground line voltage drop in high-accuracy D/A-converters. The symmetrical switching sequence suppresses the contribution to INL [Bast 98a] by a factor of four compared to the sequential switching sequence:

$$\mathrm{INL}_{sym,gnd} \approx \frac{gmR_{gnd}}{36\sqrt{3}} \tag{6.32}$$

Or a 14-bit accuracy requires once again a resistance smaller than 3.8Ω. This is *not* met with minimal-width metal lines. The cancellation of the ground line voltage thus requires additional attention. This will be discussed in subsection 6.6.2.4.

Secondly, in a matrix of cells there is a certain edge effect [Pava 94, JoMa 97, Hast 01]. The processing of a silicon device within an array of identical devices is different from a device situated at the edge of the array. This is because etching processes have a different activity at these different positions [Vit 85, Malo 94, Pava 94, Hast 01]. To avoid this sudden effect a row or column of *dummy* devices is added to the array of identical devices [Vit 85, Malo 94, Pava 94, Hast 01]. These devices will have different electrical properties but are unused. This error source is thus compensated.

Thirdly, in [Tuin 97] the effect of metal coverage on the matching of MOS transistors is described. A substantial mismatch error has been reported for MOS transistors not covered by the same metal layers. It is thus preferable to cover every single unit in the current source array with the same metal layers. This error source can thus be compensated if a layout is generated with this requirement.

The last error sources are thermal gradients and technology-related errors (e.g. doping, oxide thickness gradients, distance effect, ...). The size of these errors is not known without characterization. Nevertheless they can be approximated by a Taylor series expansion around the center of the current source array:

$$\Delta I_{\text{Temp, technology}}(x, y) \approx b_0 + b_1\,x + b_2\,y + b_3\,xy + b_4\,x^2 + b_5\,y^2 + \ldots \tag{6.33}$$

where (x,y) are the coordinates of the unit in the current source array.

The current source array thus contains units with errors which are (to first order) *linear* and *quadratic* in spatial distribution. Let us call these spatial error profiles $\epsilon_{sp}^{(1)}(x, y)$ and $\epsilon_{sp}^{(2)}(x, y)$ for first and second order respectively. In [Miki 86, Lin 98] every current source is implemented as one single unit (as shown in figure 6.11(a) and (b)), concentrated at one position, having a total residual error $\epsilon_{res}(x, y)$ equal to the spatial error:

$$\epsilon_{res}^{\text{unsplit}}(x, y) = \epsilon_{sp}^{(1)}(x, y) + \epsilon_{sp}^{(2)}(x, y) \tag{6.34}$$

In the case of 8- and 10-bit D/A-converters this error is sufficiently low. The 10-bit D/A-converter presented in [Lin 98] already uses systematic error compensation by applying biasing separately for each quadrant of the current source array. In the 12-bit D/A-converter presented in [Bast 98b], every current source is split into four units of 1/4 the value in four

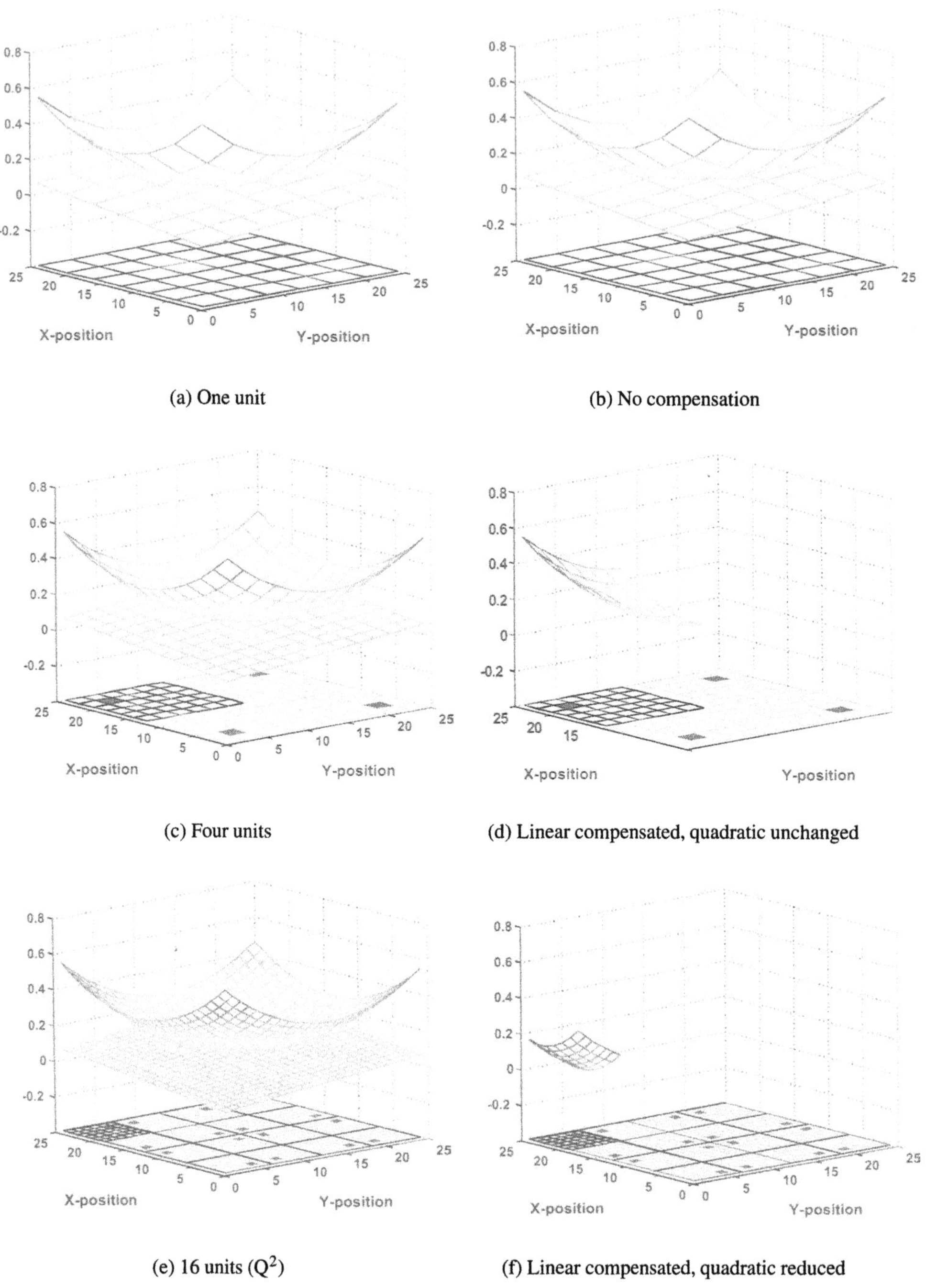

(a) One unit

(b) No compensation

(c) Four units

(d) Linear compensated, quadratic unchanged

(e) 16 units (Q^2)

(f) Linear compensated, quadratic reduced

Figure 6.11: Relative current errors.

different locations (as shown in figure 6.11(c) and (d)). By splitting the current source, a spatial averaging of the error is achieved. When the distribution of the current source transistors is symmetric around the **X** and **Y** axes, the linear terms are compensated (as is the case with all odd higher-order terms of the Taylor series expansion). However the quadratic errors are left unaltered (as is the case with all even higher-order terms of the Taylor series expansion):

$$\epsilon_{res}^{4\text{ units}}(x, y) = \epsilon_{sp}^{(2)}(x, y) \tag{6.35}$$

The residual error distribution for a basic segment is shown in figure 6.11(c) and (d) on the right-side plot. In order to suppress the quadratic error, the current source must be split in a higher number of current source units. By splitting the current source in 16 units as depicted in figure 6.11(e) and (f), the systematic and graded errors are suppressed by a factor of four in the **X** direction and a factor of eight in the **Y** direction:

$$\epsilon_{res}^{16\text{ units}}(x, y) = \frac{\epsilon_{sp}^{(2)}(x)}{4} + \frac{\epsilon_{sp}^{(2)}(y)}{8} \tag{6.36}$$

where the quadratic spatial errors have been split in an x and y component. This switching scheme will be referred to as Quad Quadrant (Q^2) as four (quad) units in every quadrant all together compose one current source.

A test chip was fabricated to investigate the different layout-degrading effects. The results of this test chip will now be discussed first. Using this test chip a second implementation has been successfully designed.

6.6.2.1 Floorplan of the Test Chip's Current Source Array

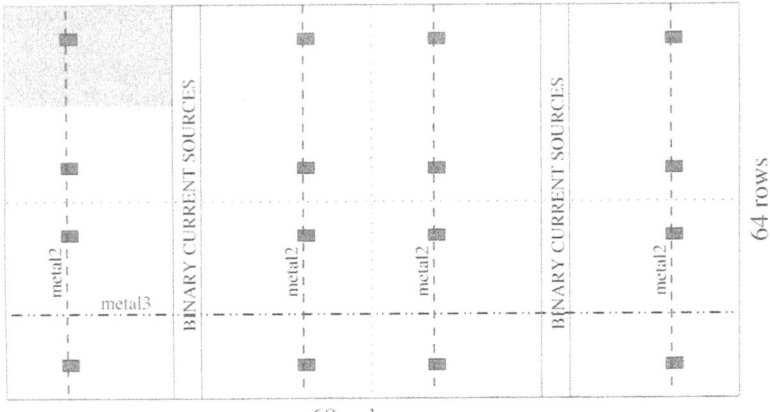

Figure 6.12: Floorplan of the current source array of the 14-bit D/A-converter test chip.

The current source array is implemented as one large, uniform array of units. The floorplan of the array is shown in figure 6.12. Its size is 68 columns by 64 rows. The 16 units per unary current source are connected as indicated on the figure. The power and biasing is provided with horizontal metal1 lines. The units are flipped every next row to share the power and biasing lines between two rows. The units forming one unary current source are connected with metal2 lines vertically and with metal3 lines horizontally. The unary units are completely covered with metal1, metal2 and metal3.

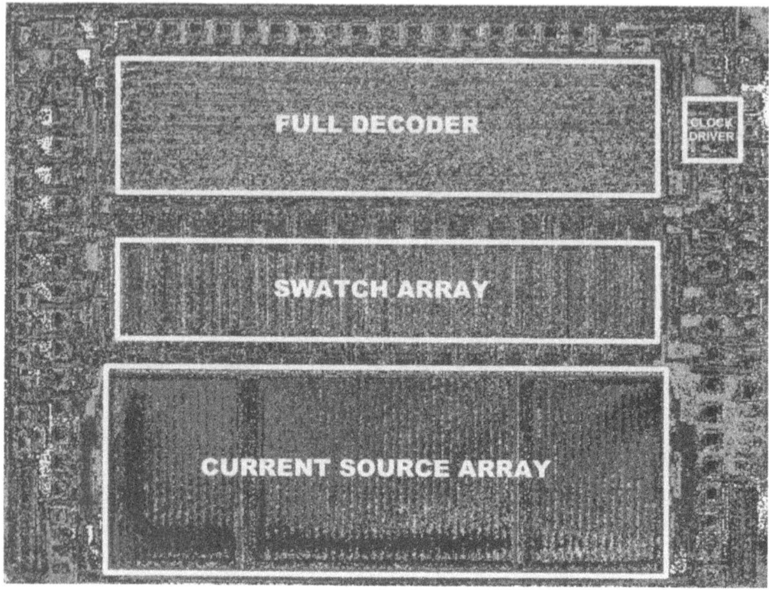

Figure 6.13: Microphotograph of the 14-bit D/A-converter test chip.

The binary units are spread across four columns at the positions indicated: two columns in the middle of the left half of the matrix, two columns in the middle of the right half. The binary units are connected through metal2 and metal3 lines. Only in this case less metal2 lines are required. This results in less coverage of the binary current sources by metal2 lines. This can clearly be seen in the lower array on figure 6.13: the lower density of metal2 lines is visually observable.

On the chip photo in figure 6.13, the decoder can be seen at the top of the chip. In the middle the swatch array is situated. A clock driver (in the top-right corner) completes the chip, to make it a fully functional D/A-converter.

6.6.2.2 Test Chip Measurements

In figure 6.14, a differential nonlinearity (DNL) measurement is shown of this 14-bit D/A-converter. From this plot the errors of individual unary current sources can be extracted, and associated with their location on the silicon. So using the measurement results shown in figure 6.14 and the used switching scheme, the individual errors of the *unary* current sources are extracted. It must be noted that the current errors relate to the sum of 16 individual units spread across the matrix as indicated on figure 6.12. The extracted profile is shown in fig-

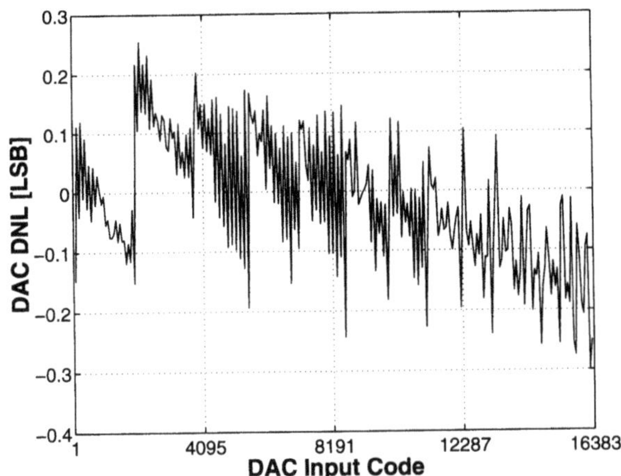

Figure 6.14: DNL measurement of the 14-bit D/A-converter test chip.

ures 6.15(a) and (b). The virtual location of the sources on these figures is the location of the top left quadrant shown in grey on figure 6.12.

As can be clearly seen on the error profiles, the errors are not at all caused by purely random mismatch. There is a strong correlation between position and error. In fact the noise seen on the plots is more related to measurement noise than to actual mismatch.

The data is now analyzed as in [Pava 94]. Therefore we average the errors of the current sources in both the horizontal and vertical direction. The resulting error profiles are shown in figures 6.15(c) and (d).

Consider now figure 6.15(c). It shows the average error of the current sources in column 1 up till column 16. In reality the current in column 1 of this plot is the sum of all current units in columns 1, 34, 35 and 68. It can clearly be seen that the first three *virtual* columns of the matrix suffer from what is known as the edge effect. Since beyond columns 1 and 68 no dummy sources are laid out, the etching of the devices deviates from the etching inside the array. This effect is felt up till column three. Expressed as a distance this is about 100μm. As predicted in [Pava 94], for NMOS transistors the current in the sources at the edges is lower than the current in the bulk of the matrix.

On the right side of the plot also a drop in current is noticeable. The current plotted there is the one generated by the neighbors of the binary current sources, the units in columns 16, 19, 50 and 53. This is explained by the fact that the metal coverage of the binaries is different (less metal2 wires), and was predicted in [Tuin 97]. The matching of identical MOS transistors is adversely affected by metal coverage.

The vertical dimension of the current source matrix is smaller. This is because the unit is flat and the matrix is approximately square: 64 by 68 units. Therefore the error profile is less pronounced, see figure 6.15(d). The edge effect is now only visible on one side. This can be explained by the fact that on the center of the rows no binary devices have been inserted. There is only one *virtual* edge. What however remains unexplained is the fact that a drop is noticed at the edge, followed by an increase in the average current for row two. This is not

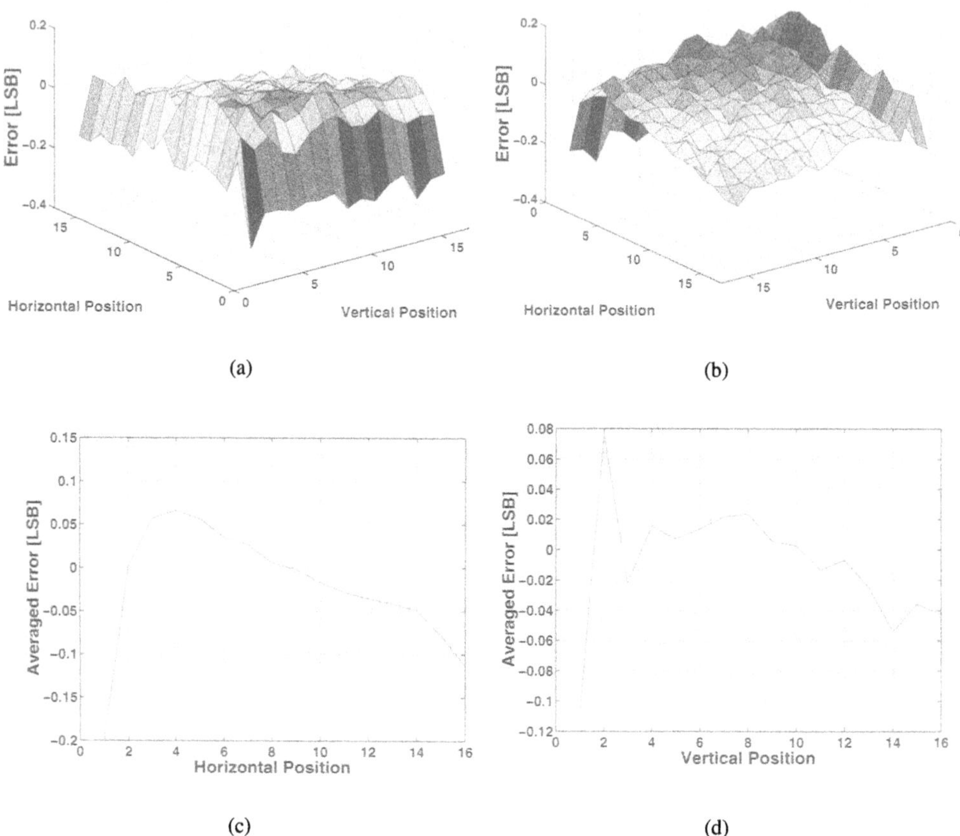

Figure 6.15: The errors of the unary current sources in the matrix: (a) error surface, (b) opposite angle error surface, (c) averaged horizontal error and (d) averaged vertical error.

predicted by [Pava 94] and no obvious explanation could be found. The distances are also much lower for the row edge effect, although also the third row could be considered to have edge effect related errors. This distance amounts to about 50μm, compared to the 100μm of the columns.

Finally, on the horizontal error, when the edges are not considered, half of a parabola curve is visible. This is exactly the signature of the quadratic error discussed in equation (6.36): $\epsilon_{sp}^{(2)}(x)$. In the vertical direction this error is not visible. This is explained by the much smaller height of the current source array (note also the difference of the scale on figures 6.15(c) and (d); the vertical error is much smaller than the horizontal error).

6.6.2.3 Revised Guidelines and Conclusions

In Table 6.5 the matching rules proposed by [Vit 85] are summarized. These rules of course apply for high-accuracy applications, as for instance the D/A-converters that are the subject of this work, and could also be of use in other high-accuracy MOS applications.

1.	Same structure
2.	Same temperature
3.	Same shape, same size
4.	Minimum distance
5.	Common-centroid geometries
6.	Same orientation
7.	Same surroundings
8.	Non minimum size

Table 6.5: Rules for optimum matching.

A few additional remarks can be formulated when the measurement results of the test chip are taken into account:

- *Same surroundings* has often been interpreted as being a rule which is equivalent to adding *one* row and *one* column of dummy devices around a matrix. This is not always sufficient. In fact it depends on the requested accuracy, technology and probably orientation of the devices to determine how far the edges of a matrix are felt (due to unequal surroundings) and thus how many rows and columns of dummy cells are required. In our case the results of figures 6.15(c) and (d) indicate that at least three dummy rows/columns would be required to avoid the *same surroundings* effect, irrespective of the direction.

- Same metal coverage has been reported as being important for matching in [Tuin 97]. In this test chip this is confirmed. The absence of metal2 wires on the neighbors of the binary current cells is being felt. So the same surroundings rule should be complemented with same metal coverage across the complete matrix.

- The use of common-centroid geometries [LakSan 94b] can be extended with the following remark. There is an optimum splitting for matching equal devices. If the sources are split in too few units, the systematic effects will cause large mismatches. By splitting in more units, all these (spatial) systematic effects are spatially averaged. Splitting in too much units does not bring any additional improvement, while the cost (extra wiring and parasitic resistance/capacitance) goes up. There is thus an optimal splitting and spreading of current sources for D/A-converters.

These revised guidelines are taken into account for generating the layout of the current source array in our final design. The extracted errors of figure 6.15 will be used as an estimation of the size of the error profiles for this design.

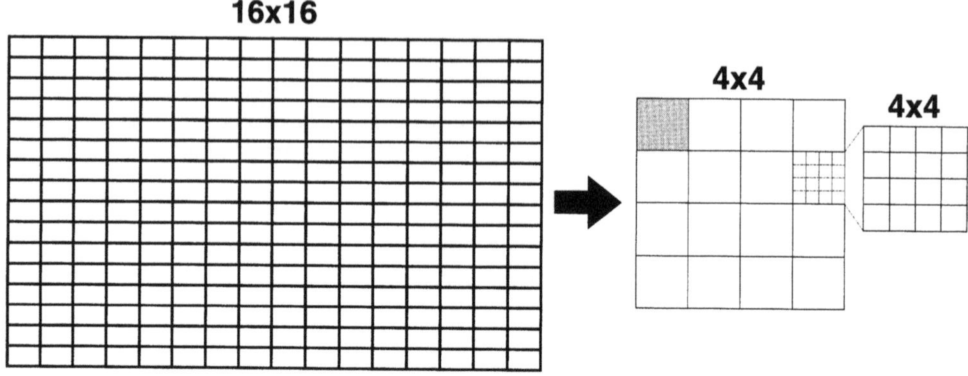

Figure 6.16: Hierarchical approach to optimize the switching sequence of 256 sources.

6.6.2.4 The Optimized Switching Sequence

The linearity of the D/A-converter is now determined by the accumulation of the residual errors when the current sources are switched on one by one. It is essential to keep the accumulated error as low as possible, or in other words to turn on current sources in a sequence such that the systematic error residues are not accumulating. Note that some current sources have a residual error higher than average (positive DNL) while others have a residual error below the average (negative DNL). This leads us to the choice of the switching sequence for the 8–6 segmented 14-bit D/A-converter. If quadratic errors are taken into account and using the Quad Quadrant scheme of figure 6.11(e) and (f), an error residue as shown in figure 6.11(f) is found in every quadrant (adapted to the extracted measurement results). Only 255 current sources are required for the D/A-converter function. So one of the 256 current sources is used as biasing circuit.

The switching sequence of the 255 unary current sources is an important design parameter to limit the INL. Therefore, to select the sequence of the current sources and determine the best switching scheme (256! possible solutions), an optimization has been undertaken. The goal is to *randomize* the different error contributions (positive and negative) so that no error accumulation occurs. The large number of possible solutions (256!) makes direct optimization infeasible. A *divide and conquer* approach has been chosen: divide the problem into two more tractable problems. The 16×16 current source matrix of cells with the above quadratic-like error residue (which is calculated from the assumed error profile), is divided into sixteen 4×4 regions as shown in figure 6.16. The switching sequence of these regions of current sources (A–P) will be optimized to compensate for the quadratic-like residual errors. Since the sixteen current sources in every 4×4 region do not have exactly the same residue, there still is a remaining small second-order residue within every 4×4 region. This can be approximated as linear and the switching sequence within each 4×4 region therefore will be optimized to compensate for these linear-like second-order residues.

The problem of the switching sequence has thus been reduced to two lower complexity problems. The first one is the optimization of the sequence of sixteen current source regions in a 4×4 matrix subject to quadratic errors. This problem has 16! different solutions. The second is the optimization of the switching sequence of sixteen current sources in a 4×4 matrix subject to linear error profiles and also has 16! possible solutions.

Let's first concentrate on the quadratic sequence optimization problem. Assume that every current source region has an absolute error which is quadratically dependent on its position:

$$\epsilon^{(1)}(x, y) = a_0 + a_1 x^2 + a_2 y^2 \tag{6.37}$$

where a_0 has been added to ensure the average error of all current source (regions) is zero. If the problem would be in one dimension (for instance x only, $a_2 = 0$), the size or sign (a_1) of the error doesn't matter for the optimization: the error is suppressed as good as possible, its INL contribution will depend on the size and the sign of the errors only:

$$\mathrm{INL}^{(1)}_{systematic} = f(a_1) \tag{6.38}$$

Unfortunately it has been found in the test chip that in both directions a residual, systematic error is found. The error in the vertical direction is much smaller than the error in the horizontal direction. There is however no reason to believe that the error profiles will always be exactly like the ones measured on the test chip. Therefore the only reasonable assumptions that can be made are the following (these have been taken into account to define the cost function of the optimization problem):

- the horizontal error will be larger than the vertical one, at least a factor of two
- the size and sign of the vertical error is unknown, relative to the horizontal error — they can have the same sign or not, with a preference for equal sign

The cost function of the optimization is then defined as follows. Look for the switching sequence that minimizes the INL of the two-dimensional error profile whereby the sign of the errors is the same and where the size of the vertical error is half the size of the horizontal error, and within these profiles look for one that minimizes the INL of the error profiles with the same sizes but having opposite signs.

The optimization algorithm then generates all 16! sequences and searches for the sequences obeying this criterion. The search tree is bounded as soon as the INL exceeds the already obtained minimal value. This can be done since the intermediate INL can be calculated when k sources have been selected:

$$\mathrm{INL}(i) = \sum_{j=0}^{j=i} \epsilon^{(1)}(x_j, y_j) \tag{6.39}$$

$$\mathrm{INL}^{pos}_{intermediate}(k) = \max(\mathrm{INL}(i)) \quad \text{for } i : 1 \rightarrow k \tag{6.40}$$

$$\mathrm{INL}^{neg}_{intermediate}(k) = \min(\mathrm{INL}(i)) \quad \text{for } i : 1 \rightarrow k \tag{6.41}$$

$$\mathrm{INL}_{intermediate}(k) = \max(\mathrm{INL}^{pos}_{intermediate}(k), -\mathrm{INL}^{neg}_{intermediate}(k)) \tag{6.42}$$

As soon as the $\mathrm{INL}_{intermediate}$ exceeds the already obtained value, the search algorithm does a backtracking step and this branch is not further explored. The optimization run takes approximately 12 hours of CPU time on a SUN Ultra-1/170 workstation.

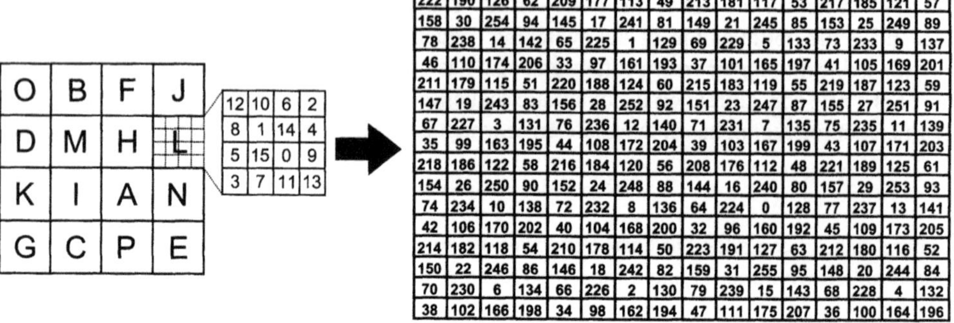

Figure 6.17: Switching sequence of the Q^2 Random Walk switching scheme.

In [Cong 00] new methods and algorithms have been proposed to solve this sequence optimization problem. It must be noted that, although the cost function is slightly different, the switching sequence obtained with the branch and bound approach resulted in an INL-bounded sequence (as defined in [Cong 00]), which could not be improved upon by [Cong 00].

The second sequence optimization has a linear error profile. Since it compensates a second-order residual error, less care has been taken to optimize this sequence (the assumption of linearity is not correct for all regions anyway). Therefore a manually derived symmetrical switching sequence has been chosen. It visits symmetrically the current sources of the 4×4 region. This linear switching sequence is thus not optimal, as has been found in [Cong 00] and could potentially be improved upon (albeit the manually derived sequence is only approximately 30% worse than the reported optimal linear switching scheme of [Cong 00]).

This leads to the overall switching sequence of the unary current sources:

1. current source 0 in region A
2. current source 0 in region B
3. ...

17. current source 1 in region A
18. current source 1 in region B
19. ...

254. current source 15 in region N
255. current source 15 in region O

This switching sequence is shown graphically in figure 6.17.

By *random walking* through the 255 current sources, the residual error is not accumulated but rather *randomized*, hence the name *Q^2 Random Walk* switching scheme. Figure 6.18 compares simulations of the resulting INL, for the same error profiles extracted from test structures, in case of the classical switching scheme used in [Miki 86] and the presented Q^2 Random Walk switching scheme [Vdbus 99a, VdPlas 99b]. The resulting INL is about 10 times smaller using the Q^2 Random Walk switching scheme, although in both cases a quad quadrant (Q^2) current source array was used. The overall nonlinearity suppression thus equals

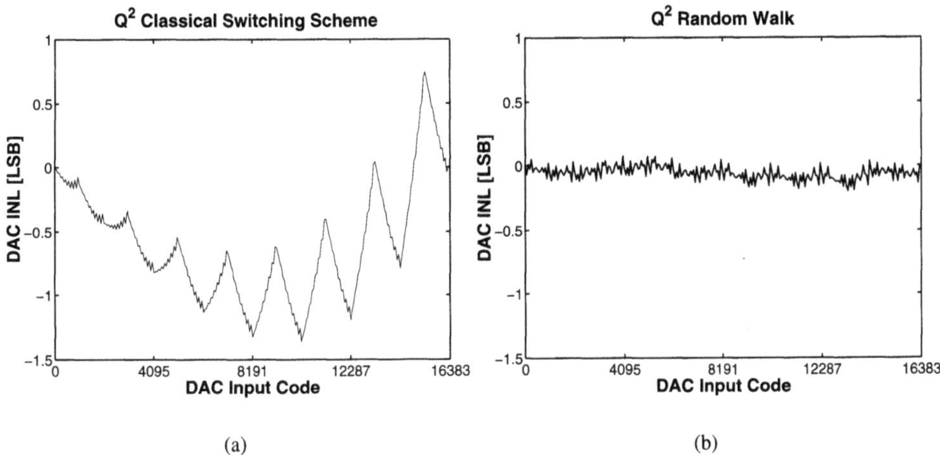

(a) (b)

Figure 6.18: Simulation of INL for the same error profiles using: (a) Q^2 classical sequential switching scheme [Miki 86], (b) Q^2 Random Walk switching scheme [Vdbus 99a, VdPlas 99b].

4×10 in the X direction and 8×10 in the Y direction (a factor of 4 and 8 due to Q^2 spatially averaging and a factor of 10 due to the Random Walk switching sequence), overcoming the technology limits and resulting in the first CMOS D/A-converter with intrinsic 14-bit accuracy.

Current source 15 in region P is not used as a current source. It is configured as a diode and used as a biasing reference for the current source array. Since it is spread across the array in the same way as any other unary current source, it tracks these sources accurately.

6.6.2.5 Current Source Array Layout Generation

The placement of the basic units in the current source array has been determined. The current source array layout is now generated automatically with **Mondriaan** ([VdPlas 98] or chapter 5 of this work).

The basic current source unit is laid out manually and is symbolically shown in figure 6.19. As can be seen on the figure, the device has been folded. This has been done to obtain approximately the wire pitch determined in equation(6.28) and the correct aspect ratio for the current source array. The *final* wire pitch of the 14-bit D/A-converter core is 11.6μm. This value is used later on to generate the layouts of the swatch array and digital decoder and the buses connecting these modules.

In **Mondriaan**'s flow then the first step is floorplanning. In this case the floorplan contains a fixed assignment of the basic cells, this is the optimized sequence/placement of the unit current sources (as explained in the previous section). The binary units are placed such that their respective centers of gravity are at the center of the array. The pin assignment is derived as follows: the basic cells are scanned column by column and pins are allocated to the lowest numbered units that are not yet brought out to a pin. This arranges the pin wires in a sequence

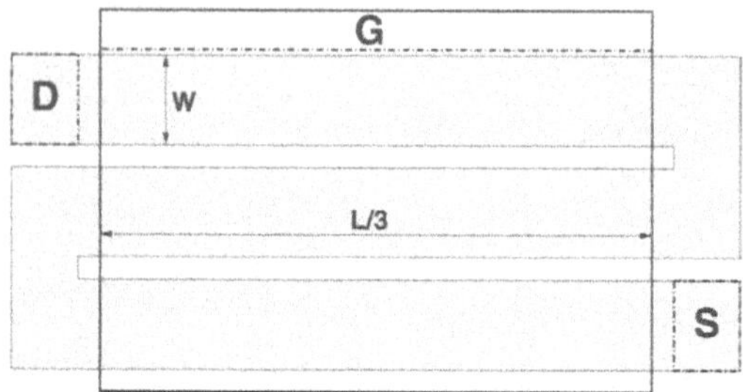

Figure 6.19: Layout (cell outline) of the current source transistor.

such that in the first quadrant the first 64 unary current sources are connected, the second quadrant connects the next 64 unary current sources and so on.

During the symbolic route phase the wires are routed to connect the parallel current source units. Furthermore, **Mondriaan** ensures that equal metal coverage of the unit current sources is maintained (this is a matching requirement), by inserting dummy metal strips in the routing. The technology mapping phase outputs a completed, DRC-correct layout and a mask-level pin list in the used 1P3M 0.5μm CMOS process.

6.6.3 Swatch Array Layout Generation

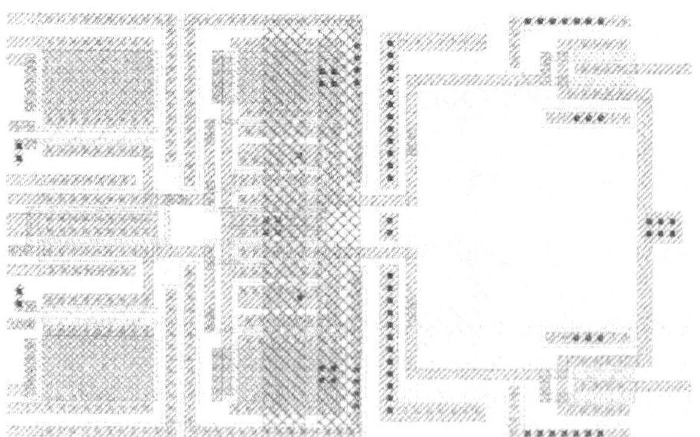

Figure 6.20: Layout of the swatch (switch/latch) cell.

The basic swatch cell has been laid out manually as shown in figure 6.20. The placement and routing of the swatch array is then done automatically with the **Mondriaan** tool (chapter 5). Inputs to the tool are the pin list of the current source array, the netlist and the swatch cell. The floorplanning in this case consists of determining the pin assignment (using the fixed pin positions of the current source array) and the cell assignment. The symbolic route and the technology mapping phase outputs again the final layout and a pin list. This time the pin list is used to derive the steering signals coming from the full decoder.

6.6.4 Full Decoder Standard Cell Place and Route

The layout of the digital full decoder is generated using a standard cell place and route tool, for instance the Cell 3 ensemble from Cadence [Cell3 Manual 95], or the tools from Avant! [Aquarius 97]. The pin list obtained from the swatch array layout is input to this layout tool. The standard cells are then placed and routed.

6.6.5 Layout Assembly

The modules are placed stacked on top of each other. The bus generators of the **Mondriaan** tool are used to generate the connections between the three modules (full decoder, swatch array and current source array). Trees are used to collect the output signals and distribute the clocking signal from the clock driver to the swatch array to have equal delay.

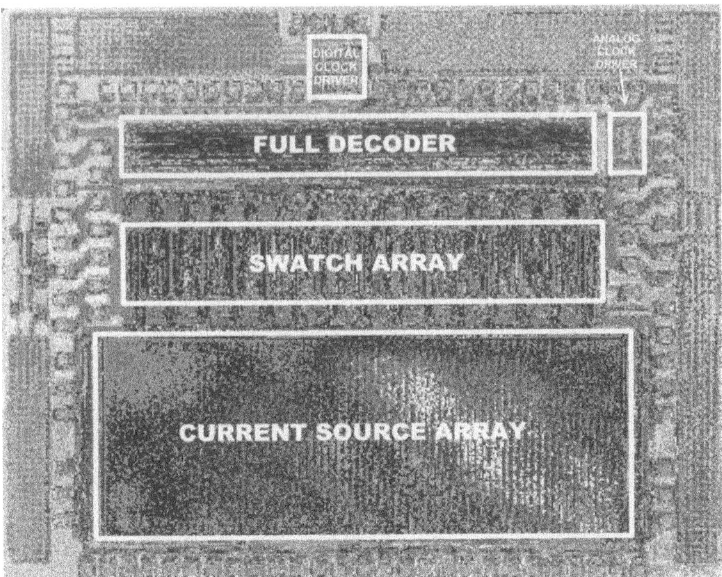

Figure 6.21: Microphotograph of the 14-bit D/A-converter [Vdbus 99a, VdPlas 99b].

The bonding pads are placed and manually connected to all the external pins of the D/A-converter. For our 14-bit D/A-converter this results in the layout shown on the microphotograph in figure 6.21. As was already stated during floorplanning, the use of a fixed pitch has resulted in an elegant chip assembly since the modules have approximately the same width.

6.7 Extraction of a Behavioral Model for Verification

After the layout is completed, a behavioral model is generated where the model parameters are extracted from the designed circuit [Vdbus 98b, Vdbus 99b], as indicated on the flow in figure 6.1. The resulting model can then be used for final system verification of systems where the D/A-converter is part of.

6.7.1 Static Behavior: INL

For modeling the static behavior, an additional stochastic term is added to the output equation (6.2). This additional term can be derived using Principal Component Analysis (PCA) [Joli 86] which has been applied in a similar way for modeling A/D-converters in [Liu 92, Gie 92].

Assume $\mathbf{q}$ is a random INL measurement (q_i denotes the INL error for code i). These samples are obtained using Monte-Carlo simulations in a numerical simulator (Hspice) with an appropriate statistical (mismatch) device model and tool, for instance MMPRE [Verha 96, Verha 97] that was discussed in section 3.5.2. After normalization, this set of correlated variables q_i is transformed into a set of uncorrelated variables $\mathbf{c} = (c_1, c_2, \ldots, c_k)$, using a linear transformation $\mathbf{c} = \mathbf{Sq}$. This is achieved by calculating the Singular Value Decomposition (SVD) of the correlation matrix (Σ):

$$\Sigma \equiv E\{\mathbf{q} \cdot \mathbf{q}^{\mathbf{t}}\} \tag{6.43}$$

The correlation matrix Σ can be estimated by obtaining a large number of samples of $\mathbf{q}$, for example utilizing Monte-Carlo analysis, as follows:

$$\overline{\mathbf{q}}_{est} = \sum^{m} \frac{\mathbf{q}}{m} \tag{6.44}$$

$$\Sigma_{est} = \frac{\mathbf{Q} \cdot \mathbf{Q}^{\mathbf{t}}}{m} \tag{6.45}$$

where $\overline{\mathbf{q}}_{est}$ is the estimated mean value of vector $\mathbf{q}$ and $\mathbf{Q}$ is the matrix containing m samples of vector $\mathbf{q} - \overline{\mathbf{q}}_{est}$.

The Singular Value Decomposition of Σ then can be calculated and it has the following properties:

$$\Sigma = \mathbf{T} \Lambda \mathbf{T}^{\mathbf{t}} \quad \text{where} \quad \Lambda = \begin{bmatrix} \lambda_1 \cdots 0 \\ \vdots \ddots \vdots \\ 0 \cdots \lambda_{2^n} \end{bmatrix} \quad \text{and} \quad \lambda_i = \text{var}\{c_i\} \tag{6.46}$$

The principal components correspond to the largest values λ_i of this decomposition, which are estimates for the variance of the independent random variables c_i. The correlated random variables q_i can then be estimated as follows. Take a random sample of the uncorrelated variables c_i and calculate q_i using the transformation matrix $\mathbf{T}$:

$$\mathbf{q}_{est} = \mathbf{Tc} + \overline{\mathbf{q}}_{est} \tag{6.47}$$

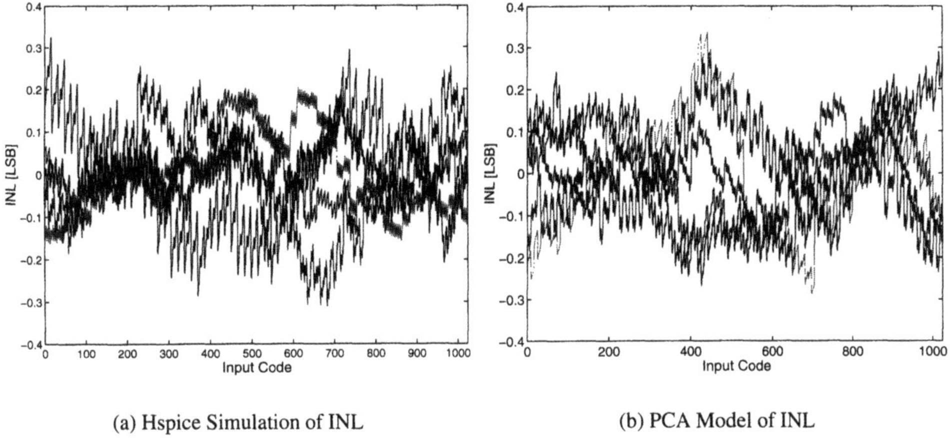

(a) Hspice Simulation of INL

(b) PCA Model of INL

Figure 6.22: Comparison of numerically simulated INL with PCA extracted model of INL.

A 10-bit segmented D/A-converter was modeled using the proposed method. The residual (non-modeled) total variance is less than 0.001%. To verify the resulting behavioral model 100 random INL samples were generated and verified against 100 (other) test samples generated by Monte-Carlo simulation using Hspice. Both Monte-Carlo simulations and behavioral model showed an INL below 0.4LSB. Five samples of each of these sets (behavioral model and Monte-Carlo simulations) are depicted in figure 6.22.

Note that in figure 6.22(a) the MMPRE statistical analysis exhibits the typical characteristics of a 6–4 segmented D/A-converter architecture. The errors of the binary sources (16 codes long) are repeated 64 times, while the unary sources cause a large-scale random variation of the INL curves. In fact the PCA method isolates the statistical independent variables, in this case the errors of the individual binary sources and the unary sources. The **T** matrix transforms these into the INL curve (which is a linear combination of these independent error sources). That can be seen in figure 6.22(b), the large-scale random variation is of course different (two identical samples are statistically unlikely), but its size is on average the same. The binary errors are also random and are repeated as small-scale variations 64 times. This is exactly what is to be expected of a 6–4 segmented D/A-converter architecture. The PCA extraction thus creates a model which is *statistically equivalent* to the actual circuit and at the same time checks (through the residual variance which should be very small) that the model is correct.

6.7.2 Dynamic Behavior: Glitch Energy

The glitch model as presented in section 6.3, is extended. Firstly, a separate damped sine is used for switching on respectively off a current source. The number of current sources that are switched on or off can be readily computed from the chosen topology (i.e. the choice of the number of bits l that steer the binary-weighted current source array). Secondly, the amplitude

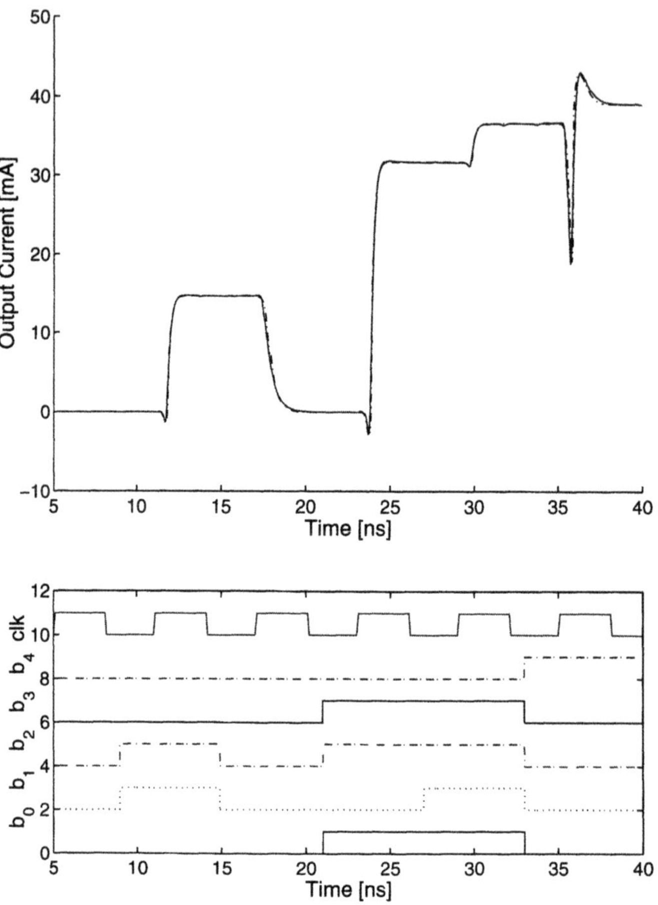

Figure 6.23: Comparison of extracted glitch model with numerical simulation, the straight line is obtained using device-level simulation, the dash dotted line is obtained by using the extracted behavioral mode and simulation. At the bottom the clock and five bit lines are shown.

and the time constant of the damped sine of the left-hand side and the right-hand side (as shown in figure 6.5) are controlled separately. This results in 8 parameters which can easily be extracted from a numerical simulation (Hspice [Hspice Manual 99]) switching one bit on and off. The comparison of a Hspice simulation and the derived model is depicted in figure 6.23. The glitch energy was modeled within 1%: both behavioral model and numerical simulation resulted in a glitch energy of 0.13pV.s. The numerical simulation required 4:37 minutes of CPU time on a HP 712/100 workstation, the behavioral model 12 seconds.

This concludes the complete design process of the D/A-converter as an embedded functional block.

6.8 Experimental Results

To evaluate the proposed systematic design methodology, a number of high-accuracy, high-speed D/A-converters have been designed, fabricated and measured. First the measurement setup is briefly described, next the measurement results of the different D/A-converters will be presented.

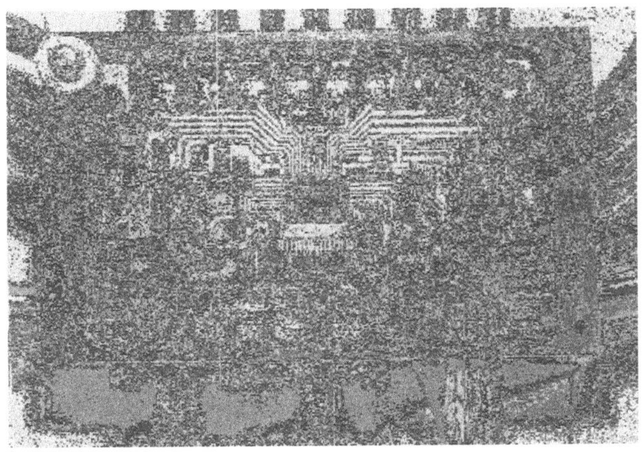

Figure 6.24: Photograph of the measurement setup.

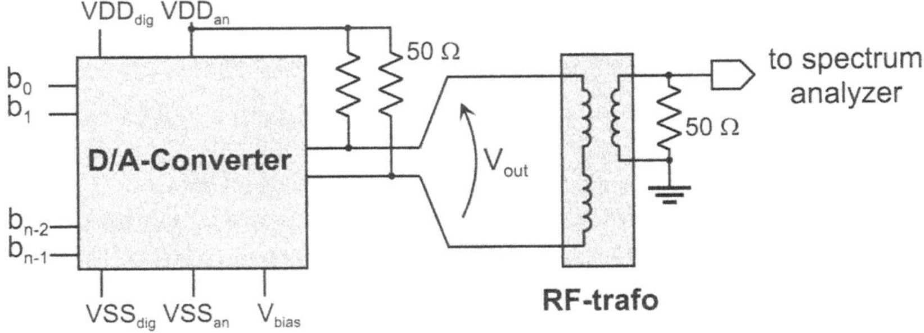

Figure 6.25: Block diagram of the dynamic measurement setup.

6.8.1 Measurement Setup

The package setup for the measurements is shown in figure 6.24: the fabricated die is mounted on a ceramic substrate, where all power supplies have been locally decoupled. The ceramic substrate is encapsulated in a copper-beryllium case to shield the circuit from external noise coupling. The static measurements are performed with a 50Ω double-terminated cable. The measurement setup for the dynamic characterization is shown in figure 6.25. Dynamic measurements were performed with an HP 3585 spectrum analyzer having a frequency range of 40MHz, and having a guaranteed dynamic range of 80dB, with a typical value of 84dB.

6.8.2 Measurement Results

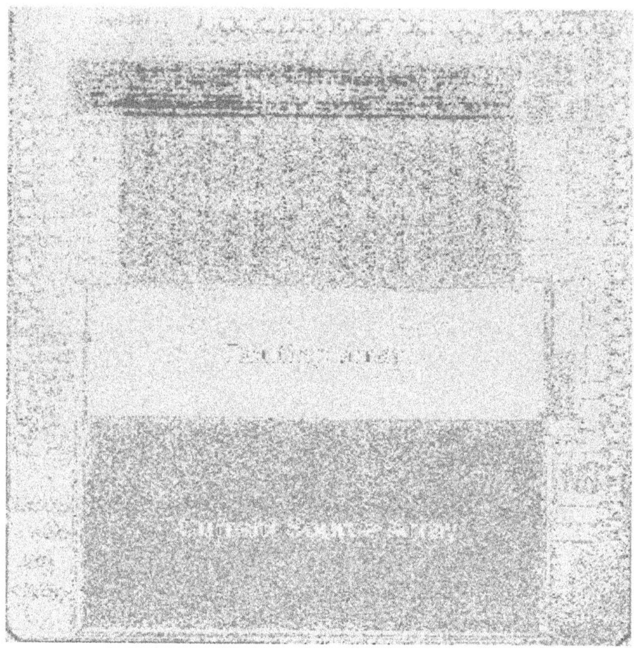

Figure 6.26: Microphotograph of the 12-bit D/A-converter [VdBosch 98].

Three designs were realized using the proposed design methodology. Firstly a 12-bit D/A-converter with a 200MSamples/s update rate was implemented [VdBosch 98]. A microphotograph of the chip is shown in figure 6.26. The chip has an INL of 0.5LSB (shown in figure 6.27(a)), a DNL of 0.8LSB (shown in figure 6.27(b)), a glitch energy of 0.8pV.s and an SFDR of 69dB@500kHz full-scale input signal. The chip runs from a single 2.7V power supply and consumes 140mW. When developing this first chip, the layout tool **Mondriaan** still lacked functionality resulting in large routing overhead, which explains the larger chip area compared to the second and third design of 14-bit D/A-converters. The worst-case glitch measurement is shown in figure 6.27(c). This glitch measurement includes both the digital coupling (clock feedthrough) and the code transition. It is measured at the transition from code 4079 to code 4080 (code 11111110 1111 to code 11111111 0000). The output spectrum of this chip is shown in figure 6.27(d) for an input signal of 500kHz. In figure 6.27(e) the SFDR as a function of output signal frequency is shown at an update rate of 200MSamples/s. In figure 6.27(f) the SFDR of a 500kHz full-scale sine-wave is shown as a function of sampling frequency.

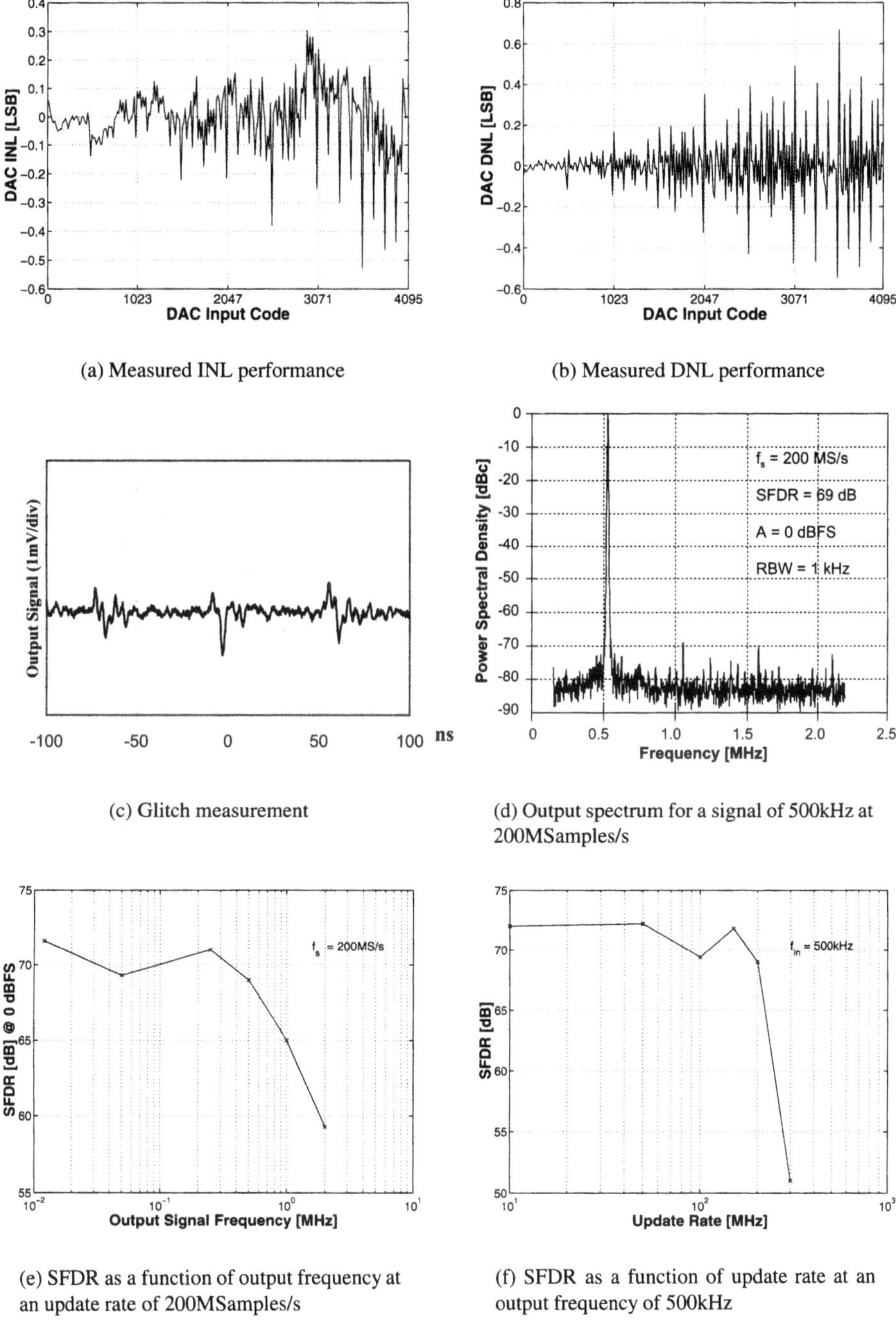

(a) Measured INL performance

(b) Measured DNL performance

(c) Glitch measurement

(d) Output spectrum for a signal of 500kHz at 200MSamples/s

(e) SFDR as a function of output frequency at an update rate of 200MSamples/s

(f) SFDR as a function of update rate at an output frequency of 500kHz

Figure 6.27: Measurement results of the 12-bit D/A-converter [VdBosch 98].

Secondly, a 14-bit D/A-converter with a 200Msamples/s update rate was implemented [VdPlas 99a]. The chip has an INL of 2.5LSB, a glitch energy of 0.3pV.s. The chip runs from a single 2.7V power supply and consumes 300mW. The chip photograph was shown in figure 6.13 and a DNL plot has been shown in figure 6.14.

Finally, a second 14-bit D/A-converter was implemented [Vdbus 99a, VdPlas 99b]. The chip photograph was shown in figure 6.21. The update rate of this converter is 150MSamples/s. The chip has an INL of 0.3LSB and a DNL of 0.2LSB. The INL and DNL curves are shown in figure 6.28(a) and 6.28(b). This proves that the approach of using an optimized switching scheme is required for 14-bit accuracy. The settling time is 0.9ns. The converter has a SFDR of 84dB@500kHz full-scale input signal, the measured spectrum is shown in figure 6.28(c). In figure 6.28(d) the spectrum at the output is shown for a full-scale input signal at 5MHz. A SFDR of 61dB is obtained. The power consumption of the third design is 300mW. In figure 6.28(e) the SFDR as a function of output signal frequency is shown at an update rate of 150MSamples/s. In figure 6.28(f) the SFDR of a 500kHz full scale sine-wave is shown as a function of sampling frequency.

The measurements of the fabricated chips are summarized in Table 6.6.

Specification	**design1**	**design2**	**design3**	**Unit**
Number of bits	12	14	14	–
Segmentation	8–4	8–6	8–6	–
INL	0.5	2.5	0.3	LSB
DNL	0.8	0.5	0.2	LSB
Glitch energy	0.8	0.3	NM[a]	pV.s
SFDR@500kHz	69	NM[a]	84	dB
Settling time (10–90%)	NM[a]	1	0.9	ns
Sample frequency	200	200	150	MSamples/s
Output range	0.5	0.5	0.5	V
Load	25	25	25	Ω
Digital levels	CMOS	CMOS	CMOS	–
Power supply	2.7	2.7	2.7	V
Technology	1P3M 0.5μm CMOS			–
Power consumption	140	300	300	mW
Area	3.5 x 4	3.5 x 3.5	3.2 x 4.1	mm^2

[a]Not Measured.

Table 6.6: Measured performance of the three systematically designed D/A-converters.

6.8.3 Breakdown of Design Time

The time spent on the different steps in the proposed design methodology have been summarized in Table 6.7. During the first design the different design trade-offs were explored and

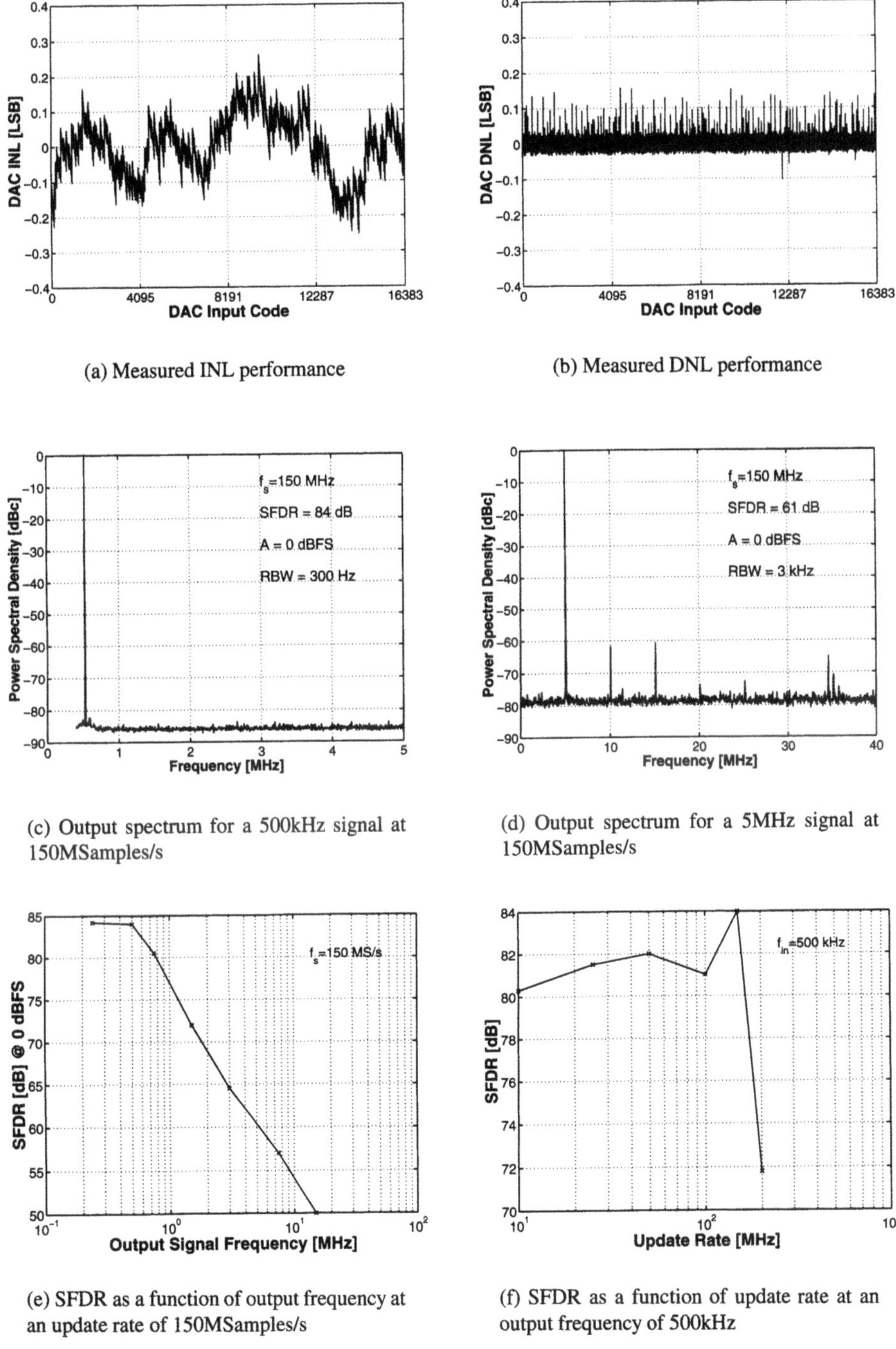

(a) Measured INL performance

(b) Measured DNL performance

(c) Output spectrum for a 500kHz signal at 150MSamples/s

(d) Output spectrum for a 5MHz signal at 150MSamples/s

(e) SFDR as a function of output frequency at an update rate of 150MSamples/s

(f) SFDR as a function of update rate at an output frequency of 500kHz

Figure 6.28: Measurement results of the 14-bit D/A-converter [Vdbus 99a, VdPlas 99b].

Design phase		**design1**	**design2**	**design3**
Sizing & synthesis	high-level	2 weeks	1 week	1 day
	current-source array	1 week	1 hour	–
	swatch array	1 week	2 days	–
	thermocoder	1 day	1 day	1 day
Layout	floorplan	2 days	1 hour	1 hour
	current-source array	3 days	1 day	1 hour
	swatch array	1 week	3 days	7 hours
	thermocoder	1 week	4 days	4 days
	assembly	4 days	3 days	3 days
Verification	sizing	1 week	1 week	1 week
	layout	1 week	1 week	1 week
Total person effort		**11 weeks**	**6 weeks**	**4 weeks**

Table 6.7: Time spent on design, layout and verification of the three designs.

embedded in the presented Matlab scripts. Using these scripts for the second and the third design, the design time could be reduced from 4 weeks to 1 week. The layout of the swatch array was done manually for the first design, as the layout tool **Mondriaan** still lacked functionality at that time. One week was needed to draw the swatch cell and swatch array manually.

In the second design the swatch cell was laid out manually in 3 days, the generation of the swatch array itself took only a few hours with **Mondriaan**. For the third design the basic cells were modified, and the arrays were generated with **Mondriaan**. Although the switching scheme was completely different, the layout generation took only 8 hours (current source and swatch array). The layout assembly of the different blocks was done manually for all designs. DRC, ERC and LVS checking was done to verify the generated layout. It must however be noted that, although LVS checks whether the layout conforms to the schematic, it cannot check that the position of the sources is correct. At this moment no verification tool is available that verifies the positions of analog cells. If analog circuits increasingly start to depend on the position of cells in layout, this will become a more severe problem. Although it would not be impossible (the position of the cells is known in layout anyway) to solve this, the open problem is how to specify the positions of the layout cells in the netlist or schematic.

Parasitics were then extracted and the sizing was verified using Hspice. As shown in Table 6.7, the overall design time was reduced from **11** weeks to **4** weeks of total person effort. This is a reduction by a factor of *3*, demonstrating the effectiveness of the systematic design methodology to increase analog design productivity.

6.9 Conclusions

In this chapter the systematic design of high-speed, high-accuracy current-steering D/A-converters has been described. This work resulted in the first 14-bit linear CMOS D/A-converter that does not require tuning or trimming. This successful result has been obtained due to the following factors:

- the systematic top-down, bottom-up design methodology. The design methodology links the performance directly to the architectural, module-level and device-level design parameters. Every design decision is verified against the requested performance.
- a novel D/A-converter architecture; this new variant of the segmented architecture class is highly flexible, while it does not sacrifice the achievable performance.
- the use of point tools to automate parts of the design. Both commercial tools for logic synthesis and standard cell place and route have been combined with in-house developed generic point tools (for instance **Mondriaan**) and dedicated programs (sizing scripts in Matlab, or switching sequence optimizer in C). These tools did not limit the designer; rather they extended the designer's capabilities in finding a more optimal solution for the design problems, leading to an overall more optimal design.
- a motivated design team, bringing together knowledge and expertise ranging from matching of MOS transistors to logic synthesis.

All these factors have contributed to realize the presented work. At the same time it has been possible to reduce the design time considerably (a factor of 3), as has been shown in the design time breakdown. This is explained by the design team approach. Many people work in parallel, each being good at what they have to do in the design process. However as with all design teams, the organization and management becomes important. The systematic design methodology and flexible architecture (where separate modules are clearly identified) greatly eased these management problems: the design naturally splits up in different parts after the architectural design phase. At the layout level a single wiring pitch links the modules that have to be laid out. Much of the design work can thus be done in parallel.

In summary, it has been proven that systematic analog design has many benefits. However systematic design is only one ingredient in the recipe for success. Other contributing factors are a suitable circuit architecture, a motivated, capable design team, and support from design automation tools. This opens up the road for successful SoC designs containing high-performance analog functionblocks.

Chapter 7

Conclusions

In the SoC era with transistor counts approaching 100Mtransistors/chip, design productivity is one of the utmost important factors of success. The (economic) profit driving the microelectronics industry is governed by the market window opportunities. Combined with the ever increasing complexity encountered in todays designs (Moore's law), designers are faced with the *productivity gap*: the capabilities offered by the deep submicron process technology can not be exploited fully by lack of design capacity. This is true both for digital and analog design. This thesis work has concentrated on potential solutions for the analog design productivity gap. Two paths have been identified; on the one hand, the design of commodity analog designs [Gie 01] (low-challenge designs) can be automated to a large extent; on the other hand, the design of star analog designs [Gie 01] (high-challenge designs) can be supported by systematic design methodologies and tools. Both paths have been explored in this work.

In part I of this work the **AMGIE** analog synthesis system has been presented. It is a synthesis system targeted to the automatic design of analog circuits, such as OPAMPs, OTAs, etc. from specification down to mask layout (i.e. transforming behavior into geometrical structure). It implements a top-down refinement, bottom-up assembly, performance-driven design methodology, employing a functionblock hierarchy. The top-down path consists of topology selection and sizing & optimization steps, followed by verification. The bottom-up path consists of layout generation followed by extraction and verification steps. The **AMGIE** system has a modular software architecture making it easily extendible with new algorithms and tools. It uses two libraries: (1) a cell library containing a number of circuit topologies that are used to create designs and (2) a technology library providing CMOS technology independence through parameterization. The five design tasks: topology selection, sizing & optimization, layout generation, verification and redesign, have been automated.

Topology selection is carried out by applying a sequence of three filters to the list of topologies available in the cell library; the first two filters (boundary checking and interval analysis) eliminate infeasible topologies from the list and perform an initial ranking, the third filter (rule-based ranking) performs a final ranking of the remaining candidates.

The sizing & optimization tool use a modified equation-based optimization approach to automate the sizing process. Included is an integrated setup environment (ISAAC and DONALD) to derive the sizing model (a declarative analytical model). Accuracy, traditionally a weak point of equation-based approaches, has been improved by using encapsulated device models, high-quality models of the active devices and high-accuracy equations modeling the behavior of the circuits. Both global (VFSR) and local (Hooke–Jeeves and SQP) optimization algorithms have been integrated in the **OPTIMAN** tool to ensure effective optimization results.

Layout generation has been implemented using the LAYLA tools [Lam 99]. LAYLA implements a direct performance-driven macro-cell place & route methodology to automate the mask-level layout generation of analog circuits.

Verification has been implemented using a black-box approach. It interfaces to commercial and non-commercial numerical device-level simulators. By using verification templates and biasing/clocking templates an automatic setup and performance extraction procedure has been created. Statistical verification for mismatch is provided with MMPRE or MIMI [Verha 97]. Technology variations and operating ranges of temperature and power supply are verified using corner analysis.

If design errors occur, that are either detected by the design tools themselves (for instance topology selection did not find any suitable topology for the requested specifications) or are detected by the verification tool (for instance after extraction the phase margin drops below the requested value), the redesign wizard proposes the (novice) designer a set of corrective procedures.

Illustrative and representative examples have been added throughout the text to more clearly demonstrate the implemented algorithms and techniques. In the third chapter three synthesis experiments have been presented in detail that test the capabilities of the **AMGIE** system.

The first experiment compared three different approaches for the sizing synthesis of a typical OTA circuit: a *manual designer's* approach, a *simulation-based optimization* approach and an *equation-based optimization* approach. The *equation-based* approach implemented in the **AMGIE** system proves to be the preferred candidate when the high setup time can be written off over many design runs, since it has the lowest run-time of the three approaches. The design quality was comparable to the manual and optimization-based results. This is explained by the use of encapsulated device models (SPICE-accuracy) and by the derivation in a systematic way of high-quality equations for small-signal and large-signal performance specifications.

In the second reported experiment the **AMGIE** system was tested for its support of non-experienced designers. A classroom of EE Master students divided into 9 groups of 3 persons each, had to design an OTA circuit for a set of performance specification values. The time was limited to 2 and a half hours (one session) and despite the inexperience of the designers both in designing circuits and in using the **AMGIE** system, the experiment proved successful: all groups designed a functional circuit.

The third experiment was the design of a charge-sensitive amplifier – pulse-shaping amplifier (CSA-PSA) circuit for space applications. The complexity of this circuit is at the limit of what the **AMGIE** system can handle: approximately 100 (active and passive) devices. Using different hierarchical techniques the design of this circuit has been automated. A setup time of less than 4 months has been achieved. A (re)design of this topology then takes approximately 2 days. A prototype has been manufactured and measured. The resulting design did not only perform within specifications but its power consumption was almost four times lower than a previous manual design with the same performance.

In part II the research work carried out in the field of *systematic design* of high-performance analog integrated circuits has been reported.

In chapter 5 a layout methodology has been presented that is targeted to the automatic layout generation of highly-regular array-type blocks. These blocks are often found in analog modules such as flash-type A/D-converters, current-steering D/A-converters, cellular neural networks, etc. The methodology uses a three-step procedure to transform the schematic into a mask-level layout: floorplanning, symbolic routing and technology mapping. The approach raises the abstraction level compared to other existing approaches by automating the last two phases in a tool called **Mondriaan**. Not only does the methodology result in a considerable design productivity boost, it also enlarges analog layout capabilities which can be exploited by the designer to surmount the technological boundaries for layout-driven analog designs. The layout synthesis problem of these regular blocks is solved in a *fast* and *technology independent way*, promoting *layout reuse*. A set of bus and tree generators completes the presented tool set. Industrial-strength examples have demonstrated the applicability and usefulness of the implemented approach.

In the last chapter the *systematic design methodology* has been applied to the design of high-accuracy current-steering D/A-converters. First the design flow has been discussed. Next the operating principle of segmented current-steering D/A-converters has been explained and a typical specification set has been presented. The novel architecture that was used to design the converter was proposed next. The novel architecture is much more flexible than the row–column-based segmented architecture traditionally used to implemented this type of converter.

The first phase in the design flow is the specification phase. Using behavioral modeling and simulation the specification of the D/A-converter functionblock have been derived. The second phase in the design flow is the synthesis of the converter. A top-down refinement, bottom-up, mixed-signal design strategy has been adopted. First the architectural sizing parameters of the design were determined, next the device-level sizing parameters. The digital thermometer decoder was synthesized from VHDL code. In the bottom-up path, **Mondriaan** was used to generate the layout of the analog modules, while a standard cell place & route tool was used to create the digital layout. The optimization of the switching sequence, one of the most important parameters of the design for obtaining the intrinsic accuracy, has been explained in detail. The result of this optimization is the novel Q^2 Random Walk switching scheme. In the last phase of the design a behavioral model is extracted that mimics the actual silicon part.

The chapter concludes with the presentation of three implementations. One of these implementations is the first 14-bit intrinsically accurate CMOS current-steering D/A-converter known to the authors that does not require any form of trimming or tuning [Vdbus 99a, VdPlas 99b]. This proves that the systematic design methodology is capable of delivering high-quality designs. Also the design time spent on the three prototypes has been reported. A comparison indicates that automating part of the design, both by using in-house developed tools (**Mondriaan**, sizing scripts, C programs to optimize switching sequence, etc.) and commercially available tools (logic synthesis, standard cell place & route, etc.), has led to a significant design productivity increase: a factor of 3 was reported. This demonstrates what this thesis set out to prove: analog design quality and productivity are compatible and achievable with analog computer-aided design methodologies and tools.

This work contributed important results to *analog synthesis*: with the **AMGIE** system was proven that fully automated synthesis of moderate-complexity analog circuits is feasible, as demonstrated by the experimental results; the *systematic design* approach, supported by tools, resulted in an improved *analog design productivity* while still allowing the designer enough flexibility to achieve high performance, as demonstrated by the design of high-accuracy D/A-converters.

There is one message that this text tries to convey: always investigate the design methodology you're using when designing analog circuits. Probably it can be improved and tools can help you to speed up the design or improve the quality of the design. This is an investigative and research work that is never finished.

Bibliography

[Aftab 94] S. Aftab and M. Styblinski, "IC variability minimization using a new Cp and Cpk based variability/performance measure", in *Proceedings IEEE International Symposium on Circuits and Systems (ISCAS)*, May 1994, pp. 149–152.

[Anta 95] B. Antao and A. Brodersen, "Behavioral Simulation for Analog System Design Verification", *IEEE Transactions on Very Large Scale Integration (VLSI) Systems*, vol. 3, no. 3, pp. 417–429, Sept. 1995.

[Aquarius 97] Avant! Corporation, 46871 Bayside Parkway Fremant, CA 94538, *Aquarius Manual*, 1997.

[Bala 99] F. Balasa and K. Lampaert, "Module Placement for Analog Layout Using the Sequence-Pair Representation", in *Proceedings Design Automation Conference (DAC)*, June 1999, pp. 274–279.

[Bas 93] B. Basaran, R. A. Rutenbar, and L. Carley, "Latchup-Aware Placement and Parasitic Bounded Routing of Custom Analog Cells", in *Proceedings IEEE/ACM International Conference on Computer Aided Design (ICCAD)*, Nov. 1993, pp. 415–421.

[Bast 96a] J. Bastos, M. Steyaert, B. Graindourze, and W. Sansen, "Matching of MOS Transistors with Different Layout Styles", in *Proceedings IEEE International Conference on Microelectronic Test Structures (ICMTS)*, Mar. 1996, pp. 17–20.

[Bast 96b] J. Bastos, M. Steyaert, and W. Sansen, "A High Yield 12-bit 250-MS/s CMOS D/A-converter", in *Proceedings Custom Integrated Circuits Conference (CICC)*, May 1996, pp. 431–434.

[Bast 98a] J. Bastos, *Characterization of MOS Transistor Mismatch for Analog Design*, PhD thesis, KULeuven, Apr. 1998.

[Bast 98b] J. Bastos, A. Marques, M. Steyaert, and W. Sansen, "A 12-bit Intrinsic Accuracy High-Speed CMOS DAC", *IEEE Journal of Solid-State Circuits (JSSC)*, vol. 33, no. 12, pp. 1959–1969, Dec. 1998.

[Been 93] G. Beenker, J. Conway, G. Schrooten, and A. Slenter, "Analog CAD for Consumer ICs", in *Analog circuit design*, J. Huijsing, R. van der Plassche, and W. Sansen, Eds. Kluwer Academic Publishers, 101 Philip Drive, Norwell, MA 02061, US, 1993.

[Bern 98] K. Bernstein, K. M. Carrig, C. M. Durham, P. R. Hansen, D. Hogenmiller, E. J. Nowak, and N. J. Rohrer, *High Speed CMOS Design Styles*, Kluwer Academic Publishers, 101 Philip Drive, Norwell, MA 02061, US, Apr. 1998.

[Bru 96] J. D. Bruce, H. W. Li, M. J. Dallabetta, and R. J. Baker, "Analog Layout Using ALAS!", *IEEE Journal of Solid-State Circuits (JSSC)*, vol. 31, no. 2, pp. 271–274, Feb. 1996.

[Carl 88] L. Carley and R. A. Rutenbar, "How to automate analog IC design", *IEEE Spectrum*, vol. 25, no. 8, pp. 26–30, Aug. 1988.

[Carl 89] L. Carley, D. Garrod, R. Harjani, J. Kelly, T. Lim, E. Ochotta, and R. A. Rutenbar, "ACACIA: The CMU analog design system", in *Proceedings Custom Integrated Circuits Conference (CICC)*, May 1989, pp. 4.3.1–4.3.5.

[Carl 96] L. Carley, G. Gielen, R. A. Rutenbar, and W. Sansen, "Synthesis tools for mixed-signal ICs: progress on front-end and back-end strategies", in *Proceedings Design Automation Conference (DAC)*, June 1996, pp. 298–303.

[Cell3 Manual 95] Cadence Design Systems, Inc., *Cell3 Ensemble Reference Manual*, 1995.

[Chang 90] Z. Y. Chang and W. M. Sansen, *Low-Noise Wide-Band Amplifiers in Bipolar and CMOS Technologies*, Kluwer Academic Publishers, 101 Philip Drive, Norwell, MA 02061, US, Nov. 1990.

[Chang 92] H. Chang, A. Sangiovanni-Vincentelli, F. Balarin, E. Charbon, U. Choudhury, G. Jusuf, E. Liu, E. Malavasi, R. Neff, and P. R. Gray, "A top-down, constraint-driven design methodology for analog integrated circuits", in *Proceedings Custom Integrated Circuits Conference (CICC)*, May 1992, pp. 8.4.1–8.4.4.

[Chang 94] H. Chang, E. Liu, R. Neff, E. Felt, E. Malavasi, E. Charbon, A. Sangiovanni-Vincentelli, and P. R. Gray, "A top-down, constraint-driven design methodology based generation of n-bit interpolative current source D/A-converters", in *Proceedings Custom Integrated Circuits Conference (CICC)*, May 1994, pp. 369–372.

[Chang 95a] H. Chang, E. Felt, and A. Sangiovanni-Vincentelli, "Top-down, constraint-driven design methodology based generation of a second order Σ/Δ A/D-converters", in *Proceedings Custom Integrated Circuits Conference (CICC)*, May 1995, pp. 533–536.

[Chang 95b] H. Chang, *A Top-Down, Constraint-Driven Design Methodology for Analog Integrated Circuits*, PhD thesis, UCBerkeley, 1995.

[Chang 96] H. Chang, E. Charbon, U. Choudhury, A. Demir, E. Felt, E. Liu, E. Malavasi, A. L. Sangiovanni-Vincentelli, and I. Vassiliou, *A Top-Down, Constraint-Driven Design Methodology for Analog Integrated Circuits*, Kluwer Academic Publishers, 101 Philip Drive, Norwell, MA 02061, US, 1 edition, 1996.

[Chang 99] H. Chang, L. Cooke, M. Hunt, G. Martin, A. McNelly, and L. Todd, *Surviving the SOC revolution — A guide to platform-based design*, Kluwer Academic Publishers, Dordrecht, the Netherlands, Nov. 1999.

[Chang 00] C.-Y. Chang and S. M. Sze, *ULSI Devices*, John Wiley & Sons Ltd., May 2000.

[Char 94a] E. Charbon, E. Malavasi, D. Pandini, and A. Sangiovanni-Vincentelli, "Imposing Tight Specifications on Analog ICs through Simultaneous Placement and Module Optimization", in *Proceedings Custom Integrated Circuits Conference (CICC)*, May 1994, pp. 525–528.

[Char 94b] E. Charbon, E. Malavasi, D. Pandini, and A. Sangiovanni-Vincentelli, "Simultaneous Placement and Module Optimization of Analog ICs", in *Proceedings Design Automation Conference (DAC)*, June 1994, pp. 31–35.

[Chen 93] J. Chen and M. Styblinski, "A Systematic Approach of Statistical Modeling and its Application to CMOS Circuits", in *Proceedings IEEE International Symposium on Circuits and Systems (ISCAS)*, May 1993, vol. 3, pp. 1805–1808.

[Chou 90a] U. Choudhury and A. Sangiovanni-Vincentelli, "Use of Performance Sensitivities in Routing of Analog Circuits", in *Proceedings IEEE International Symposium on Circuits and Systems (ISCAS)*, May 1990, vol. 1, pp. 348–351.

[Chou 90b] U. Choudhury and A. Sangiovanni-Vincentelli, "Constraint Generation for Routing Analog Circuits", in *Proceedings Design Automation Conference (DAC)*, June 1990, pp. 561–566.

[Chou 90c] U. Choudhury and A. Sangiovanni-Vincentelli, "Constraint based Channel Routing for Routing Analog and Mixed Analog/Digital Circuits", in *Proceedings IEEE/ACM International Conference on Computer Aided Design (ICCAD)*, Nov. 1990, pp. 198–201.

[Chua 93] L. Chua and T. Roska, "The CNN Paradigm", *IEEE Transactions on Circuits and Systems I: Fundamental Theory and Applications*, vol. 40, no. 3, pp. 147–156, Mar. 1993.

[Cla 80] D. Clary, R. Kirk, and S. Sapiro, "SIDS (A Symbolic Interactive Design Systems)", in *Proceedings Design Automation Conference (DAC)*, June 1980, pp. 292–295.

[Claas 00] T. Claasen, "First-Time-Right Si but to the Right Specification", keynote session at DAC, June 2000.

[Cohn 91] J. M. Cohn, D. J. Garrod, R. A. Rutenbar, and L. Carley, "KOAN/ANAGRAMII: New tools for device-level analog placement and routing", *IEEE Journal of Solid-State Circuits (JSSC)*, vol. 26, no. 3, pp. 330–342, Mar. 1991.

[Cong 00] Y. Cong and R. L. Geiger, "Switching Sequence Optimization for Gradient Error Compensation in Thermometer-Decoded DAC Arrays", *IEEE Transactions on Circuits and Systems II: Analog and Digital Signal Processing*, vol. 47, no. 7, pp. 585–595, July 2000.

[Curr 01] L. J. Curran, "Mixed-signal ICs: One name, many definitions", http://www.ebnonline.com/story/OEG20010521S0036, May 2001.

[Debyser 98a] G. Debyser, F. Leyn, G. Gielen, W. Sansen, and M. Styblinski, "Efficient Statistical Analog IC Design using Symbolic Methods", in *Proceedings IEEE International Symposium on Circuits and Systems (ISCAS)*, May 1998, vol. 6, pp. 21–24.

[Debyser 98b] G. Debyser and G. Gielen, "Efficient Analog Circuit Synthesis with simultaneous Yield and Robustness Optimization", in *Proceedings IEEE/ACM International Conference on Computer Aided Design (ICCAD)*, Nov. 1998, pp. 308–311.

[Debyser 00] G. Debyser, "Final routines for analog design plan generation", Tech. Rep. S4.1f-48, MEDEA A409: SADE, KULeuven ESAT-MICAS, Dec. 2000.

[Degra 87] M. Degrauwe, O. Nys, E. Dijkstra, J. Rijmenants, S. Bitz, B. Goffart, E. Vittoz, S. Cserveny, C. Meixenberger, G. van der Stappen, and H. J. Oguey, "IDAC: an interactive design tool for analog CMOS circuits", *IEEE Journal of Solid-State Circuits (JSSC)*, vol. 22, no. 6, pp. 1106–1116, Dec. 1987.

[DeRant 00] C. De Ranter, B. De Muer, G. Van der Plas, P. Vancorenland, M. Steyaert, G. Gielen, and W. Sansen, "CYCLONE: Automated Design of Received Frequency LC Oscillators", in *Proceedings Design Automation Conference (DAC)*, Los Angeles, June 2000, pp. 11–14.

[Don 97] S. Donnay, G. Gielen, W. Sansen, W. Kruiskamp, D. Leenaerts, and W. van Bokhoven, "High-level synthesis of analog sensor interface front-ends", in *Proceedings European Design and Test Conference (ED&TC)*, Mar. 1997, pp. 56–60.

[Don 98] S. Donnay, *Analog High-Level Design Automation in Mixed-Signal ASICs*, PhD thesis, KULeuven, Dec. 1998.

[Duff 67] R. J. Duffin, E. L. Peterson, and C. Zener, *Geometric Programming : Theory and Applications*, John Wiley & Sons Ltd., 1967.

[EDTN 99] P. McGoldrick, "Philips TDA935X/6X/8X One Chip Television", http://www.edtn.com/analog/prod329.htm, Sept. 1999.

[ElTa 89] H. El Tahawy, A. Chianali, and B. Hennion, "Functional Verification of Analog Blocks in Fideldo: a Unified Mixed-mode Simulation Environment", in *Proceedings IEEE International Symposium on Circuits and Systems (ISCAS)*, Aug. 1989, vol. 3, pp. 2012–2015.

[ElTu 89] F. El-Turky and E. Perry, "BLADES: an artificial intelligence approach to analog circuit design", *IEEE Transactions on Computer-Aided Design of Integrated Circuits and Systems*, vol. 8, no. 6, pp. 680–692, June 1989.

[Felt 93] E. Felt, E. Malavasi, E. Charbon, T. Totaro, and A. Sangiovanni-Vincentelli, "Performance-Driven Compaction for Analog Integrated Circuits", in *Proceedings Custom Integrated Circuits Conference (CICC)*, May 1993, pp. 17.3.1–17.3.4.

[Fern 98] F. V. Fernandez, A. Rodriguez-Vazquez, J. L. Huertas, and G. Gielen, *Symbolic Analysis Techniques: Applications to Analog Design Automation*, IEEE Press, NY, 1998.

[Fish 87] J. A. Fisher and R. Koch, "A Highly Linear CMOS Buffer Amplifier", *IEEE Journal of Solid-State Circuits (JSSC)*, vol. 22, no. 3, pp. 330–334, June 1987.

[Fitz 98] D. Fitzpatrick and I. Miller, *Analog Behavioral Modeling with the Verilog-A Language*, Kluwer Academic Publishers, 101 Philip Drive, Norwell, MA 02061, US, 1998.

[Fle 93] R. Fletcher, *Practical Methods of Optimization*, John Wiley & Sons Ltd., Chichester and New York, second edition edition, 1993.

[Foty 96] D. Foty, Ed., *MOSFET modeling with SPICE: principles and practice*, Prentice-Hall, Inc., Fletcher, Vermont, first edition edition, 1996.

[Gar 88] D. Garrod, L. Carley, and R. A. Rutenbar, "Automatic Layout of Custom Analog Cells in ANAGRAM", in *Proceedings IEEE/ACM International Conference on Computer Aided Design (ICCAD)*, Nov. 1988, pp. 544–547.

[Getr 90] I. Getreu, "Behavioral Modeling of Analog Blocks using the SABER Simulator", in *Proceedings Midwest Symposium on Circuits and Systems (MWSCAS)*, Aug. 1990, pp. 977–980.

[Ghar 96] R. Gharpurey and R. G. Meyer, "Modeling and Analysis of Substrate Coupling in Integrated Circuits", *IEEE Journal of Solid-State Circuits (JSSC)*, vol. 31, no. 3, pp. 344–353, Mar. 1996.

[Gie 89] G. Gielen, H. Walscharts, and W. Sansen, "ISAAC: a Symbolic Simulator for Analog Integrated Circuits", *IEEE Journal of Solid-State Circuits (JSSC)*, vol. 24, no. 6, pp. 1587–1597, Dec. 1989.

[Gie 90] G. Gielen, H. Walscharts, and W. Sansen, "Analog circuit design optimization based on symbolic simulation and simulated annealing", *IEEE Journal of Solid-State Circuits (JSSC)*, vol. 25, no. 3, pp. 707–713, June 1990.

[Gie 91a] G. Gielen, *Symbolic Analysis for Automated Design of Analog Integrated Circuits*, PhD thesis, KULeuven, Apr. 1991.

[Gie 91b] G. Gielen, P. Wambacq, and W. Sansen, ISAAC *version 4.0 – user manual*, Katholieke Universiteit Leuven, Belgium, Dept. Elektrotechniek — ESAT, Karsteelpark Arenberg 10, B-3001 Leuven-Heverlee, 1 edition, Apr. 1991.

[Gie 91c] G. Gielen and W. Sansen, *Symbolic analysis for automated design of analog integrated circuits*, Kluwer Academic Publishers, 101 Philip Drive, Norwell, MA 02061, US, Nov. 1991.

[Gie 92] G. Gielen, E. Liu, A. Sangiovanni-Vincentelli, and P. R. Gray, "Analog behavioral models for simulation and synthesis of mixed-signal systems", in *Proceedings European Design Automation Conference (EDAC)*, Sept. 1992, pp. 464–468.

[Gie 95a] G. Gielen, G. Debyser, P. Wambacq, K. Swings, and W. Sansen, "Use of symbolic analysis in analog circuit synthesis", in *Proceedings IEEE International Symposium on Circuits and Systems (ISCAS)*, Apr. 1995, vol. 3, pp. 2205–2208.

[Gie 95b] G. Gielen, G. Debyser, K. Lampaert, F. Leyn, K. Swings, G. Van der Plas, W. Sansen, D. Leenaerts, P. Veselinovic, and W. van Bokhoven, "An Analogue Module Generator for Mixed

Analogue/Digital ASIC Design", *International Journal of Circuit Theory and Applications*, vol. 23, no. 4, pp. 269–283, July 1995.

[Gie 95c] G. Gielen, G. Debyser, S. Donnay, K. Lampaert, F. Leyn, K. Swings, G. Van der Plas, P. Wambacq, and W. Sansen, "Comparison of Analog Synthesis using Symbolic Equations and Simulation", in *Proceedings European Conference on Circuit Theory and Design (ECCTD)*, Aug. 1995, pp. 79–82.

[Gie 00] G. Gielen and R. A. Rutenbar, "Computer-Aided Design of Analog and Mixed-signal Integrated Circuits", *Proceedings of the IEEE*, vol. 88, no. 12, pp. 1825–1852, Dec. 2000.

[Gie 01] G. Gielen, "Panel: When Will the Analog Design Flow Catch Up With the Digital Methodology ?", panel session at Design Automation Conference (DAC), July 2001.

[Harj 89] R. Harjani, R. A. Rutenbar, and L. Carley, "OASYS: a framework for analog circuit synthesis", *IEEE Transactions on Computer-Aided Design of Integrated Circuits and Systems*, vol. 8, no. 12, pp. 1247–1266, Dec. 1989.

[Harj 96] R. Harjani and J. Shao, "Feasibility and Performance Region Modeling of Analog and Digital Circuits", *Analog Integrated Circuits and Signal Processing*, vol. 10, no. 1–2, pp. 23–43, June 1996.

[Harv 92] J. P. Harvey, M. I. Elmasry, and B. Leung, "STAIC: An interactive framework for synthesizing CMOS and BiCMOS analog circuits", *IEEE Transactions on Computer-Aided Design (TCAD)*, vol. 11, no. 11, pp. 1402–1415, Nov. 1992.

[Hast 01] A. Hastings, *The Art of Analog Layout*, Prentice-Hall, Inc., Dec. 2001.

[Hend 93] R. Henderson, L. Astier, A. El-Khalifa, and M. Degrauwe, "A Spreadsheet Interface for Analog Design Knowledge Capture and Re-use", in *Proceedings Custom Integrated Circuits Conference (CICC)*, May 1993, pp. 13.3.1–13.3.4.

[Hers 98] M. del Mar Hershenson, S. P. Boyd, and T. H. Lee, "GPCAD: A Tool for CMOS Op-Amp Synthesis", in *Proceedings IEEE/ACM International Conference on Computer Aided Design (ICCAD)*, Nov. 1998, pp. 296–303.

[Hers 99] M. del Mar Hershenson, S. S. Mohan, S. P. Boyd, and T. H. Lee, "Optimization of Inductor Circuits via Geometric Programming", in *Proceedings Design Automation Conference (DAC)*, June 1999, pp. 994–998.

[Hooke 61] R. Hooke and T. A. Jeeves, "Direct Search", *Solution of Numerical and Statistical Problems, JACM*, vol. 8, no. 2, pp. 212–229, Feb. 1961.

[Hspice Manual 99] Avant! Corporation, 46871 Bayside Parkway Fremont, CA 94538, *Star-Hspice Manual*, release 1999.2 edition, June 1999.

[Ing 00] M. Ingels, *CMOS Interface Circuits for Optical Communication*, PhD thesis, KULeuven, 2000.

[Ingb 89] L. Ingber, "Very Fast Simulated Re-annealing", *Mathematical Computer Modelling*, vol. 12, no. 8, pp. 967–973, Aug. 1989.

[ITRS 99] "International Technology Roadmap for Semiconductors", http://public.itrs.net/Files/1999_SIA_Roadmap/Home.htm, 1999.

[ITRS 00] "International Technology Roadmap for Semiconductors 2000 Update", http://public.itrs.net/Files/2000UpdateFinal/2kUdFinal.htm, 2000.

[Joh 79] D. Johannsen, "BRISTLE BLOCKS: A Silicon Compiler", in *Proceedings Design Automation Conference (DAC)*, June 1979, pp. 310–313.

[Joli 86] I. Joliffe, *Principal Component Analysis*, Springer-Verlag, New York (USA), 1986.

[JoMa 97] D. A. Johns and K. Martin, *Analog Integrated Circuit Design*, chapter Processing and Layout, pp. 105–118, John Wiley & Sons Ltd., New York, 1997.

[King 95] P. Kinget and M. Steyaert, "A programmable analog cellular neural network CMOS chip for high speed image processing", *IEEE Journal of Solid-State Circuits (JSSC)*, vol. 30, no. 3, pp. 235–243, Mar. 1995.

[King 96a] P. Kinget, *Analog VLSI Integration of Parallel Signal Processing Systems*, PhD thesis, KULeuven, May 1996.

[King 96b] P. Kinget and M. Steyaert, "Impact of Transistor Mismatch on the speed–accuracy–power trade-off of Analog CMOS Circuits", in *Proceedings Custom Integrated Circuits Conference (CICC)*, May 1996, pp. 333–336.

[Koh 90] H. Koh, C. Séquin, and P. Gray, "OPASYN: a compiler for CMOS operational amplifiers", *IEEE Transactions on Computer-Aided Design of Integrated Circuits and Systems*, vol. 9, no. 2, pp. 113–125, Feb. 1990.

[Kras 99] M. J. Krasnicki, R. Phelps, R. A. Rutenbar, and L. Carley, "MAELSTROM: Efficient Simulation-Based Synthesis for Analog Cells", in *Proceedings Design Automation Conference (DAC)*, June 1999, pp. 945–950.

[Kuhn 87] J. Kuhn, "Analog Module Generators for Silicon Compilation", *VLSI System Design*, vol. 8, no. 5, pp. 74–80, May 1987.

[LakSan 94a] K. R. Laker and W. M. Sansen, *Design of Analog Integrated Circuits and Systems*, chapter Operational Amplifier Design, pp. 486–535, McGraw-Hill, New York, 1994.

[LakSan 94b] K. R. Laker and W. M. Sansen, *Design of Analog Integrated Circuits and Systems*, McGraw-Hill, New York, 1994.

[Laksh 86] K. Lakshmikumar, R. Hadaway, and M. Copeland, "Characterization and Modeling of Mismatch in MOS transistors for Precision Analog Design", *IEEE Journal of Solid-State Circuits (JSSC)*, vol. 21, no. 6, pp. 1057–1066, June 1986.

[Lam 95] K. Lampaert, G. Gielen, and W. Sansen, "A Performance-Driven Placement Tool for Analog Integrated Circuits", *IEEE Journal of Solid-State Circuits (JSSC)*, vol. 30, no. 7, pp. 773–780, July 1995.

[Lam 96a] K. Lampaert, G. Gielen, and W. Sansen, "Analog routing for manufacturability", in *Proceedings Custom Integrated Circuits Conference (CICC)*, May 1996, pp. 175–178.

[Lam 96b] K. Lampaert, G. Gielen, and W. Sansen, "Thermally constrained placement of analog and smart power integrated circuits", in *Proceedings European Solid-State Circuits Conference (ESSCIRC)*, Sept. 1996, vol. 22, pp. 160–163.

[Lam 98] lampaert, *Analog Layout Generation for Performance and Manufacturability*, PhD thesis, KULeuven, Jan. 1998.

[Lam 99] K. Lampaert, G. Gielen, and W. Sansen, *Analog Layout Generation for Performance and Manufacturability*, Kluwer Academic Publishers, Dordrecht, the Netherlands, Apr. 1999.

[Lau 99] E. Lauwers and G. Gielen, "A Power Estimation Model for High-speed CMOS A/D Converters", in *Proceedings Design, Automation and Test in Europe Conference (DATE)*, Mar. 1999, pp. 401–405.

[Lau 00] E. Lauwers and G. Gielen, "ACTIF: A high-level power estimation tool for Analog Continuous-Time Filters", in *Proceedings IEEE/ACM International Conference on Computer Aided Design (ICCAD)*, Nov. 2000, pp. 193–196.

[Leen 90] D. M. W. Leenaerts, "Application of Interval Analysis for Circuit Design", *IEEE Transactions on Circuits and Systems (TCAS)*, vol. 37, no. 6, pp. 803–807, June 1990.

[Leyn 97a] F. Leyn, W. Daems, G. Gielen, and W. Sansen, "Analog Circuit Sizing with Constraint Programming Modeling and Minimax Optimization", in *Proceedings IEEE International Symposium on Circuits and Systems (ISCAS)*, June 1997, vol. 3, pp. 1500–1503.

[Leyn 97b] F. Leyn, W. Daems, G. Gielen, and W. Sansen, "A Behaviorla Signal Path Modeling Methodology for Qualitative Insight in and Efficient Sizing of CMOS Opamps", in *Proceedings IEEE/ACM International Conference on Computer Aided Design (ICCAD)*, Nov. 1997, pp. 374–381.

[Leyn 98] F. Leyn, G. Gielen, and W. Sansen, "An efficient DC root solving algorithm with guaranteed convergence for analog integrated CMOS circuits", in *Proceedings IEEE/ACM International Conference on Computer Aided Design (ICCAD)*, Nov. 1998, pp. 304–307.

[Liang 98] J. Liang, "Mixed-signal IC market to surpass $10 billion in 1997 and $22 billion by 2001", Tech. Rep., Dataquest, Jan. 1998.

[Lin 98] C.-H. Lin and K. Bult, "A 10b 500MSample/s CMOS DAC in $0.6mm^2$", *IEEE Journal of Solid-State Circuits (JSSC)*, vol. 33, no. 12, pp. 1948–1958, Dec. 1998.

[Liu 92] E. Liu, G. Gielen, H. Chang, A. Sangiovanni-Vincentelli, and P. R. Gray, "Behavioral Modeling and Simulation of Data Converters", in *Proceedings IEEE International Symposium on Circuits and Systems (ISCAS)*, May 1992, vol. 5, pp. 2144–2147.

[Mak 95] C. Makris and C. Toumazou, "Analog IC design automation: Part II — Automated circuit correction by qualitative reasoning", *IEEE Transactions on Computer-Aided Design of Integrated Circuits and Systems*, vol. 14, no. 2, pp. 239–254, Feb. 1995.

[Mala 93] E. Malavasi and A. Sangiovanni-Vincentelli, "Area Routing for Analog Layout", *IEEE Transactions on Computer-Aided Design of Integrated Circuits and Systems*, vol. 12, no. 8, pp. 1186–1197, Aug. 1993.

[Mala 96] E. Malavasi, E. Charbon, E. Felt, and A. Sangiovanni-Vincentelli, "Automation of IC layout with analog constraints", *IEEE Transactions on Computer-Aided Design of Integrated Circuits and Systems*, vol. 15, no. 8, pp. 923–942, Aug. 1996.

[Malo 94] F. Maloberti, "Layout of Analog and Mixed Analog-Digital Circuits", in *Design of Analog-Digital VLSI Circuits for Telecommunication and Signal Processing*, J. Franca and Y.Tsividis, Eds. Prentice-Hall, Inc., Englewood Cliffs, NJ, second edition, 1994.

[Maly 86] W. Maly, A. J. Strojwas, and S. W. Director, "VLSI Yield Prediction and Estimation: A Unified Framework", *IEEE Transactions on Computer-Aided Design (TCAD)*, vol. 5, no. 1, pp. 114–130, Jan. 1986.

[Matlab 99] Mathworks, *Matlab User Manual*, 1999.

[Mats 01] S. Gotoh, T. Takahashi, K. Irie, K. Ohshima, N. Mimura, K. Aida, T. Maeda, T. Yamamoto, K. Sushihara, Y. Okamoto, Y. Tai, M. Usui, T. Nakajima, T. Ochi, K. Komichi, and A. Matsuzawa, "A Mixed-Signal 0.18μm CMOS SOC for DVD Systems with 432MSample/s PRML Read Channel and 16Mb Embedded DRAM", in *Proceedings International Solid-State Circuits Conference (ISSCC)*, Feb. 2001, pp. 182–183.

[MeCo 80] C. Mead and L. Conway, *Introduction to VLSI Systems*, Addison-Wesley Publishing Company, 1980.

[Med 94] F. Medeiro, F. V. Fernandez, R. Castro-Dominguez, and A. Rodriguez-Vazquez, "A statistical optimization-based approach for automated sizing of analog cells", in *Proceedings IEEE/ACM International Conference on Computer Aided Design (ICCAD)*, Nov. 1994, pp. 594–597.

[Med 95] F. Medeiro, B. Perez-Verdu, A. Rodriguez-Vazquez, and J. L. Huertas, "A vertically-integrated tool for automated design of $\Sigma\Delta$ modulators", *IEEE Journal of Solid-State Circuits (JSSC)*, vol. 30, no. 7, pp. 762–772, July 1995.

[Medea 00] –, "The MEDEA Design Automation Roadmap, Design Automation Solutions For Europe", Tech. Rep. 2nd release, MEDEA Applications Steering Group, May 2000.

[Mentor-Graphics 98] Mentor Graphics Corporation, 8005 S.W. Boeckman Road, WilsonVille, Oregon 97070, *Mentor Graphics ICstation manual*, 1998.

[Mey 93] V. Meyer zu Bexten, C. Moraga, R. Klinke, W. Brockherde, and K. G. Hess, "ALSYN : Flexible Rule-Based Layout Synthesis for Analog IC's", *IEEE Journal of Solid-State Circuits (JSSC)*, vol. 28, no. 3, pp. 261–268, Mar. 1993.

[Miki 86] T. Miki, Y. Nakamura, M. Nakaya, S. Asai, Y. Akasaka, and Y. Horiba, "An 80-MHz 8-bit CMOS D/A Converter", *IEEE Journal of Solid-State Circuits (JSSC)*, vol. 21, no. 6, pp. 983–988, June 1986.

[Mont 97] P. D. N. Montford, "Piet Mondriaan", http://www.cogapp.demon.co.uk/piran/mondrian/, 1997.

[Nagel 75] L. Nagel, "SPICE2: a computer program to simulate semiconductor circuits", Memo UCB/ERL M520, University of California, Berkeley, Electronics Research Laboratory, May 1975.

[Naka 91] Y. Nakamura, T. Miki, A. Maeda, H. Kondoh, and N. Yazawa, "A 10-b 70-MS/s CMOS D/A-converter", *IEEE Journal of Solid-State Circuits (JSSC)*, vol. 26, no. 4, pp. 637–642, Apr. 1991.

[Neff 95] R. R. Neff, *Automatic Synthesis of CMOS Digital/Analog Converters*, PhD thesis, UCBerkeley, Apr. 1995.

[Neff 96] R. R. Neff, P. R. Gray, and A. Sangiovanni-Vincentelli, "A Module Generator for High-Speed CMOS Current Output Digital/Analog Converters", *IEEE Journal of Solid-State Circuits (JSSC)*, vol. 31, no. 3, pp. 448–451, Mar. 1996.

[Och 96] E. Ochotta, R. A. Rutenbar, and L. Carley, "Synthesis of high-performance analog circuits in ASTRX/OBLX", *IEEE Transactions on Computer-Aided Design of Integrated Circuits and Systems*, vol. 15, no. 3, pp. 273–294, Mar. 1996.

[OtEy 01] F. O. 't Eynde, J. Schmit, V. Charlier, R. Alexandre, C. Sturman, K. Coffin, B. Mollekens, J. Craninckx, S. Terrijn, A. Monterastelli, S. Beerens, P. Goetschalckx, D. Joos, S. Guncer, and A. Pontioglu, "A Fully-Integrated Single-Chip SOC for Bluetooth", in *Proceedings International Solid-State Circuits Conference (ISSCC)*, Feb. 2001, pp. 196–197.

[Owen 95] B. R. Owen, R. Duncan, S. Jantzi, C. Ouslis, S. Rezania, and K. Martin, "BALLISTIC: An Analog Layout Language", in *Proceedings Custom Integrated Circuits Conference (CICC)*, May 1995, pp. 41–44.

[Pang 00] Y. Pang, F. Balasa, K. Lampaert, and C.-K. Cheng, "Block Placement with Symmetry Constraints Based on the O-Tree Non-Slicing Representation", in *Proceedings Design Automation Conference (DAC)*, June 2000, pp. 464–467.

[Pava 94] A. Pavasovic, A. G. Andreou, and C. R. Westgate, "Characterization of Subthreshold MOS Mismatch in Transistors for VLSI Systems", *Journal of VLSI Processing*, vol. 8, no. 1, pp. 75–85, July 1994.

[Pel 89] M. Pelgrom, A. Duinmaijer, and A. Welbers, "Matching properties of MOS transistors", *IEEE Journal of Solid-State Circuits (JSSC)*, vol. 24, no. 5, pp. 1433–1439, Oct. 1989.

[Pel 90] M. Pelgrom, "a 10-b 50-MHz CMOS D/A-converter with 75Ω buffer", *IEEE Journal of Solid-State Circuits (JSSC)*, vol. 25, no. 6, pp. 1347–1352, Dec. 1990.

[Phel 99] R. Phelps, M. J. Krasnicki, R. A. Rutenbar, L. Carley, and J. R. Hellums, "ANACONDA: Robust Synthesis of Analog Circuits Via Stochastic Pattern Search", in *Proceedings Custom Integrated Circuits Conference (CICC)*, May 1999, pp. 567–570.

[Phel 00] R. Phelps, M. J. Krasnicki, R. A. Rutenbar, L. Carley, and J. R. Hellums, "A Case Study of Synthesis for Industrial-Scale Analog IP: Redesign of the Equalizer/Filter Frontend for an ADSL CODEC", in *Proceedings Design Automation Conference (DAC)*, June 2000, pp. 1–7.

[Rab 96] J. Rabaey, Ed., *Digital Integrated Circuits – A Design Perspective*, Prentice-Hall, Inc., Englewood Cliffs, NJ, 1996.

[Ran 97] N. Randazzo, G. V. Russo, D. L. Presti, S. Panebianco, C. Petta, and S. Reito, "A four-channel, low-power CMOS charge preamplifier for silicon detectors with medium value of capacitance", *IEEE Transactions on Nuclear Science (TNS)*, vol. 44, no. 1, pp. 31–35, Feb. 1997.

[Raz 95] B. Razavi, Ed., *Principles of Data Conversion System Design*, IEEE Press, 1995.

[Reyn 96] P. Reynaert, L. Callewaert, D. Orton, S. Boardman, J. Stent, J. Agaesse, J. Fischer-Binder, J. Riihiaho, K. Tukkiniemi, G. Gielen, G. Debyser, K. Lampaert, F. Leyn, G. Van der Plas, and W. Sansen, "ADMIRE: advanced mixed signal design environment", in *IEEE International Conference on Electronics, Circuits and Systems (ICECS)*, Rodos, Greece, Oct. 1996, pp. 428–431.

[Rijm 89] J. Rijmenants, T. Schwartz, J. Litsios, and R. Zinszer, "ILAC: An automated layout tool for analog CMOS circuits", *IEEE Journal of Solid-State Circuits (JSSC)*, vol. 24, no. 2, pp. 417–425, Apr. 1989.

[Rijnd 88] L. Rijnders, P. Six, and H. J. D. Man, "Design of a Process-Tolerant Cell Library for Regular Structures Using Symbolic Layout and Hierarchical Compaction", *IEEE Journal of Solid-State Circuits (JSSC)*, vol. 23, no. 3, pp. 714–721, June 1988.

[Rijns 93] J. J. F. Rijns, "54MHz switched-capacitor video channel equaliser", *Electronics Letters*, vol. 29, no. 25, pp. 2181–2182, Dec. 1993.

[Roov 96] R. Roovers, *High Speed A/D Converters in Standard CMOS Technology*, PhD thesis, KULeuven, Mar. 1996.

[Sale 96] R. Saleh, B. Antao, and J. Singh, "Multi-level and Mixed-domain Simulation of Analog Circuits and Systems", *IEEE Transactions on Computer-Aided Design of Integrated Circuits and Systems*, vol. 15, no. 1, pp. 68–82, Jan. 1996.

[Sam 99] H. Samueli, "Broadband Communications ICs: Enabling High-Bandwidth Connectivity in the Home and Office", in *Proceedings International Solid-State Circuits Conference (ISSCC)*, Feb. 1999, pp. 26–30.

[Sans 94] W. Sansen, G. Gielen, G. Van der Plas, K. Swings, S. Donnay, and K. Lampaert, "Analog Module Generation for Mixed A/D ASIC Design", in *IEEE International Conference on Electronics, Circuits and Systems (ICECS)*, Cairo, Egypt, Dec. 1994, pp. –.

[Schwe 99] R. Schwencker, J. Eckmueller, H. Graeb, and K. Antreich, "Automating the Sizing of Analog CMOS Circuits by Consideration of Structural Constraints", in *Proceedings Design, Automation and Test in Europe Conference (DATE)*, Mar. 1999, pp. 323–327.

[Sher 95] N. A. Sherwani, *Algorithms for VLSI Physical Design Automation*, Kluwer Academic Publishers, 101 Philip Drive, Norwell, MA 02061, US, June 1995.

[SIA 97] –, "The National Technology Roadmap For Semiconductors", Tech. Rep., SIA (Semiconductor Industry Association), 1997.

[Snoey 01] W. Snoeys, M. Burns, M. Campbell, E. Cantatore, V. Cencelli, R. Dinapoli, E. Heijne, P. Jarron, P. Lamanna, D. Minervini, M. Morel, V. O'Shea, V. Quiquempoix, D. San-Segundo-Bello, B. Van-Koningsveld, and K. Wyllie, "Pixel readout chips in deep submicron CMOS for ALICE and LHCb tolerant to 10 mrad and beyond", *Nuclear Instruments & Methods in Physics Research, Section A (Accelerators, Spectrometers, Detectors and Associated*, vol. 466, no. 2, pp. 366–375, July 2001.

[SpectreHDL 98] Cadence Design Systems, Inc., 555 River Oaks Parkway, San Jose, CA 95134, USA, *Spectre Reference Manual*, 4.4.3 edition, 1998.

[Spel 98] P. Spellucci, "An SQP method for general nonlinear programs using only equality constrained subproblems", *Mathematical Programming*, vol. 82, no. 3, pp. 413–448, Mar. 1998.

[Stey 91] M. Steyaert, P. Kinget, and W. Sansen, "Full integration of extremely large time constants in CMOS", *Electronics Letters*, vol. 27, no. 10, pp. 790–791, May 1991.

[Stey 93] M. Steyaert, *MOS Transistor Model for Hand Calculation*, KULeuven ESAT-MICAS, 1993.

[Su 93] D. K. Su, M. J. Loinaz, S. Masui, and B. A. Wooley, "Experimental Resuls and Modeling Techniques for Substrate Noise in Mixed-Signal Integrated Circuits", *IEEE Journal of Solid-State Circuits (JSSC)*, vol. 28, no. 4, pp. 420–430, Apr. 1993.

[Swi 90] K. Swings, G. Gielen, and W. Sansen, "An intelligent analog IC design system based on manipulation of design equations", in *Proceedings Custom Integrated Circuits Conference (CICC)*, May 1990, pp. 8.6.1–8.6.4.

[Swi 91] K. Swings and W. Sansen, "DONALD: a Workbench for interactive design space exploration and sizing of analog circuits", in *Proceedings European Design Automation Conference (EDAC)*, Mar. 1991, pp. 475–479.

[Swi 94] K. Swings and W. Sansen, *Constraint Programming using* DONALD, Katholieke Universiteit Leuven, Belgium, Dept. Elektrotechniek — ESAT, Karsteelpark Arenberg 10, B-3001 Leuven-Heverlee, 2nd edition, May 1994.

[Swi 95] K. Swings, *Analog circuit design using constraint programming*, PhD thesis, KULeuven, May 1995.

[Synopsys 98] Synopsys, inc., *Synopsys Reference Manual*, 1.0 edition, Aug. 1998.

[ThoLoo 97] S. Thoen and S. Loos, "Ontwerp van een hoog performante 8-bit Analoog-Digitaal Convertor in CMOS 0.5 μm technologie", Master's thesis, KULeuven, May 1997.

[Tou 95] C. Toumazou and C. Makris, "Analog IC design automation: Part I — Automated circuit generation: new concepts and methods", *IEEE Transactions on Computer-Aided Design of Integrated Circuits and Systems*, vol. 14, no. 2, pp. 218–238, Feb. 1995.

[Tscher 71] S. N. Tschernikow, "Lineare Ungleichungen", *VEB Deutscher Verlag der Wissenschaften*, 1971.

[Tuin 97] H. P. Tuinhout and M. Vertregt, "Test Structures for Investigation of Metal Coverage Effects on MOSFET Matching", in *Proceedings IEEE International Conference on Microelectronic Test Structures (ICMTS)*, Mar. 1997, vol. 10, pp. 179–183.

[Uytt 00] K. Uyttenhove, A. Marques, and M. Steyaert, "A 6-bit, 1 Ghz Acquisition Speed ADC with digital error correction", in *Proceedings Custom Integrated Circuits Conference (CICC)*, May 2000, pp. 249–252.

[Vanco 01] P. Vancorenland, G. Van der Plas, M. Steyaert, G. Gielen, and W. Sansen, "a Layout-aware Synthesis Methodology for RF Mixers", in *Proceedings IEEE/ACM International Conference on Computer Aided Design (ICCAD)*, San Jose, US, Nov. 2001, pp. 358–362.

[VdBosch 98] A. Van den Bosch, M. Borremans, J. Vandenbussche, G. Van der Plas, A. Marques, J. Bastos, M. Steyaert, and W. Sansen, "A 12 bit 200 MHz Low Glitch CMOS D/A Converter", in *Proceedings Custom Integrated Circuits Conference (CICC)*, Santa Clara, May 1998, pp. 249–252.

[VdBosch 00] A. Van den Bosch, M. Borremans, J. Vandenbussche, G. Van der Plas, M. Steyaert, G. Gielen, and W. Sansen, "Modeling and Realisation of High Accuracy, High Speed Current-Steering CMOS D/A-converter", *Measurement*, vol. 28, no. 2, pp. 128–138, Sept. 2000.

[Vdbus 95] –, "Demonstration and validation of the module generator", Tech. Rep. ASTP4-KUL-JVDB-1, KULeuven ESAT-MICAS, Oct. 1995.

[Vdbus 98a] J. Vandenbussche, S. Donnay, F. Leyn, G. Gielen, and W. Sansen, "Hierarchical top-down design of analog sensor interfaces: from system-level specifications down to silicon", in *Proceedings Design, Automation and Test in Europe Conference (DATE)*, Mar. 1998, pp. 716–720.

[Vdbus 98b] J. Vandenbussche, G. Van der Plas, G. Gielen, M. Steyaert, and W. Sansen, "Behavioral model for D/A converters as VSI virtual components", in *Proceedings Custom Integrated Circuits Conference (CICC)*, Santa Clara, May 1998, pp. 473–476.

[Vdbus 98c] J. Vandenbussche, F. Leyn, G. Van der Plas, G. Gielen, and W. Sansen, "A fully integrated low-power CMOS particle detector front-end for space applications", *IEEE Transactions on Nuclear Science (TNS)*, vol. 45, no. 4, pp. 2272–2278, Aug. 1998.

[Vdbus 99a] J. Vandenbussche, G. Van der Plas, A. Van den Bosch, W. Daems, G. Gielen, M. Steyaert, and W. Sansen, "A 14-bit, 150 MSamples/s Update Rate, Q^2 Random Walk CMOS DAC", in *ISSCC Digest of technical papers*, San Francisco, Feb. 1999, pp. 146–147.

[Vdbus 99b] J. Vandenbussche, G. Van der Plas, G. Gielen, and W. Sansen, "Behavioral Model of Reusable D/A Converters", *IEEE Transactions on Circuits and Systems II: Analog and Digital Signal Processing*, vol. 46, no. 10, pp. 1323–1326, Oct. 1999.

[Vdbus 01] J. Vandenbussche, G. Van der Plas, W. Daems, A. Van den Bosch, G. Gielen, M. Steyaert, and W. Sansen, "Systematic Design of High-Accuracy Current-Steering D/A-converter Macrocells for Integrated VLSI Systems", *IEEE Transactions on Circuits and Systems II: Analog and Digital Signal Processing*, vol. 48, no. 3, pp. 300–309, Mar. 2001.

[VdPlas 94] G. Van der Plas, G. Gielen, and W. Sansen, "Modeling and Representation of the Integrated Circuit Design Process", in *Proceedings of the European Knowledge Acquisition Workshop (EKAW)*, Hoegaarden, Belgium, Sept. 1994, p. 10.

[VdPlas 96a] G. Van der Plas, G. Gielen, and W. Sansen, **AMGIE** *Software User Manual*, Katholieke Universiteit Leuven, Belgium, Dept. Elektrotechniek — ESAT, Karsteelpark Arenberg 10, B-3001 Leuven-Heverlee, 1 edition, Mar. 1996.

[VdPlas 96b] G. Van der Plas, J. Vandenbussche, F. Leyn, K. Lampaert, M. Buckens, K. Marent, G. Gielen, W. Sansen, and C. Das, **AMGIE** *Cell Library*, Katholieke Universiteit Leuven, Belgium, Dept. Elektrotechniek — ESAT, Karsteelpark Arenberg 10, B-3001 Leuven-Heverlee, 1 edition, Mar. 1996.

[VdPlas 97] G. Van der Plas, J. Vandenbussche, G. Gielen, M. Steyaert, and W. Sansen, "EsteMate: a Tool for Automated Power and Area Estimation in Analog Top-down Design and Synthesis", in *Proceedings Custom Integrated Circuits Conference (CICC)*, Santa Clara, May 1997, pp. 139–142.

[VdPlas 98] G. Van der Plas, J. Vandenbussche, G. Gielen, M. Steyaert, and W. Sansen, "Mondriaan: a Tool for Automated Layout Synthesis of Array-type Analog Blocks", in *Proceedings Custom Integrated Circuits Conference (CICC)*, Santa Clara, May 1998, pp. 485–488.

[VdPlas 99a] G. Van der Plas, J. Vandenbussche, A. Van den Bosch, W. Daems, M. Steyaert, G. Gielen, and W. Sansen, "MOS Transistor Mismatch for High Accuracy Applications", in *Proceedings of the ProRISC IEEE Benelux Workshop on circuits, systems and signal processing (ProRISC)*, Mierlo, the Netherlands, Nov. 1999, pp. 529–534.

[VdPlas 99b] G. Van der Plas, J. Vandenbussche, W. Sansen, M. Steyaert, and G. Gielen, "A 14-bit Intrinsic Accuracy Q^2 Random Walk CMOS DAC", *IEEE Journal of Solid-State Circuits (JSSC)*, vol. 34, no. 12, pp. 1708–1718, Dec. 1999.

[VdPlas 00] G. Van der Plas, J. Vandenbussche, W. Daems, A. Van den Bosch, M. Steyaert, G. Gielen, and W. Sansen, "Systematic Design of a 14-bit 150-Msamples/s CMOS Current-Steering D/A Converter", in *Proceedings Design Automation Conference (DAC)*, Los Angeles, June 2000, pp. 452–457.

[VdPlas 01] G. Van der Plas, G. Debyser, F. Leyn, K. Lampaert, J. Vandenbussche, G. Gielen, W. Sansen, P. Veselinovic, and D. Leenaerts, "AMGIE – A Synthesis Environment for CMOS Analog Integrated Circuits", *IEEE Transactions on Computer-Aided Design (TCAD)*, vol. 20, no. 9, pp. 1037–1058, Sept. 2001.

[vdPlassche 94] R. van de Plassche, Ed., *Integrated Analog-to-Digital and Digital-to-Analog Converters*, Kluwer Academic Publishers, 101 Philip Drive, Norwell, MA 02061, US, 1994.

[Verha 96] W. Verhaegen, "Geautomatiseerde testpatroongeneratie voor analog geïntegreerde schakelingen", Master's thesis, KULeuven, May 1996.

[Verha 97] W. Verhaegen, G. Van der Plas, G. Gielen, and W. Sansen, "Automated test pattern generation for analog integrated circuits", in *Proceedings IEEE VLSI Test Symposium (VTS)*, May 1997, pp. 296–301.

[Verilog-AMS 98] IEEE Standards, *Verilog-AMS Language Reference Manual*, 1.0 edition, Aug. 1998.

[Ves 95] P. Veselinovic, D. Leenaerts, W. van Bokhoven, F. Leyn, F. Proesmans, G. Gielen, and W. Sansen, "A Flexible Topology Selection Program as part of an Analog Synthesis System", in *Proceedings European Design and Test Conference (ED&TC)*, Mar. 1995, pp. 119–123.

[Ves 97] P. Veselinovic, *Analog Design Automation — Topology selection and piecewise linear model generation*, PhD thesis, TUE, June 1997.

[VHDL-AMS 99] IEEE Standards, *1076.1 Language Reference Manual*, 1.0 edition, Mar. 1999.

[Vit 85] E. A. Vittoz, "The Design of High-Performance Analog Circuits on Digital CMOS Chips", *IEEE Journal of Solid-State Circuits (JSSC)*, vol. 20, no. 3, pp. 657–665, Mar. 1985.

[Vlad 94] A. Vladimirescu, *The Spice Book*, John Wiley & Sons Ltd., New York, 1994.

[VSI 97] –, "Virtual Socket Interface Architecture Document", Tech. Rep. 1.0, VSI Alliance, 1997.

[Wamb 95] P. Wambacq, F. Fernandez, G. Gielen, W. Sansen, and A. Rodriguez-Vazquez, "Efficient symbolic computation of approximated small-signal characteristics", *IEEE Journal of Solid-State Circuits (JSSC)*, vol. 30, no. 3, pp. 327–330, Mar. 1995.

[Wikn 99] J. J. Wikner and N. Tan, "Influence of Circuit Imperfections on the Performance of DACs", *Analog Integrated Circuits and Signal Processing*, vol. 18, no. 1, pp. 7–20, Jan. 1999.

[Wu 94] W.-C. S. Wu, W. J. Helms, J. A. Kuhn, and B. E. Byrkett, "Digital-Compatible High-Performance Operational Amplifier with Rail-to-Rail Input and Output Ranges", *IEEE Journal of Solid-State Circuits (JSSC)*, vol. 29, no. 1, pp. 63–66, Jan. 1994.

[Wu 95] T.-Y. Wu, C.-T. Jih, J.-C. Chen, and C.-Y. Wu, "A low glitch 10-bit 75-MHz CMOS video D/A-converter", *IEEE Journal of Solid-State Circuits (JSSC)*, vol. 30, no. 1, pp. 68–72, Jan. 1995.

Index

GPSR Compliance
The European Union's (EU) General Product Safety Regulation (GPSR) is a set of rules that requires consumer products to be safe and our obligations to ensure this.

If you have any concerns about our products, you can contact us on

ProductSafety@springernature.com

In case Publisher is established outside the EU, the EU authorized representative is:

Springer Nature Customer Service Center GmbH
Europaplatz 3
69115 Heidelberg, Germany

www.ingramcontent.com/pod-product-compliance
Ingram Content Group UK Ltd.
Pitfield, Milton Keynes, MK11 3LW, UK
UKHW020118200726
13856UKWH00002B/607

9781475783766